CEREAL KILLERS:

Celiac Disease and Gluten-Free A to Z

by
Dr. Ron Hoggan, Ed. D.
and
Scott Adams, Founder of Celiac.com

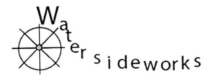
Watersideworks

and

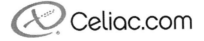
Celiac.com

ISBN: 1449918204
ISBN-13: 9781449918200

AUTHORS:

Ron Hoggan, Ed. D.

Scott Adams

Jefferson Adams

Danna Korn

Prof. Rodney Ford, M.B., B.S., M.D., F.R.A.C.P.

Janet Doggett

Cynthia Kupper, RD, CD

Roy S. Jamron

Laura Wesson

Jim Ford

Réjean Perron

Kenneth Fine, M.D.

William Dickey, Ph.D., M.D., F.A.C.G.

Dr. Scot Lewey

Kathleen LaPoint

Vanessa Maltin

Shelley Case, B.Sc., RD

Vijay Kumar, Ph.D., FACB

Antonio Tursi, M.D.

Edward R. Arnold

Carol Farmholtz

Ginny Nehring

Mike Pearson

Jules E.D. Shepard

More information about each of these authors can be located at:

http://www.celiac.com/articles/21972/1/Cereal-Killers/Page1.html

CEREAL KILLERS – CELIAC DISEASE AND GLUTEN SENSITIVITY A TO Z: TABLE OF CONTENTS

Chapter 4: Differentiating/identifying celiac disease and gluten sensitivity

Chapter 5: Analysis of important facets of celiac disease and gluten sensitivity

Chapter 6: Nutrition: The dietary, political, and economic battleground

INTRODUCTION:
WHY YOU SHOULD READ THIS BOOK

You hold in your hands the most diverse discussion of gluten sensitivity and celiac disease currently available in a single volume. <u>Cereal Killers</u> explores a wide range of sometimes contradictory perspectives on the various disease processes incited by gluten. These include the many illnesses and increased disease susceptibility to which gluten contributes, as well as ailments associated with gluten-induced illnesses. We also offer some speculations and hypotheses regarding the means by which gluten wreaks havoc on genetically vulnerable individuals.

Science is a process of making observations of events and trends, formulating a hypothesis based on those observations, then testing that hypothesis to see if it can be used to predict future observations. This is the approach that most of the authors of this book have used. Each writer/investigator has made observations that are somehow related to grains and how they interact with the human body. They then formulate and explain the hypothesis they have developed. Testing these hypotheses is often a built-in component of living or working with gluten sensitivity and/or celiac disease. We learn from excluding gluten from our diets as well as from the results of accidental or intentional ingestions. We even learn from the cravings that beset many of us following gluten ingestion. We also learn from observing the travails of others who struggle because of their genetic incompatibility with the various cereal grains that have come to be known as "gluten" grains.

Most writing about celiac disease and gluten sensitivity is laden with bias. Even those who claim objectivity by asserting indifference to their research findings bring their prior experiences, and hence, their biases to bear on their observations, the research choices they make, the procedures they follow, and the assumptions they make. By choosing the data they will collect, they implicitly choose the data they will ignore. This involves deciding prior to their investigation which observations will be relevant or important enough to record. Then the data must be interpreted. This is an enormous force in determining research outcomes. The interpretation of the data assembled cannot help but shape investigative findings.

For instance, one cereal grain researcher who specializes in the investigation of rice at the United States Department of Agriculture (U.S.D.A.) recently asserted, at the national conference of CSA/USA (Celiac Sprue Association of the United States of America) in Buffalo, NY, that he is confident that he doesn't have any bias when it comes to his research. Yet he was quick to challenge the grouping of rice with more allergenic grains such as wheat, rye, and barley. Clearly, he believes that rice is, at least in some respects, a superior food to these other grains. Although I agree with him, that's still a bias. It is a presumption based on some, perhaps many, relevant facts combined with a personal matrix of prior beliefs and experiences. Bias is a preference or dislike for something in the absence of **all** relevant information, and sometimes, in the presence of pre-conceived notions about a particular subject. For instance, we did not discuss the tendency that rice has for absorbing and retaining significantly more arsenic than the gluten grains. Had I been aware of this at the time of that discussion in Buffalo, it certainly would have changed my perception of rice as a 'safe' food. I did point out that rice is highly glycemic which is also a negative feature of this grain.

It is biases that shape and inform how we see our world. For instance, to a teenager, a shaved head or pink and green streaks in her/his hair may be considered very chic. That person's parents, on the other hand, may have an entirely different set of biases regarding those same colorful streaks or razor-induced baldness.

Each of us experiences our world in a subjective manner. We have prior learning and experiences that shape how we feel and think about the things we encounter today. Only objects can be objective. Feeling, thinking beings can only experience the world as feeling, thinking beings – not objects. Thus, the notion of objectivity is, at the very least, questionable when applied to a person or group of people.

Because of our human limitations, bias is impossible to escape. We can't know everything about even one single phenomenon in our world. Each of our pre-conceived notions about our world, and our place in it, is based on what we've been taught, what we have observed, our experiences, our professional training, and in very special cases, our imaginations. Through all of that experience, we come to expect specific pairings and outcomes. Those expectations are colored by our consciousness. Whether we are aware of our biases or not, we can't help infusing them into our observations of our world and specific events in it. Thus, a claim of objectivity is a highly questionable assertion.

Many of the perspectives expressed in this book are biased against gluten grains. It isn't that we are unaware that grains were probably a huge factor in the birth of civilization.

Neither are we unaware of the huge numbers of people who might starve without the products of grain cultivation. Our collective bias lies somewhere between the extremes of trying to rid the planet of this poison and the belief that gluten grains may be beneficial to some people but they are potentially devastating to a small but significant portion of the population.

Ours is a loose-knit, grass roots investigative group of people who composed the essays that form this book. We work independently but see further because we are "standing on the shoulders of giants" (Sir Isaac Newton). Not one of the contributors to this book is exempt from bias. In fact, individual biases are celebrated here. In <u>Cereal Killers</u>, we offer diverse, often competing, sometimes clashing ideas regarding many facets of current understandings of gluten sensitivity and celiac disease, along with some radically new ideas drawn from the peer reviewed medical and scientific literature and/or personal and/or professional experience. Some of the notions herein are even based on intuitive leaps that are not obviously grounded in the scientific method but are deemed by the editors to have merit.

It is this mix of perspectives, insights, experiences, and beliefs that add up, in this volume, to provide the reader with a rich understanding of many minority and dominant views of gluten sensitivity in its various manifestations. Thus, while we make no claim to objectivity, this blend of individual perspectives amounts to something much richer, more diverse, and more informative than so called "objective" reports can possibly offer, even if they could achieve some level of objectivity.

Realistically, any scientific proposition may soon be displaced by newer understandings. In short, most of what we know now will soon be replaced because it will be shown to be, at least partly, incorrect. All of us have so much to learn. Humanity moves, from one generation to the next, through a dark tunnel. We sometimes develop an inflated view of our own knowledge of physiology and imagine it to be huge. Yet what we do not know is vastly greater than what is already known. And some of what is known is, to one degree or another, incorrect.

As the world's burgeoning population taxes natural resources at all levels, each of us is pressed more tightly into smaller and smaller spaces. Most of us are now urbanites who can no longer grow our own vegetables, fruits, and berries. Most of our meat is raised in impossibly cramped conditions. Some animals are force-fed to address a variety of economic objectives and culinary preferences. At the very least, these animals are fed growth hormones aimed at enhancing profits through rapid, unnatural growth. Such crowded conditions inevitably result in the transmission of infectious ailments as many of these animals are forced to stand in their own feces. Ruminants, such as cattle, naturally graze on whatever is on the ground. In saner times, that would be grass. All too often now, they are munching on their neighbor's excrement. This necessitates extensive use of antibiotics, creating a perfect breeding ground for antibiotic resistant strains of bacteria. Modern poultry and hog operations are moving in similar directions.

Our supplies of vegetables and fruits are no less problematic. They are farmed in the same fields year after year, depleting the very minerals we need to absorb from these vegetables. Pesticides and fungicides are sprayed on these plants to reduce damage and losses, ultimately enhancing profits. Those same chemicals can thereby find their way onto our plates and into our bodies.

To make matters worse, the comparatively healthy foods mentioned above are being displaced by refined sugars, excessively starchy vegetables, and highly glycemic grains. These three food groups are poised to decimate the industrialized world through causing epidemic rates of autoimmunity, insulin resistance, both types of diabetes, and the host of accompanying ailments that include cardiovascular disease, many cancers, and cognitive decline. The many facets of our self destructive dietary practices are converging quite rapidly.

All of the above mentioned, nutrition-related hazards to human health pale in comparison to those posed by our escalating consumption of the gluten-containing grains, wheat, rye, and barley. This is, in large part, due to our socially misguided belief that gluten, and the grains from which it is derived, are healthful. Even among those who are not genetically susceptible to the immune disruptions caused by gluten induced subtle injuries that mar the quality and length of our lives gluten grain consumption is displacing much healthier foods.

Nowhere is our collective ignorance more pervasive than in our widespread, dangerously mistaken beliefs about healthful nutrition. Our consumption of these foods poses an enormous threat to our physical and mental health. From increasing susceptibility to various autoimmune diseases, to increasing our risk of obesity, to causing vitamin and/or mineral deficiencies, to increasing our risk of various cancers, to altering blood flow patterns in our brains, and hence, inducing behavioral abnormalities and/or psychiatric illness, gluten grains are the authors of, or major contributors to many, perhaps most diseases of civilization.

Yet the pseudo-scientific government committees, driven by politics, economic considerations, lobbyists, and greed, publish eating guides that continue to advocate the very foods that are making us increasingly ill. At the peak of the Roman Empire's power, around 200 A.D., many Romans were aware that their lead-glazed wine cups were poisoning them. Because they preferred the taste of leaded wine, they continued to drink from these cups despite the common suspicion that this practice was causing widespread birth defects.

We are similarly self indulgent, but we lack even the basic knowledge the Romans had. Many of us may continue to imagine that gluten grains are a healthful food. Most of our archaeologists, anthropologists, and a small group of medical professionals and researchers, on the other hand, know otherwise. It is the common misconception that grains are a healthful food that poses the greatest threat to our wellbeing. Unfortunately, only a few of us have just begun to realize the importance of the threat posed by gluten grains. This has mostly come through our own experiences, after excluding these grains from our diets. Even then, the common mistaken belief is that gluten is only harmful to a small segment of the population.

Unlike any story you've ever heard or read before, this is an uplifting tale of the human struggle to survive an enormous environmental threat to humanity as we now know it. It is also about a small, dedicated group of medical researchers who have been exploring the nuances and unlocking the mysteries of the hazards posed by gluten for more than half a century. This story is written by a group of investigators, both amateur and professional, who have come together to contribute to the growing body of knowledge about one important pathogen – gluten.

As we press at the boundaries of human knowledge, the looming question is whether our research is too late to help those who are currently, and often, unknowingly being trimmed from the human gene pool because of an unrecognized susceptibility to the ravages of gluten. Our hopeful answer is aimed at stemming the tide of this insidious force as it threatens to extinguish future generations of much of humanity. Nowhere has the threat to human survival posed by gluten been more strongly asserted than in the pages of *The Journal of Gluten Sensitivity*, from which many of these articles are drawn.

Each of the voices raised here, in each of the following articles, reflects professional research, amateur investigation, and/or considerable and unique personal experience, or some combination thereof. We are shouting our warnings from the rooftops of the world. We offer insight into scientific, metabolic, and dietetic issues. We explore medical research. We offer our own, unique experiences, and we celebrate new breakthroughs and discoveries. We wish to bring everyone into the light - understanding the other side of gluten's double-edged impact on civilization.

In the following pages, we explore how eating a gluten-free diet is different from a standard American diet (SAD) and what happens when we begin to follow this better way of eating. Some of the essays explore the dynamics that take place in the gut, the nervous system, the brain, the skeletal structures, and beyond. Other essays suggest what these anecdotes and experiences imply for others.

The first in this series of essays explores some of the mixed perceptions that often accompany beginning a gluten-free diet. The next asks and answers the question of whether a gluten-free diet is a just a treatment or a cure for celiac disease and gluten sensitivity. It explores the personal meaning of the diet through a survey of gluten sensitive individuals. It reaches to the very heart of the matter and feels the pulse of the various converging research projects and individual quests for wellness. The next essay offers information for those who wish to safely dine at restaurants.

CHAPTER 1:
CELIAC DISEASE AND GLUTEN SENSITIVITY

Life with Celiac Disease or Gluten Sensitivity

by Dr. Ron Hoggan, Ed. D.

What it means to have celiac disease or non-celiac gluten sensitivity, in a nutshell, is to face a limited life expectancy for those not compliant with a gluten free diet. Yet most people with celiac disease or gluten sensitivity will never know they have it. Diagnoses of these gluten-induced conditions continue to be fraught with problems borne of practitioners' ignorance of celiac disease and frequently held strong biases that gluten sensitivity is an insignificant finding. Even those individuals with celiac disease or non-celiac gluten sensitivity, who are compliant with the diet, face a greater risk of developing some types of cancers, particularly non-Hodgkin's lymphomas[1], especially during the first 6 to 12 months after they begin to follow a gluten free diet[2].

Frankly, gluten sensitivity and celiac disease are also associated with symptoms of neurological and psychological illness[3, 4]. This topic is examined in much greater detail in chapter 3, but in the interim, it is important to recognize that gluten exposure places individuals with celiac disease or gluten sensitivity at a disadvantage on multiple levels. Who, in poor health, with disturbing, and sometimes obvious, neurological or psychiatric symptoms, and frightened for their lives, is well equipped to debate testing and diagnostic protocols with their doctor? Few of us are.

What it means to have celiac disease or gluten sensitivity, in many cases, is to be at the mercy of practitioners while simultaneously being suspicious that we are dealing with one of the many practitioners who are woefully misinformed, ill informed, or uninformed about gluten sensitivity and celiac disease. There are even some medical practitioners who are knowledgeable about celiac disease but ignorant of gluten sensitivity, or vice versa. Patients with either celiac disease or gluten sensitivity are sometimes given dangerous medical advice. Some of these practitioners who refuse to countenance the possibility that they could be in error default to blaming patients, often labeling them as emotionally disturbed or as hypochondriacs. Either way, the patient suffers – both from a missed diagnosis and from a misdiagnosis. On second thought, perhaps it is correct to label them 'disturbed'. They certainly have good cause to be disturbed.

Adding to this problem, the medical opinions expressed by some of these individuals are often parroted by journalists and others, leading to situations where gluten sensitive and celiac patients are further victimized. Quality of life issues, in the context of diagnosed celiac disease, have been examined. There can be little doubt that we face many physical and psychological challenges beyond our diagnosed condition of celiac disease[5].

To further compound the problem, the dietary treatment of celiac disease can be quite challenging at the grocery store, when eating out, and when eating at friends' and relatives' homes. The impact of this situation can take many shapes.

In this chapter, we provide some positive and encouraging advice, opinions, and directions.

Gluten-Free Diet: Curse or Cure?

by Scott Adams

I recently reviewed the results of a celiac.com survey and was surprised to learn that 37 percent of 472 respondents do not believe that there will ever be a cure for celiac disease, while 32 percent think there will be, and 31 percent are unsure. After re-reading the question I realized that it might be a loaded question. Does the gluten-free diet count as a cure? Some people may think so. Others think that the diet is a curse or, at best, just a treatment. With the vast improvement that has taken place during the last few years in the quality of gluten-free foods I like to think of the diet as a really good tasting cure. Of course the diet isn't really a cure but the diet has allowed my body to become healthy again and make me feel as though I am cured and that is what counts, isn't it?

Like most people, however, I still hold out hope that future celiac disease research will yield a complete cure - one that does not include a special diet. On the other hand, if you're like me, we should be careful what we wish for because our diet is probably healthier now than it ever was, mostly due to the necessary avoidance of most fast and processed foods. Perhaps the diet is really a blessing in disguise for many of us and we will actually live longer and healthier lives due to our improved diet in spite of having a "disease."

You may think that the current small rate of spending on celiac disease research there will never be a cure! However, after reading a proclamation by Dr. Alessio Fasano that celiac disease is "by far the most frequent genetic disease of human kind," I have renewed confidence that there will be much more money spent on research in the future and eventually a cure will be found.

More surprises in the survey results came when 6.5 percent of respondents said spelt was safe on a gluten-free diet, while 32.3 percent were unsure. I like to interpret this result as 38.8 percent of respondents were just diagnosed and are on their first visit to Celiac.com—but this is wishful thinking. Unfortunately this result means that we have more work to do. **Spelt is not safe!**

The most surprising response however, was the number of people who cheat on their diets—a full 43 percent! Some 13 percent actually cheat more than 20-40 times per year. The main excuses given for cheating: 1) People missed a particular item too much to go without it, and; 2) Gluten-free foods are not always available or are too expensive. These were the same folks who got the spelt question wrong—the ones who were just diagnosed ...... right? We have a lot of work to do.

There are just too many great alternatives out there. We should not knowingly eat gluten. After learning so much over the years about food ingredients and preparation I like to think that I could walk into a restaurant called "House of Gluten" and order a gluten-free meal. Educating ourselves about how food is prepared and which ingredients are safe or not safe is really the key to enjoying life while on this diet. Remember, the next time you are tempted, say to yourself over and over—this diet is a really good tasting cure—and don't cheat! Oh no...65 percent of respondents don't know that buckwheat is safe, and 58 percent don't know that Quinoa is safe...time for me to get back to work.

For more information on safe and forbidden foods for a gluten-free diet visit http://www.celiac.com/categories/Celiac-Disease-Information/

Taking charge of your meal when eating out

The results of the latest Celiac.com survey indicate that 71 percent of 983 respondents dine out less often now than before they went on a gluten-free diet. Further, 74 percent of those who do eat out are now more nervous and uncomfortable during their dining experience, and 50 percent of them feel this way because it is either too much trouble to explain their diet, or because they feel that restaurant employees are in too big a hurry to worry about their special needs. As a resident of San Francisco, a city that is reputed to have enough table space in its restaurants to seat everyone in the city at once, these results disappoint me. Not because I eat out less due to my gluten-restricted diet, or am uncomfortable when I do so, but because I believe that anyone with celiac disease who is armed with the proper knowledge and approach need not fear or avoid eating out.

In order to eat out safely the first thing to check before going into a restaurant is your attitude. If you are the type of person who is too embarrassed to send your meal back because they didn't follow your instructions or if you are the opposite type and are so demanding that you often annoy the staff—you will need to find some middle ground. It took me a while to reach this point but I can now go into a restaurant with confidence and I consider getting a good gluten-free meal there as a personal challenge that begins when I walk through their door.

On entering a restaurant the first thing to notice is how busy the place is, including how stressed out the workers seem to be—the more stressed out they are, the more tactful you will need to be to get what you want—a safe meal. One rule that has served me well in all situations is to keep it simple—both your order and how you place it. I never try to give a scientific discourse on celiac disease to restaurant workers as I have found that it only serves to frustrate or confuse them. Tell them only what they need to know—that you have an allergy to wheat (using the term gluten will typically lead back into long explanations) and need to make sure that your dish is wheat-free. I wouldn't tell them that you'll get violently ill if ANY wheat ends up in your meal, as some people recommend, because they probably won't want to serve you. I would also avoid going into detail about hidden ingredients that contain wheat—it will take too long to explain and you will again run the risk of scaring them into not serving you.

I usually don't approach the chef unless it's very slow because he is probably the busiest person in a restaurant. When it's busy I always ask the waiter to give the chef special order instructions, both verbally and in writing on the order ticket. Rather than try to educate the staff and make them experts on gluten, it's far more efficient if you are the one who becomes more educated with regard to the dishes you like to eat so that you can order them in a manner that will ensure your safety. I strongly believe that our diet is ultimately our responsibility and not a restaurant's (with the exception of any mistakes they might make).

The key to ordering a gluten-free meal is your prior knowledge of its ingredients and how it is prepared. Most people who have cooked have a basic understanding of how certain dishes are prepared and whether they could contain gluten. Even if you aren't a cook you might have had a particular meal often enough to know something about its ingredients and preparation methods. You need only know enough about the meal to ask the right questions and alter any preparation methods that might cause it to contain gluten.

For example, whenever I order a salad I always tell them no croutons, and to bring me olive oil and vinegar for dressing. When ordering fried rice in a Chinese restaurant, I order it without soy sauce, or I give them my own bottle to cook with. If you order something properly and it arrives incorrectly, send it back!

I recently ordered Chinese food with my family and did everything correctly — I told them about my wheat allergy, gave them my bottle of soy sauce, and told the waitress that I wanted to make sure that there was no wheat flour in or on anything that I ordered (but that corn starch is fine—if you don't clarify this point it might unnecessarily eliminate or alter many Chinese dishes). When our food arrived the chicken I ordered was breaded. After inquiring about it I found out that they used wheat flour so I sent it back, the waitress apologized, and it was no big deal.

I recommend that you purchase and read basic cookbooks for the types of foods you like to eat so you can place your order with confidence. For example, I own several cookbooks for my favorite cuisines, including ones that cover Mexican, Chinese, Thai, Italian, Vietnamese, Indian and American foods. I typically look over the relevant cookbook before I go to a particular restaurant so I can get an idea of what I want to order and how to order it. The more knowledge you have about how the dishes you like are prepared, the easier it will be for you to order them in a manner that ensures they are safe. Having these books around is also great should you begin to cook more at home, which, according to my survey, 65 percent of respondents already do. This is also something that I highly recommend.

Generally speaking I try to avoid large chain restaurants as much as possible because many of their items are highly processed and contain a huge number of ingredients. Their employees typically have no idea what's in the foods they are serving. I think that many of the survey respondents are with me on this, as 70 percent of them also eat less processed and junk foods due to their gluten-free diets. I only eat at chain restaurants if I am able to check their Web sites in advance for safe items. If I can't do this, I am extra careful about what I order. I try to eat at smaller, family-owned establishments because they usually know the ingredients and preparation methods for all of their dishes. Additionally, authentic ethnic foods such as Mexican, Vietnamese, Thai, Indian, Indonesian, Japanese and Korean typically use little wheat, so I lean more towards these types of restaurants when I eat out.

The transition to a gluten-free diet isn't easy—74 percent of survey respondents found it difficult or very difficult. Like many things in life, it took some preparation work to make the successful transition to a gluten-free diet, and the same is true for eating out. I like to think that what you put into it, you will get out of it—the more you learn about cuisine and various methods of preparation, the more pleasant and care-free your dining experiences will be, and the more likely you will enjoy a safe meal. Life is too short to not enjoy the basic pleasure of eating out. So the next time you get the urge, do your homework first, then take charge of your meal at the restaurant!

Editor's note:
As awareness of celiac disease and gluten intolerance grows, it is becoming much easier to find gluten-free selections at restaurants. Many fast food chains are also making efforts to accommodate our dietary needs.

Talking to Others About the Gluten-Free Diet

By Danna Korn

"To talk to someone who does not listen is enough to tense the devil."–Pearl Bailey

No matter what your reason for your dietary restriction, one of the hardest things about this diet is talking to people about why you must be gluten-free, and trying to explain the diet itself. Responses range from complete understanding (sorry, this is extremely rare) to people who *think* they understand but don't ("Oh, this is just like when I gave up liver for Lent!") to those who don't care an iota about your diet, to the other 95 percent of the population who really *want* to understand, but just don't get it.

There is an art to talking to people about your condition and the diet, but first there are a few basic ground rules you should know and follow.

Attitudes Are Contagious
When you're talking with other people about your diet, especially close family members who will be "in this" with you for the rest of your life and who may also someday

learn they must go gluten-free, remember that attitudes are contagious. If you give the impression that this diagnosis has ruined your life and that the diet is worse than astronaut food, others will feel that way, too.

First, these things aren't true, even if it seems that way at first. Second, you don't want your husband, wife, or kids to feel this way, especially if they're the ones on the diet. Be careful what you say. Even when they appear to be tuned out, kids and spouses often hear what you're saying. Feelings can be hurt, and lasting impressions can be made. If possible, portray a positive attitude about the diet; you may even find it rubs off on you.

Everyone's a Doctor

Before you begin talking to people about your medical condition, you should know that nearly everyone, regardless of education (or lack thereof) is a doctor. Especially when it comes to gastrointestinal distress, a subject that nearly everyone on the planet is at least vaguely familiar with.

Once you get past the squeamish introduction, you're likely to be cut off by people who want to tell *you* what you have. "It's lactose intolerance," your best friend assures you. "No, I think you have all the warning signs of colon cancer," argues Doctor Dad. "You just need acupuncture in your butt," advises your eight-year-old wanna-be doctor son who just learned the word (acupuncture, not butt).

You may have trouble getting everyone to stop with the advice and listen, but try to get through your dissertation. Then you can look forward to one of several responses (percentages are based on personal experience, not scientific findings):

- Complete understanding (0.1%): These people will listen intently as you discuss villi, bowel movements, gluten, and modified food starch, barely moving a muscle as they hang on your every word, taking careful notes so as not to poison you at your next get-together. These saints have also been known to hang flyers in their kitchens, listing safe and forbidden foods in case you drop by for an unexpected visit. Worship the ground these people walk on, because they're few and far between.
- Pseudo-understanding (they think they get it but they don't) (0.9%): These people are easily identifiable, because they nod much too quickly when you explain the situation to them. Staccato-type nodding of the head is usually accompanied by rapid-fire successive affirmative phrases such as, "Uh-huh, sure, mm-hmm, yep, gotcha, sure, yep, of course, mm-hmm." Don't burst their bubble; these people

are *used* to knowing everything, and usually can't be told otherwise. I recommend that you bring your own food to get-togethers with these people.

- Absolute and unveiled lack of interest and concern (4.0%): Gotta hand it to 'em, these folks are honest. Don't try to push a rope.
- Desire is there, but they just don't get it (95.0%): These people mean well, but either lack the ability or don't want to take the time to understand. Don't be annoyed, offended, or otherwise put off. Their attitude can't change the fact that you feel a lot better now that you've eliminated wheat or gluten, and *that's* what really counts. Don't disown them, especially because most of your friends and family will fall into this category, but don't berate them, either. Your diet isn't their concern, even if you think they should care more than they appear to.

When Those Closest to You Just Don't Get It

By Danna Korn

Obviously, dealing with this last, vast category of folks who just don't get it can be difficult. Already, you're saddled with the extra responsibilities and challenges inherent to the diet, and it may not sit well with you that some of the people closest to you are those who put forth the least effort to understand. We expect family and friends to support us, show concern, offer assistance, and make things that are important to us important to them, yet often it is exactly those people who disappoint us the most.

In this situation, we have the additional challenge of dealing with the fact that we're around them frequently, and food is often a part of social situations. Trusting them to provide foods that are safe (or worse yet) dealing with the anger and resentments that arise when they don't even bother, can test the most solid of relationships.

If they just don't get it because they're simply not capable, forgive them and move on. Some people are set in their ways, and others are intellectually incapable of grasping the intricacies of the diet. Be aware and be prepared with your own foods when getting together.

When loved ones are capable but just don't want to bother taking the time to learn about the diet and your condition, you may experience feelings of hostility and resentment. It's okay to be mad, but don't wallow in the anger; it serves no purpose and will provide no benefit because they're not going to change, and you can't force them to want to care.

It's important to avoid falling into the role of the victim. You may have some serious medical conditions, and you could be getting some sort of reinforcement from feeling victimized, both by the condition and the people around you. It gets you nowhere, except into a rut of negativity.

People who just don't get it aren't going to suddenly show interest in you, your condition, and the diet. Just as they don't *have* to cater to your diet, you don't need to cater to their insensitivity and thoughtlessness. Forgive them for their lack of sensitivity, their narcissism, and their indifference (but unless you want to start a family feud, do it in your heart rather than out loud) and move on. They may be sensitive, generous, caring people in many ways, or maybe they're not. In either case, you can't force them to care or learn about your condition or diet, and as frustrating as it can be, your only choice is to accept that fact. Don't allow yourself to get mired in the negativity that their apathy can create, and don't lower yourself to their level either by caring less about their situations.

Need-to-Know Rating Criteria

HIGH: Will these people prepare food for me? If so, it's important for them to understand which foods and ingredients are safe and which are forbidden. If you can narrow it down for them, do so. For instance, don't go to a restaurant and ask them what they have that's wheat or gluten-free and expect to get a good answer. Instead, peruse the menu, and figure out what looks as though it is safe, or could be made wheat or gluten-free. Then you can get into the intricacies of cooking procedures, contamination issues, and ingredients.

Sometimes it's easiest to explain your condition in terms of an allergy, even if your condition is celiac disease (which is not an allergy). People understand, for instance, that peanut allergies can be severe, and even a little peanut can cause some people to have a serious reaction. Sometimes it's necessary to explain that you have a "severe toxic reaction" to wheat or gluten before people will take your condition seriously. Otherwise, they may think that it's okay just to pluck the croutons off the salad after the fact.

MEDIUM: Are they asking out of curiosity or nosiness? Most people who ask about your diet do so out of genuine curiosity rather than abject obnoxiousness. Maybe they have their own dietary restrictions, and want to compare notes. Maybe they're nutritionists, or maybe they're just genuinely curious. In any case, don't be offended, but don't feel as though you have to give a dissertation on the advantages of a wheat or gluten-free diet either. Offer as much information as you're comfortable giving, and as much as it looks like they're truly interested in hearing.

A good response is usually generic at first, adding information as the listeners seem to want it. "I have a condition that makes me unable to tolerate gluten, so I eat a gluten-free diet" is usually a good start. If they want to know more, they'll ask.

LOW: Do they warrant a response? When the 16-year-old kid wearing a paper cap and taking your order at the drive-up window asks with a strong Valley Girl accent, "Like, what's wrong with the bun, dude? How come you ordered, like, all your burgers without, like, the bun?" your best response is to bite your tongue. No response is needed, unless you can muster a good, "Like, what-EVER, dude, I like 'em that way."

When Friends, Family or Loved Ones Just Don't Get it

By Danna Korn

The gluten-free lifestyle is a big part of who we are. So when friends, relatives, and loved ones don't get it—I should clarify—when they seem to *choose* not to get it—we sometimes get a little cranky.

I know—I was reminded of how it feels when loved ones don't choose to get it this past Thanksgiving when one of my relatives who shall remain nameless glutenized the mayo jar. Now I realize it may seem petty to get tweaked about someone dipping a knife in a mayo jar—but it had *gluten* all over it, and worse yet, she did the same thing *last* Thanksgiving, and I threw a tizzy about it *then*.

Realizing the first dip alone contaminated the entire jar (of course it was the club-sized jar that is the size of a small Volkswagen) there was no point in stopping her from doing it again. But I watched incredulously as she taunted me, dipping the knife into the jar—then onto the (gluten) bread—over, and over, and over again. How many *gobs* of mayo does one need on a piece of bread?!? I found myself seething, and my blood boiled with every dip-and-spread motion; I *swear* she was doing it intentionally.

Yes, I know I should have had a squeeze bottle handy, and I even write about that in my books. My mistake, but I also write about doing the "gob drop," which is—as the name implies—the process of taking a gob of (insert condiment here) and dropping it onto said piece of gluten. Using a separate knife, you spread. It's really not that tough.

The bigger point here is that it made me wonder why, after *fourteen* years of going through this, she didn't care more about our gluten-free lifestyle. I spent about six minutes pondering this when I remembered that it's not that she doesn't care—maybe she does, and maybe she doesn't. The bigger point is that she wasn't thinking about it at that moment—and that's okay.

This is *our* lifestyle, and we love it. Those friends and family who *do* care enough to call and make sure the meal they're serving us is gluten-free are to be cherished. Those who make a special trip to the health food store to buy a mix and make gluten-free cookies are to be downright hailed as saints. Even those who make a beautiful gluten-free meal and then top it with teriyaki sauce (of the gluten-containing variety) because they don't know any better are to be adored for trying.

I write about this stuff in my books, and it surprised me a little to find myself getting miffed about such a petty thing. I thought I had outgrown those feelings 14 years ago. I guess my point is that we all face certain challenges from time to time, and we need to put our brightest face forward and meet those challenges with a good attitude, lest they get the best of us.

The most important thing that helps keep me on track, for what it's worth, is to remember that the gluten-free lifestyle is the key to our health and ultimate happiness. We're blessed to know that a simple change in lifestyle is all it takes to be perfectly healthy—and that's worth a lotta mayo.

Editor's note:
You will discover in a later chapter that wheat, rye, and barley have properties that make them quite addictive. Thus, many who have given up eating gluten will be able to attest to some of the elements of the following personal story.

I Dream of Bagels: A Personal Narrative about Being Diagnosed with Celiac Disease

By Janet Doggett

When I was six years old, I lived in Dallas, Texas and I had a best friend named Judy. It was at her house that I first ate a bagel. I fell in love with its chewy, crusty texture. I didn't know much at that age, but I knew that I loved eating those bagels—I couldn't get enough.

I also knew, from a very young age, that something was wrong with me — something that doctors would one day discover and name after me. I had stomachaches all the time. I can't remember a time when my stomach didn't hurt at least a little bit.

"You were so healthy when you were young," my mother is fond of saying. Painfully shy and uncomplaining? Yes. Healthy? No! We were just blissfully unaware of what lay in wait for future doctors to discover.

In high school, I was anemic, and experienced several bouts of tachycardia that were written off to anxiety. Then, after I was married, I twice struggled with infertility. Later, the "stomachaches" returned and worsened. Doctors removed my gallbladder thinking that stones were to blame, then my uterus, thinking hormones might be causing my symptoms.

Along the way, in trying to diagnose me, doctors discovered insulin-dependent diabetes, low thyroid and high cholesterol. I also have bipolar disorder. I take a combination of 13 medications a day for my health maintenance, and I've been to the hospital at least 18 times in the past year. Still, I felt that they hadn't hit upon that one thing that was really wrong, the thing that was causing my stomach to hurt so badly.

Then, two years ago, I added "severe bone pain" to my ever-growing list of symptoms, and consulted a rheumatologist. He refused to believe it was a simple case of arthritis and tested me for malnutrition. I had no Vitamin D in my blood—a telltale sign that something was wrong with my gut. Next came the antibody test, then a biopsy. They proved that the tiny villi that lined my intestines were indeed "flattened." We had a diagnosis after only 10 years of actively seeking one. I had celiac disease, an autoimmune disease where one can't digest wheat or gluten, the protein in wheat, rye, and barley.

What? I can't eat bread? I can't have bagels?"

I was sure I would starve to death when I heard that removal of all glutens from the diet was the only treatment for this disease in which a person's intestinal lining is badly damaged. If left untreated, it can lead to malnutrition, brain ataxia, osteopenia, and eventually a cancer called lymphoma.

More specifically, what was happening was the lining of my intestines was shriveling; shrinking in reaction to the gluten in the bread or other products made with wheat, rye, or barley. The damaged intestines repair themselves with the removal of gluten from the diet, but it must be strictly avoided for life. Even the smallest taste of wheat or gluten would immediately return my intestinal villi to a flattened mass.

At first I was afraid to eat anything. All day long, gluten loomed at me from dark corners. At night I dreamt of bagels and pizza. The problem is that gluten is hidden in many foods. Obviously it is in bread, bagels, pizza, pasta, most fried foods (all wheat flour-based products) but it also is in many processed foods like canned soups and salad dressings, ice creams, foods made with caramel color, malt, barley, rye, HVP, spelt, and the list goes on. It also means that I must use separate utensils to butter my gluten-free bread, separate pots and pans to cook my food and separate colanders to drain my corn or rice-based pastas. Even certain toothpastes and lipsticks are suspect.

To have celiac disease means that you can no longer rely on the convenience of ordering take-out or eating fast food. It means being prepared *each and every time* you eat, bring-ing gluten-free sauces, dressings, buns, and breads with you.

You learn, too, that part of the reason bread is bread is because of the gluten. It is what holds it together and gives it its chewy texture. Breads made from rice and corn and the like are mealy and fall apart. They must be kept frozen and then toasted, and even then are just not the same.

Eating out is risky. You must carefully research a restaurant before you go, finding out if they offer any gluten-free foods and often speaking to the manager and the chef. I usually go to one of two restaurants that I know to have gluten-free menus. Even then there is a risk of cross-contamination or accidents.

The other day, I found a crouton in the bottom of my salad bowl. This can be disastrous to a person with celiac disease. It signaled all things dark and dastardly. Later that night, it started: a gnawing and clawing from the inside out. It is something akin to severe hunger, but more raw. Then it settled into the pit of my stomach and churned into a piece of broken glass. A reaction to gluten can feel as though every time you move you're stabbed by a shard of glass until you're bleeding from the inside out. This can result in severe projectile vomiting and other gastrointestinal symptoms that are mostly unmentionable.

The Other Celiacs

There are those people who have celiac disease and are really upbeat, even perky, about it all. There are also celiac patients who have mild or no symptoms of the disease. I'm not one of them. They will tell you that we are among the lucky ones, the ones who know they have the illness, the ones who have been diagnosed and now have all this healthy good-for-you food at our disposal. They laud the nature of the illness whereby the only treatment is dietary and does not require surgery or other invasive treatments. But if you ask me, I would much rather have one surgical procedure that would "cure" me and be able to digest wheat the rest of my life than to have to make such a lifestyle overhaul. To have celiac disease is to be socially awkward at best and to be in constant pain at worst. It is not something one wishes for.

The worst part is that no one (other than another celiac sufferer) understands. From the family member who wants you to try "just one bite" of her homemade streusel, to the restaurateur who mistakes white flour for a non-gluten product because it has been "bleached," to the medical professional who thinks it's a simple allergy rather than an autoimmune disease. The lack of awareness of celiac disease is astounding given that nearly three million Americans are said to suffer from it. One problem is that celiac disease is widely under-diagnosed. One in 133 Americans are said to have celiac disease but only one in 2000 knows they have it.

Lack of Awareness

When we are little kids, we are taught that doctors are there to help us. I have had very few doctors who actually helped me. I had one doctor, an endocrinologist, say that they would figure it all out at the autopsy. To have a chronic illness is to realize that you will not be cured. You will learn to live with some pain and illness.

This general lack of awareness of the disease and its effects, even among medical professionals, is unnerving. I've shown up at hospitals vomiting blood, writhing in pain with blood pressure so low I should be crawling, yet I've been told nothing was wrong with me, that all of my blood work was "perfectly normal" and therefore I should just go home and rest.

Of course, had they checked my gluten antibodies, they would have found them to be twice as high as normal, pointing to an accidental ingestion of gluten, which sent my body into a tailspin of auto-immune hell. Yet there is no "auto-immunologist" I can turn to for help.

What's even more frustrating is that celiac disease is not a rare illness. It is estimated that it affects three million Americans!

Lessons Learned

It is not a simple thing to just "eliminate gluten" from one's diet. Gluten, the wheat, barley and rye protein, is in many, many foods, some obvious, yes, but many hidden, too.

I dream of bagels that I can digest and that taste good. I dream of hospitals where treatment comes without skepticism and care comes with respect. And I dream of a place I can go and be welcomed where "everybody knows the name" of celiac sprue. In the meantime, I'm learning to eat to live and not the other way around. And I'm enjoying the simple things in life—the friends who will drive far enough to find a gluten-free restaurant; the same friends who won't devour the bread basket in front of you!

Editor's note:

The preceding personal stories and suggestions reflect a range of reactions to the gluten-free diet. Each expresses a unique perspective. While I feel fortunate and blessed to have been given a diagnosis and to have recovered my health through a gluten-free diet, I must admit that I don't always feel that way. Sometimes, the diet is inconvenient, expensive, and frustrating. However, I'm pleased to say that most of the time my own feelings about the diet are dominated by gratitude. I hope this attitude will continue to dominate my thinking as I suspect that it makes compliance a great deal easier. There are important health reasons for complying with the diet, as the next chapter explores in depth.

CHAPTER 2:
HOW GRAINS CAUSE HEALTH
PROBLEMS AND FATIGUE

Celiac Disease—Gluten Sensitivity: What's the Difference?

By Dr. Ron Hoggan, Ed.D.

We begin this chapter by explaining the important difference between celiac disease and gluten sensitivity (also called intolerance). Some people still struggle with this distinction. Rodney Ford's proposal of the name "gluten syndrome" is a great device for limiting this confusion. Nonetheless, it is important to understand the distinction. If nothing else, it helps us understand the origins of many of the conflicting notions in this realm.

Celiac disease is, by definition, a condition in which the intestinal wall is damaged as a result of eating gluten. It is a chronic illness, in which the symptoms wax and wane[1] for reasons that are not yet understood. Celiac disease is partly a result of genetic and environmental factors. We now know two HLA markers (DQ2 and DQ8) that predispose an individual to celiac disease[2]. One environmental factor is, of course, the consumption of gluten, but there may be other environmental contributors. Some researchers have been exploring viral infections as additional possible environmental contributors, while others have been looking at individual variations in the friendly bacteria that colonize our intestines. Recent research reveals that about 1% of the population suffers from celiac disease[3] although most remain undiagnosed.

On the other hand, gluten sensitivity is characterized by antigliadin antibodies. This condition afflicts at least 12% of the general population[4] and is found in patients with a wide variety of autoimmune diseases, including celiac disease. In one study of neurological diseases of unknown origin, a majority of patients show signs of gluten sensitivity[4]. These patients are mounting an immune response to the most common food in our western diet, yet many practitioners consider gluten sensitivity to be a non-specific finding, frequently counseling patients to ignore these test results. This is particularly unfortunate since a strict gluten-free diet has repeatedly proven helpful to patients who are fortunate enough to consult a practitioner who is versed in gluten sensitivity and its connection with autoimmunity.

Untreated celiac disease carries an elevated risk for a wide variety of autoimmune diseases. The most likely cause of this predisposition to additional autoimmune disease is a condition sometimes referred to as 'leaky gut syndrome.' We know that gluten causes intestinal damage. We also know that this damage allows large undigested and partly digested proteins to leak into the bloodstream through the damaged intestinal wall. This leakage results in immune system production of antibodies to attack these foreign proteins as if they were invading microbes. The result is the production of a huge variety of selective antibodies, and each type recognizes a particular short chain of amino acids located somewhere in the protein's structure. Unfortunately, our own tissues can contain very similar or identical sequences of amino acids. Hence, by a process called molecular mimicry, we are producing antibodies that attack both the foreign food proteins that are leaked into our blood through the damaged intestinal wall, and similar amino acid sequences in our own tissues, often resulting in an autoimmune disease[5].

Recently, in one of the few studies of cancer and mortality in association with gluten sensitivity, Anderson, et al. report a significantly higher risk of malignancy and mortality than either the general population or their small group of subjects with celiac disease[6]. Gluten sensitivity has also been reported in almost one quarter of schizophrenic patients studied, and celiac disease was found more frequently than in the general population, among the same schizophrenic patients[7]. There is an abundance of reports of elevated anti-gliadin antibodies in the context of a variety of bowel diseases, as well.

The allegedly non-specific antigliadin antibodies in gluten sensitivity provide two important pieces of information: 1) That the intestinal wall has been damaged and is permitting leakage of food proteins into the bloodstream 2) That the dynamic contributing to increased autoimmunity in celiac disease may well be an important contributing factor in non-celiac gluten sensitivity[5]. The current, common view is that celiac disease is a serious illness, while gluten sensitivity is meaningless. This is a dangerous misconception, especially for those sensitive to gluten.

This bias is also a divisive element in the gluten-sensitive/celiac community. Whether or not a person has "biopsy proven" damage to the intestinal wall, if this person gets sick from eating gluten, or mounts a measurable immune response to gluten, we are all in the same leaky boat (please pardon the pun). We need to work together to get a better understanding of gluten sensitivity in all its forms, including celiac disease. As a community, we need to discourage any kind of dismissal of illnesses that are partly or wholly mediated by gluten. If we can stand together in our quest for widespread recognition of the damaging impact of gluten consumption, we can all enjoy a healthier life. Our descendants will also inherit a healthier, more gluten-savvy world.

The Gluten Syndrome—Gut, Skin and Brain

By Prof. Rodney Ford, M.D.

The Gluten Syndrome refers to the cluster of symptoms that you experience if you react to gluten. Gluten can affect your gut, your skin, and your brain. *The Gluten Syndrome* applies to any reaction that is caused by gluten. It includes celiac disease, along with the myriad symptoms that can be experienced throughout your gastro-intestinal tract in response to gluten. It also includes many other symptoms that do not stem from your gut. These include brain and behavior disorders, irritability and fatigue, skin problems, muscular aches and pains and joint problems.

The effects of gluten are wide ranging and are now brought together under the term *'Gluten Syndrome.'* In most instances, a simple blood test (the IgG-gliadin antibody test) can identify those people who are affected.

10% Affected by Gluten

The Gluten Syndrome affects about one in ten people. However, most people who are affected are unaware that their life is being hindered by gluten. The gluten-triggered symptoms are most likely to be caused by damage to the nerves and brain. The earlier the problem is identified, the better the response to a gluten-free diet will be.

Tummy Pains and not Growing

Jonti is 3 years old. His gluten story is typical. His mother brought him to see me because she was concerned about his poor growth, and his distressing abdominal pains. His blood tests showed high gluten antibodies. His IgG gliadin was 94 units. (This test result is usually less than 15 units at this age). Other tests, including the gene test for celiac disease, showed that he did not have celiac disease.

I suggested that he go on a gluten-free diet. Within days he began to eat better, and his tummy pains went away. He is now growing again on a gluten-free diet. His mum wrote:

"I really haven't found the gluten-free diet that difficult. I found people to be incredibly helpful actually, both in the supermarket and in restaurants. In the supermarket there is a lot of normal type food that is gluten-free and it is all clearly labeled that it is gluten-free. Even if you go to the delicatessen department they will tell you which luncheon sausage is gluten-free. There are gluten-free sausages all labeled and it's normal food that tastes great.

For the baking mixes and bread mixes, you don't even have to go to the specialist health food shops. I go to no shops other than the supermarket to get food for him and I haven't really found it that difficult."

Amazed how Jonti has adapted

"I have been amazed, actually, by how easily Jonti has adapted to the gluten-free diet. I tell him it is special food for him and that it won't hurt his tummy. We have got nice biscuits from a bakery and he is allowed to choose which one he wants for morning tea. He still has normal foods like chips and sweets. He is not missing out and the other biscuits he hasn't even really asked for. The only thing is the bread! I have yet to perfect the making of the bread. Toast is about the only thing he asked for. You can get specialist cornflakes and cereals, porridge he loves, again, at the supermarket. It has been surprisingly easy actually

I'm so pleased that he is now well again. Gluten-free has made such a huge difference."

The Main Points

- *The Gluten Syndrome* refers to the cluster of symptoms that you experience if you react to gluten. It can affect your gut, skin and nerves.
- Medical practitioners accept that gluten causes celiac disease (gut damage), but often resist the notion that gluten can cause a wider spectrum of illness.
- Celiac disease, gluten intolerance and gluten sensitivity are all part of *The Gluten Syndrome*.
- Rapidly accumulating medical evidence shows that gluten is now creating a massive health problem throughout the Western world. However, woefully few people are aware of the catalogue of harm that gluten is causing. *The Gluten Syndrome* affects about one in ten people—many millions in all.
- Gluten could be responsible for one-third of all cases of chronic illness and fatigue. People suffering from these conditions are currently just tolerating their symptoms, unaware that gluten is the culprit. This is because the medical community does not yet recognize the link to gluten.

- Gluten-containing products are being added to our food chain in increasing amounts. Our wheat is being engineered to have even higher gluten content. This gluten overload is occurring without our communities being unaware of the harm that this is causing.
- Gluten can cause malfunctions of the brain and neural networks of susceptible people. The incidence of mental, neurological and brain disorders is on the rise. However, the diagnosis of gluten-sensitivity is seldom made.
- The community is already embracing the notion of gluten-sensitivity. More and more people are opting for a gluten-free lifestyle. These people are looking for a term to identify their illness. Their search is over. They have been affected by *The Gluten Syndrome*.
- A strong gluten-free movement is developing globally in response to the knowledge that going gluten-free can be so beneficial to so many people. What has been missing up until now is a name that captures the gluten problem. The missing name is *The Gluten Syndrome*.

Get Your Blood Tests

The Gluten Tests

Gluten is a protein that is found in wheat grains. This protein has a number of components, one of which is called **gliadin**. People who get sick from gluten are usually reacting to the gliadin component.

You are a Long Tube

To understand what the blood tests mean, first you need to know a little more about your immune system. It is the job of your immune system to protect you from the outside world. It protects you from the invasion of microbes (viruses and bacteria), and it also protects you from the toxins and poisons in the food that passes through your gut. Your gut is a long tube inside you that travels from your mouth to your anus. This is your gastrointestinal tract, also called your bowel. Even though it is inside your body, the contents of this tube are still on the 'outside' from your body's point of view. Lots of your immune cells coat the skin (called the mucosa) of this tube and work hard to protect you from anything that might prove to be harmful.

Gluten (Gliadin) can be Toxic

Gliadin, the toxic component of the gluten protein, is one such harmful substance. Your immune system defends your body strongly against gliadin using weapons called

antibodies and the gliadin is repelled. The outcome of your immune system's fight against gliadin is the production of antibodies that are specifically targeted towards gliadin: these are called anti-gliadin antibodies.

Gliadin Antibodies

Anti-gliadin Antibodies (commonly called the **IgG-gliadin** antibody) are weapons that have been made specifically to fight against gluten in the diet. Remember, gliadin is a component of the gluten protein. This antibody is very sensitive. It is made very specifically by your immune system to fight against gliadin. However, a high level of this antibody does not necessarily mean that you have any gut damage, so it is not very accurate in assisting the identification of patients with celiac gut damage. On the other hand, tests for this antibody are nearly always strongly positive in people with celiac disease who are not on a gluten-free diet. Once people are placed on a strict diet, these antibodies will fall to normal levels within a period ranging from few months to a year or two.

Gluten Tests Not Getting Done

There is a problem. Unfortunately, this gluten blood test, called the IgG-gliadin antibody test, is no longer available from most community laboratories. Many laboratories have decided to discontinue this test. Their opinion is that it is worthless—for detecting celiac disease.

I disagree with their decision. My latest data shows that huge numbers of people remain undiagnosed with serious symptoms because of the misinterpretation of this gluten test result. At the moment it is difficult to get the medical labs to do your gluten test. They are unwilling to consider that gluten causes a wide spectrum of illness that has been written up in the international medical literature. They have turned a blind eye to the problem. If you can't test for gluten reactions, then you will not be able to make the diagnosis!

A Diagnosis at Last!

Mandy wrote this letter to me: "Hi Dr Rodney Ford. For many, many, years I have been to doctors complaining of a bloated tummy, extreme cramping pains, and diarrhea (to the point I had no time to get to the toilet). I have recently had some blood tests for celiac done by my GP. My results showed: the tTG was negative; and the IgG-Gliadin result strongly positive. He could not explain it to me, but he said that I did not have celiac disease."

"I have no idea what these tests mean. Although I got no answers, I had to try something. I was at the end of my nerves! My bad health has always been upsetting my social and working life. I often have to rush home to the toilet."

Amazing on a Gluten-free Diet

"So I decided to try a gluten-free diet! I have now been gluten-free for a month. It is amazing! Already I feel like a different person! No more bloating, just the odd stomach cramp. Also, all my headaches have gone. But I still feel really tired and not sure how to overcome this. Can you help me please by explaining my blood test results—and should I have any more tests? What else I can do to help myself? I hope you can help me Dr Ford. Gluten, up to now, seems to have made my life a misery. Even though I feel so much better already, I want to get even better. Kind regards, Mandy."

The Gluten Syndrome

I replied: "Thanks. I am glad that you are feeling a lot better off gluten. From your story and your blood test results, you have gluten-sensitivity. You do not have celiac disease (your low tTG level shows that you do not have any gut damage from gluten). But you are still getting sick from gluten (your high IgG-gliadin level shows that your body reacts to gluten). The good news is that it takes many months to get the full benefits of a gluten-free diet. I expect that you will continue to feel better over the next few months. You should be taking some additional iron and a multivitamin supplements because you will be relatively iron deficient—that will be making you tired."

The Time has Come

The history of science and medicine is littered with vehement arguments against any new idea that runs contrary to traditional beliefs. Ironically however, it takes new ideas to make progress. It was George Bernard Shaw who said:

> The reasonable man adapts himself to the world: the unreasonable one persists in trying to adapt the world to him. Therefore, all progress depends on the unreasonable man.

Thousands Convinced

Many people are joining the ranks of the gluten-free. There are thousands of people like you who have read this information and who are concerned about how gluten might be affecting them. There a millions of people who are sick and tired of being ignored and who are looking for more energy and vitality. There are the practitioners in the field of complementary medicine who are aware of the concept of gluten-sensitivity. There are the laboratories that have developed the gliadin antibody test and know that their tests are specific for gluten reactions. There are the gluten-free food manufacturers who have recognized that there is an ever-increasing demand for gluten-free products. There are the networks of people in the health food industry who appreciate the value of high-quality food and a gluten-free diet. Lastly, there are the supermarkets and grocery stores that are sensitive to the demands of their customers.

Who Might Oppose this Trend?

As previously discussed, medical practitioners are wary of overturning tradition. They do not want to be seen as alternative and want to avoid acting outside of the recommended clinical guidelines. In addition, there are the grain-growers and the bread-makers who make their living from gluten, and the pharmaceutical companies who make their living from the sick and unwell.

Bad Behavior on Gluten

Kimberley is 12 years old. She has *The Gluten Syndrome* and her behavior gets disturbed with gluten. She does not have celiac disease, but she does have a high gluten test. (Her IgG-gliadin level was 55 units—It should be less than 20.)

Her mum said: "It is interesting about how behavior troubles are linked to gluten! Our youngest, Kimberley, is now 12 years old. She had her IgG-gliadin measured and it was high. She was clearly a lot better when she was off gluten. However then she decided to 'try' gluten again. Rodney suggested a small amount but she went for it—big time!"

By the end of a week, two other parents had asked what was wrong with her. Another parent asked "what on earth's the matter with her" she seemed so different and stroppy. She admitted she felt "absolutely awful" but really didn't want to admit it as she knew it meant she'd have to completely give up gluten."

Anyway, after a lot of talking, she agreed it wasn't in her best interests to eat gluten. From that day she has been gluten-free ever since, with the odd very long envious glance at French bread! With our support she's very compliant with being GF now, which I think is remarkable for her age. Clearly, she now understands and gets the benefits of GF. But I was really shocked at how affected her behavior was after a reintroduction of gluten."

Could You Have The Gluten Syndrome?

One in every ten people is affected by gluten. If you have chronic symptom (feeling sick, tired and grumpy) then you should get checked for *The Gluten Syndrome*.

Ironing Some Wrinkles Out of Gluten Sensitivity

By Dr. Ron Hoggan, Ed. D.

Close to one quarter of the world's population, in both industrialized and developing countries, suffer from iron deficiency and/or iron deficiency anemia. As mentioned by Dr. Ford in the previous article, iron deficiency is a common companion of gluten sensitivity. Although it is a widespread problem, those who are gluten sensitive should be particularly careful to monitor their iron status regularly. Iron deficiency is not only an important sign of undiagnosed celiac disease, it may also reflect some degree of intestinal damage—and most of our iron is absorbed in the same part of the intestine as calcium and other minerals. The jejunum is the site of most of the damage caused by gluten, which may explain the significant overlap between gluten sensitivity and iron deficiency.

The two primary causes of iron deficiency, in adults, are either inadequate absorption of iron or excessive blood loss, and intestinal bleeding is common in the gluten syndrome. Iron deficiency can also result from certain vitamin deficiencies, which can also be a feature of celiac disease.

Several years after I began following a gluten-free diet, a blood test that was part of a regular physical exam revealed that I was mildly anemic. By now you may be wondering, just as I did, what the difference is between iron deficiency and iron deficiency anemia. Simply put, iron deficiency anemia is where the hemoglobin content of one's blood is below normal. This means that there are fewer blood cells that carry oxygen to be distributed throughout the body. Iron deficiency, on the other hand, is where iron stores are lower than they should be.

My greatest concern with my own inclination to anemia is that iron deficiency can impair memory and reduce learning acuity. Most of this impact occurs prior to the development of anemia. Iron deficiency first depletes iron stores in a wide range of tissues and organs before it causes significant losses to hemoglobin. Iron is needed to make several neurotransmitters including dopamine, serotonin, and norepinepherine. These neurotransmitters are involved in a wide range of brain activities related to alertness, attention, remembering, learning, and a variety of other brain functions. Iron stores are so important that some researchers at the University of Maryland have reported that iron deficient adolescent girls (without anemia) show a significant improvement in IQ test scores after only 8 weeks of taking iron supplements.

There are many other symptoms of iron deficiency anemia, including shortness of breath, light-headedness, lethargy, and pale skin. However, it is important not to just rush out and start taking iron supplements. Iron overdose can cause damage to the liver, the heart, or the pancreas. The body must maintain an exquisitely careful balance for optimal function and good health. Further, a significant number of celiacs also suffer from hereditary hemochromatosis which is a condition in which the body is overly thrifty, storing too much iron. Supplementing iron in such a case could have some very serious consequences. Regular testing is an important strategy.

Iron deficiency and/or iron deficiency anemia is less likely to be given the attention it warrants simply because of the frequency with which it occurs. However, it is a particularly important issue to those who are gluten sensitive, if only from a quality-of-life perspective. Even if peace of mind is the only result of getting regular check-ups that include a complete blood count, ferritin, and transferrin, our reward is large.

Similarly, early detection and reversal of iron deficiency before it causes memory disturbances and other unwanted symptoms, and before it develops into anemia, could be a huge dividend to collect from paying careful attention to our iron levels. Anemia in celiac disease is discussed more extensively in the next article.

The Anemia and Celiac Disease Connection

By Cynthia Kupper, RD, CD

Anemia is one of the most common presentations in adults with newly diagnosed celiac disease. In 1996 approximately 3.4 million Americans were diagnosed with anemia, according to the Centers for Disease Control, and out of these 2.1 million were under the age of 45. Celiac disease can present with classic and/or atypical symptoms. Atypical symptoms of celiac disease are associated with malabsorption and can include iron deficiency anemia in both adults and children.

Celiac disease was once thought to be a childhood disease. However the average age at diagnosis today is 40 to 50 years old. It is more commonly seen in women than men.

Celiac disease is a disease that can begin in infancy with gastrointestinal symptoms, in childhood, or even late in life. Many persons diagnosed later in life may have no gastro-intestinal symptoms. Often, in older adults, routine health checks discover silent celiac disease, because of undefined anemia or bone disease[3].

Anemia can be a symptom of many conditions, including excess blood loss from bleed-ing or surgery; autoimmune diseases such as celiac disease; chronic infections, or from the use of some medications. There are different types of anemia. Blood studies are used to help determine the type of anemia, its possible cause, and the correct treatment. *Macrocytic anemia* is usually caused by a folate or vitamin B12 deficiency. *Microcytic ane-mia* is caused from iron deficiency. Inflammation, either chronic or acute, can alter fer-ritin levels in persons with iron-deficiency anemia. When inflammation is present, iron levels can appear either normal or elevated in iron deficiency.

Folate deficiency should be considered in persons who have both celiac disease and anemia. Folate is absorbed in the jejunum, the upper part of the small intestine. This is the part of the small intestine that is largely damaged in untreated or undiagnosed celiac disease. Celiac disease is a disease of malabsorption due to inflammation and damage of the microvilli and villi of the small intestine. The microvilli and villi normally increase the absorption capacity of the small intestine by expanding its surface area by nearly 500 times. When there is damage to the jejunum and duodenum, the absorption of many nutrients, including iron, is altered. Celiac disease is not often suspected when a person is diagnosed with persistent anemia that does not respond well to traditional therapies, even though iron absorption can be significantly altered by the damage to the intestine.

Studies suggest that persons with celiac disease may present with anemia as a single symptom or one of many symptoms. The incidence of anemia in the patients with newly diagnosed celiac disease ranges from 4% in the United States, to 24% in Romania, and over 66% in East Indian patients. In surveys of members of national celiac support groups in Canada and the U.S., anemia is a common pre-celiac diagnosis. Three recent studies in the United Kingdom screened men and women with anemia for celiac disease and found undiagnosed celiac disease in 2.3 to 6.7 percent of subjects. Another study in the UK screened 1,200 people in the general population and found celiac disease in one percent, a frequency similar to that of the U.S. study.

It is possible to conservatively estimate that 78,000 people Americans with anemia could have celiac disease as the cause of their anemia. Clearly, physicians treating patients with anemia should consider screening them for celiac disease, especially if the anemia is unresponsive to traditional therapy.

Anemias Found in Celiac Disease

Several conditions can contribute to the development of anemia, including blood loss, poor diet, genetic disorders, chronic illnesses, and damage to the bone marrow from radiation or chemotherapy. Gastrointestinal conditions, such as Crohn's disease or celiac disease, that decrease the absorption of iron, folate, or vitamin B12 can also cause anemia. Iron-deficiency anemia is the most common type of anemia found in women. The most common causes of iron-deficiency anemia are blood loss due to menstruation or pregnancy, and poor absorption of iron from foods[15]. Iron deficiency is uncommon in postmenopausal women. If iron-deficiency anemia is discovered in postmenopausal women, it is generally the result of bleeding in the gastrointestinal tract or malabsorption.

Both iron-deficiency anemia and B12 deficiencies are common in celiac disease. Iron-deficiency anemia is the most common type of anemia found with celiac disease. Decreased iron and folate absorption are often seen in untreated celiac disease. Many physicians overlook iron and folate malabsorption as a cause of anemia. As part of the evaluation process for iron-deficiency anemia endoscopic procedures are often per-formed, generally without taking biopsies of the small intestine. If biopsies are not taken, celiac disease would be overlooked as the cause of the anemia.

Generally, anemia develops slowly with symptoms worsening over time. Common symptoms of anemia include extreme fatigue, pale skin, weakness, shortness of breath, lightheadedness, and cold hands and feet. Iron-deficiency anemia symptoms may also include cracks at the sides of the mouth, complaints of inflamed or sore tongue, brittle nails, pica, headaches, decreased appetite, and increased infections. Some people may also experience Restless Leg Syndrome. If not treated, iron-deficiency anemia can lead to other severe health problems, such as heart irregularities; complications with pre-mature and low-birth-weight infants; and delayed growth and development in children. Symptoms of Vitamin B_{12} deficiency can cause yellowing or darkening of the skin, col-orblindness to yellow-blue colors, and confusion or forgetfulness. Signs of vitamin B12 deficiencies such as neurological problems, peripheral neuropathy, mental confusion and forgetfulness can be seen before anemia is diagnosed.

The most likely cause of vitamin B12 deficiency in celiac disease is due to damage in the small intestine, which makes it difficult to adequately absorb B12. Bacterial over-growth in the small intestine is another possible cause of B12 deficiency. Anemia, as a result of vitamin B12 deficiency is considered to be uncommon in celiac disease that is diagnosed early.

In a small study of 39 patients, Dahele, *et al.*, 16 (41 percent) were found to have vitamin B12 deficiency and 16 were anemic. After four months on a gluten-free diet all patients with B12 deficiency had B12 levels that normalized. Only five patients with combined folate and B12 deficiencies received B12 therapy.

Dickey found in screening celiac patients with low serum vitamin B12 levels that low B12 is common in celiac disease without having pernicious anemia, and may be the only presenting manifestation of celiac disease (14). Studies by Dahele and Dickey suggest that vitamin B12 deficiency is a common condition in untreated celiac disease, however their studies do not support that pernicious anemia is associated with celiac disease. Dahele and Dickey indicate the vitamin B12 deficiency usually resolves on a gluten-free diet, without vitamin B12 replacement.

Treating Anemia in Celiac Disease

The most important issue in anemia, resulting from celiac disease, is to follow a strict gluten-free diet. The small intestine must heal in order to absorb nutrients correctly and adequately. Studies indicate that it can take several months to years to heal the small intestine in persons with celiac disease and it is imperative that all persons with celiac disease have regular follow-up visits with a dietitian to check the adequacy of their diet.

A gluten-free diet alone has been shown to reverse signs of anemia in most newly diagnosed celiac patients. In otherwise healthy individuals, it takes six to 12 months of diet therapy to correct anemia. Reversing anemia in persons with celiac disease may take several months longer, even with supplementation. Iron replacement therapy may not be necessary in mildly depleted persons. In these cases a gluten-free diet high in iron-rich foods and a good gluten-free multi-vitamin supplement should be tried for six to 12 months before further therapy options are considered. Persons taking iron supplements should take iron with vitamin C-rich foods, such as citrus juice, which will help increase iron absorption. They should also avoid calcium and dairy products within an hour of eating iron-rich foods, as calcium binds with iron and neither nutrient is absorbed well. Iron-rich foods including fish, poultry, and red meats should be included at each meal. Use of coffee and tea should be restricted.

Iron supplementation therapy recommendations for persons with celiac disease vary by physician. Recommendations of up to one gram of iron per day, with close monitoring for clinical and blood level improvement are sometimes recommended. In severe situations, blood transfusions are used to boost the patient's initial iron and hemoglobin levels. As with other medications, all supplements used must be gluten-free.

Foods rich in iron that are naturally gluten-free include: lean red meats, liver, kidney, clams, oysters, shrimp, chicken, haddock, crab, tuna, salmon, turkey, broccoli, parsley, leafy greens, peas, dried beans, lentils, peaches, pears, dates, raisins, dried prunes, and blackstrap molasses. Many of the special seeds and flours used in the gluten-free diet are rich in iron, including amaranth, buckwheat, Montina™, quinoa, and teff. These foods are also high in other nutrients, including calcium, amino acids, magnesium, zinc and fiber. When compared to whole wheat and enriched all-purpose white wheat flours (iron content 4.7 mg and 5.8 mg, respectively), many of the gluten-free flours are nutritionally equal or superior to wheat flour. Amaranth, buckwheat, flax, garfava, millet, Montina™, quinoa, rice bran and soy all have higher iron content than wheat flours. In gluten-free baking, a blend of flours is required for best results.

Many of the flours mentioned above are used as secondary ingredients in the flour blends, in combination with refined starches such as rice flour, potato starch and tapioca or corn starch, all of which are much lower in iron than wheat flour. Using the whole seed or groat of these seeds in cooking can significantly increase the iron content of the gluten-free diet. Many of these products make wonderful side dishes and starches in casseroles or soups. Teff is used as a staple food in Ethiopia. It is extremely high in iron and it is speculated that it is the extensive use of teff that keeps the incidence of iron-deficiency anemia low in Ethiopia. For persons with celiac disease who are also lactose intolerant or choose to follow a vegetarian diet, inclusion of these seeds helps to assure adequate nutrient intake.

Anemia is common in the general population and even higher in celiac disease. Malabsorption is a common cause of anemia. Persons with anemia are at risk for celiac disease. Patients with anemia from unknown reasons or those who do not respond to traditional treatments require further evaluation, which should include screening for celiac disease. If celiac disease is discovered, appropriate treatment with a gluten-free diet that includes foods that are rich in iron is normally all that is necessary to treat anemia in most cases.

The Dietary Reference Index (RDI) for Iron:

7 to 10 mg/day for young children
8 to 11 mg/day for males

15 to 18 mg/day for females of menstrual age

8 mg/day for older females

27 mg/day during pregnancy

Editor's note:

The following articles explore some of the health concerns that are often seen in connection with celiac disease. From fibromyalgia, to food cravings, to interstitial cystitis, thyroid disease and various nutrient deficiencies, to autoimmunity, celiac disease either underlies or accompanies many of these conditions and complaints. While some of the following reports may not yet be congruent with mainstream Medicine, some unique and intriguing insights are offered in the articles that form the remainder of this chapter.

Unraveling Fibromyalgia

By Roy S. Jamron

Fibromyalgia frequently occurs among those with celiac disease but, to my knowledge, no published study to date provides prevalence data. However, one survey found that in cases of celiac disease that were initially misdiagnosed by physicians, 9% were initially diagnosed as having fibromyalgia[1,2,3].

Fibromyalgia is defined as a chronic widespread pain lasting more than three months in all four body quadrants with pain present in at least 11 of 18 specific tender point sites. Fibromyalgia does not cause joint pain or swelling, as arthritis does, but produces pain in soft tissues around joints, in skin, and in organs throughout the body. A wide variety of symptoms and syndromes are usually associated with fibromyalgia. These include fatigue, stiffness (especially upon awakening), disturbed sleep, dry mouth, dry eyes, dry skin, headaches, frequent urination, cold sensitivity, mental fog, dizziness, irritable bowel syndrome, restless leg syndrome, and more. Pain location and severity, as well as the severity of symptoms and syndromes, can vary in an individual from day to day. The characteristics of fibromyalgia differ widely from individual to individual. The condition can be long-term and extremely debilitating, affecting quality of life and limiting one's employment options. People with chronic fatigue syndrome suffer many of the same symptoms of fibromyalgia suggesting a possible relationship[4,5].

There is no laboratory test for fibromyalgia. Diagnosis is a process of ruling out other possible conditions through medical history, physical examination, and finally, evaluating the 18 tender points. A skilled examiner determines the number of tender points, by applying pressure to the points, as the patient reports whether pain is experienced. As the number of tender points can vary from day to day, and the test relies on the skill of the examiner and the patient's pain perceptions.

Rheumatologists are recognizing the shortcomings of this diagnostic protocol. In fact, the number of tender points does not even correlate to the severity of the pain experienced by fibromyalgia patients. An emerging view is that those with 11 out of 18 tender point criteria simply fall on one end of a spectrum of fibromyalgia-like chronic widespread pain.

Some 80% of those diagnosed with fibromyalgia are women. Across different countries, the prevalence rate of fibromyalgia ranges from 0.5% to 5%. Chronic widespread pain that falls short of the minimum 11 tender points, affects 7.3% to 12.9% of the general population[6]. This means there are many more people who suffer fibromyalgia-like pain and symptoms without technically meeting the diagnostic criteria for fibromyalgia. This discussion is meant to include those people. Thus, when fibromyalgia is mentioned here, it includes all those with fibromyalgia-like symptoms regardless of the number of tender points.

Medical science is still grappling with the exact cause and nature of fibromyalgia. First thought to be an inflammation of the muscles and soft tissue, studies have not found inflammation and have found normal muscle response in patients[7,8]. Now, most researchers suspect that abnormalities of the brain and central nervous system are responsible for the disorder. Initiation or triggering of fibromyalgia has been attributed to injuries, stress, infections, or toxins, and frequently accompanies a number of autoimmune diseases. Conventional medical treatment of fibromyalgia is limited to over-the-counter and prescription pain medications, including analgesics, anti-inflammatory medications, narcotics, and pain patches. Anti-depressants, muscle relaxants, anti-spasm and anti-convulsive medications, sleep medications and sedatives, and some newer neurological drugs are also prescribed. Additional therapies include physical rehabilitation and nutrition. The effectiveness of these treatments varies widely among individuals, and none offers a cure. Many people turn to alternative medicine when conventional medicine fails to provide relief. Magazine and newspaper ads and Internet web sites target the desperate, and sufferers may be more likely to be relieved of their money than their pain.

My Symptoms

I don't know how many tender points I have had or may have had, but I have fibromyalgia-like chronic widespread pain and symptoms that became so bad I had to quit my job a few months ago. I am a self-diagnosed celiac and am gluten-free for more than six years. Over a year ago I developed a pain in my left shoulder, which eventually shifted to the right shoulder. Then the pain moved into my legs, especially the right leg. I was fatigued. My mouth and throat were dry at night. I had to urinate frequently. I felt colder than normal. My right leg ached when lying in bed. I was extremely stiff in the morning. Bowel discomfort was already present from celiac disease but fibromyalgia may have made it worse. There was often swelling in my ankles and feet. It became painful to walk or put on a shirt or a coat. My symptoms continued to worsen, affecting both arms and shoulders, both legs and my right hip. Any small chore or physical activity became a challenge. Turning the steering wheel of my truck hurt. I dreaded grocery shopping.

I suspect that my condition may have been triggered by years of exposure to chemicals and cleaning solvents present in the environment at my job in the automotive industry—chemicals I did not work with directly, but which were used in quantity near my work area. This would not be the first time chemicals or toxins caused fibromyalgia-like pain.

Seven years ago I underwent surgical repair of a right inguinal hernia (a tear in the tissue near the groin allowing the intestine to protrude beneath the skin), followed six months later by a repair of a left inguinal hernia. In each case, I was given an intravenous antibiotic, local anesthetic and sedation. After the first surgery, I experienced a sharp pain in the right leg that made it too painful to even move my leg or bend the knee. The pain diminished after a day, but it took more than a month to fully regain movement in my right leg without pain.

After the second surgery, I did not experience any leg pain, but I did experience a strange dry, metallic cotton-like sensation in my mouth lasting more than a day. These two sensations would later come back to haunt me when I engaged in a self-experiment.

After diagnosing myself with celiac disease, I wondered if an overabundance of bacteria could be responsible for continuing bowel discomfort. I wanted to try an antibiotic to see if it could provide relief. On the internet, I found that over-the-counter Pepto-Bismol tablets (bismuth subsalicylate) have antibiotic properties. It has been used to treat microscopic colitis and, in combination with other antibiotics, helicobacter pylori infection. Label instructions state that up to eight doses of Pepto-Bismol may be taken in a 24-hour period (for adults, a dose is two tablets.) The treatment for microscopic colitis is eight tablets a day for eight weeks, and I decided to try this treatment. It seemed safe enough. No warnings, no adverse reactions were indicated. Millions of people use Pepto-Bismol without any problems.

From the beginning, Pepto-Bismol made me uncomfortable. I could only tolerate six tablets a day, instead of eight. After one week, I began to experience stiffness in my legs in the morning. At the end of two weeks I felt so bad that I decided to end the experiment—but it was too late. Even after stopping, the stiffness in the legs continued to worsen.

A few days later, I experienced the same intense pain in my right leg and the strange, dry metallic cotton-like mouth sensation I had experienced after the hernia surgeries, only this time it was much worse. I was bed-ridden and unable to walk or go to work for three days. The pain was at first localized to my right leg, my right wrist, and a finger, which had received stitches for a cut when I was seven years old, but after a few days the pain began to spread out.

Eventually the pain spread to both shoulders and both legs and looked very much like fibromyalgia. The pain finally remained primarily in the right leg. Other symptoms included frequent urination, night chills, and night sweats that left my sheets soaked. After four months, the pain and symptoms finally went away, and I resumed "normal" activities, hoping never to experience such pain again.

In both cases of surgery, and the Pepto-Bismol episode, the trigger of the pain was clear and certain. Two weeks of Pepto-Bismol exposure resulted in four months of pain. I can only speculate about what chemical exposure may have caused my current condition or how long I may have been exposed to the chemicals. I have no idea how long the current symptoms may last. I wonder why I am overly sensitive to these chemicals and drugs? And exactly what is the mechanism that causes my fibromyalgia pain? Medical science offers no answers at this time. It therefore falls on me to find an explanation for my fibromyalgia and, hopefully, find a treatment. What follows is a hypothesis, which I believe offers just that.

In this process, there are some assumptions I have to make. For instance, I have to assume that the nature of the chronic, widespread pain I feel is similar to the pain experienced by other fibromyalgia sufferers. I can only know my own pain. I cannot know theirs. I am also assuming that whatever mechanism is causing my own pain is the same mechanism that causes pain in other fibromyalgia victims.

Fibromyalgia: Neuropathy or Inflammation?

The current dominant medical belief is that abnormal brain and central nervous system response is behind fibromyalgia pain—I do not agree. My pain exists at specific body locations and intensifies with certain stretching and extension movements of the limbs. It feels to me like multiple local inflammations. If the central nervous system or brain is generating abnormal pain signals, then why is the pain coming from specific points and limb movements instead of everywhere in my body? Additionally, why would I have swelling in my ankles and feet? Finally, at times, I hear and feel "squishing" at the sites of pain when I move my limbs. The brain is certainly not creating this "squishing". All signs point to a physical abnormality and if inflammation is not present in the muscle tissue, then it must be somewhere else.

In a review of medical publications, I became intrigued by a reference to two Spanish sisters with alpha1-antitrypsin (AAT) deficiency and fibromyalgia. The liver produces alpha1-antitrypsin, an important anti-inflammatory and proteinase inhibitor that circulates in serum impregnating most body tissues. An in-vitro study found that a low level of alpha1-antitrypsin induces human monocytes (white blood cells) to release pro-inflammatory substances. In those with AAT deficiency, a genetic flaw prevents liver cells from secreting alpha1-antitrypsin, and it builds up within the liver instead of being circulated. The risk of liver and lung disorders is increased in AAT deficient patients. The two Spanish sisters underwent AAT replacement therapy, and, strikingly, their fibromyalgia symptoms vanished. During a worldwide commercial shortage of AAT replacement therapy, their therapy was halted for 4-6 months a year during each of 5 years of treatment. Each time therapy was halted and resumed, their fibromyalgia symptoms reappeared and vanished. This led their doctors to propose a hypothesis suggesting that fibromyalgia may be related to an imbalance between inflammatory and anti-inflammatory substances[9,10,11].

A review of AAT deficiency websites and discussion sites did not provide any prevalence data for fibromyalgia among AAT deficient patients, nor was fibromyalgia a significant topic of discussion, which I interpreted as suggesting that fibromyalgia requires more than just AAT deficiency. Low levels of AAT are found in patients who test positive for human immunodeficiency virus (HIV). Studies have found rates of fibromyalgia, based on tender points, in HIV positive patients at 11% and 29%[12,13,14,15]. Interestingly, low levels of AAT were found in a significant percentage of a group of children living in an area with industrial air pollution, relative to AAT levels in children from an unpolluted area. AAT levels were restored to normal in most of the children after a year and a half[16]. This suggests that chemicals in the environment may have an adverse affect on liver function, in turn, reducing AAT production, thus increasing the risk of developing fibromyalgia symptoms.

The Liver Connection

At this point, my attention turned to liver function. Could abnormal liver function be a factor contributing to fibromyalgia? Liver dysfunction of any type in celiac disease, at time of diagnosis, has been reported in up to 42% of adults and 54% of children. The most common irregularity is raised levels of transaminase enzymes (released by damaged liver cells), which usually normalize on a gluten-free diet. Chronic hepatitis, fibrosis, cirrhosis, fatty liver, primary biliary cirrhosis, primary sclerosing cholangitis, and autoimmune hepatitis have all been found present in celiac disease patients, usually remitting following treatment and a gluten-free diet. Increased intestinal permeability and gluten toxicity have both been proposed as mechanisms leading to liver dysfunction[17,18,19].

The liver plays a number of crucial roles in maintaining the body. It regulates serum levels of glucose and synthesizes and regulates cholesterol. It synthesizes and secretes numerous blood proteins. Bile, necessary for the digestion of fats, is also synthesized and secreted by the liver. The liver stores glucose, minerals such as copper and iron, fat-soluble vitamins (vitamins A, D, E, and K), vitamin B12, folate, and other substances. Through processes of purification, transformation and clearance, the liver removes harmful substances from the blood (such as ammonia and toxins) breaking them down or transforming them into less harmful compounds. The liver metabolizes most hormones and ingested drugs into either more or less active substances. Many toxins or chemicals inhaled, digested, or absorbed through the skin are fat soluble, and it is the liver that can transform fat soluble toxins into water soluble compounds, permitting their elimination by the kidneys. The liver also removes dead cells, various debris, and microorganisms including bacteria, viruses, fungi, and parasites. Pre-existing liver disease or dysfunction can compromise liver function causing hormonal imbalances, blood protein deficiencies, and inhibit the liver's ability to remove or transform toxins. The very same chemicals and toxins the liver is attempting to remove may cause liver dysfunction or damage beginning a vicious cycle where the liver is unable to fight back, ultimately allowing the chemicals and toxins to accumulate in the liver and do increasingly more harm.

To the best of my knowledge, there are no published data on liver function and fibromyalgia. Yet there is good reason to suspect such a relationship. A relationship to alpha1-antitrypsin, synthesized and secreted by the liver, has already been discussed. Growth hormone deficiency has been linked to at least a subset of fibromyalgia patients. Some 30% of fibromyalgia patients have a low level of insulin-like growth factor-1 (IGF-1)[20]. As it happens, the liver produces IGF-1 Glutathione depletion has been suggested as factor in chronic fatigue syndrome, and thus, by implication, a possible factor in fibromyalgia[21]. Glutathione is most concentrated in the liver where it is both produced and stored. Thyroid hormone disorders have also been linked to fibromyalgia. In addition to the thyroid gland, the liver plays an important role in the regulation and circulation of thyroid hormones. And, of course, the liver removes chemicals and toxins, a suspected trigger of fibromyalgia.

The Thyroid Connection

Thyroid hormones are a key to stimulating many of the body's metabolic activities. They increase protein synthesis in virtually every body tissue and regulate oxygen consumption. They are essential for normal growth, development, and the regulation of cellular energy metabolism. Neuromuscular complaints are extremely common in patients with thyroid dysfunction[22]. There is a high rate of thyroid disorder among celiac disease patients[23].

Thyroid function was tested in a small group of fibromyalgia patients. While basal thyroid hormone levels were in the normal range, when injected with thyrotropin-releasing hormone (TRH), the fibromyalgia patients responded with a significantly lower secretion of thyrotropin and thyroid hormones[24]. One chiropractic doctor, Dr. John C. Lowe, has been studying the thyroid status in fibromyalgia patients, coming to the conclusion that some form of thyroid disease may be present in up to 89% of fibromyalgia patients. He has been administering therapeutic dosages of T3 to his fibromyalgia patients who test normal for thyroid status with up to 75% showing improvement in fibromyalgia symptoms. He theorizes that these normal thyroid fibromyalgia patients may have "thyroid hormone resistance[25,26]."

The thyroid gland secretes the hormones thyroxine (T4) and tri-idothyronine (T3) with T3 secreted in very small quantities compared to T4. T3, however, is the more active hormone, with ten times more T4 needed to produce the same physiological effect. Since T4 is the inactive hormone and the major product of the thyroid gland, it needs to be converted into the active T3 hormone. The liver accounts for a large percentage of T4 to T3 activation. Conversion of T4 to rT3 and T3 to T2, both inactive metabolites, also takes place in the liver. T3 and T4 are not water soluble, and, in order to circulate in the blood, must bind with plasma proteins. These binding proteins consist of thyroxin-binding globulin, thyroxin-binding prealbumin, and albumin, all of which are produced in the liver. The binding proteins also serve to protect T3 and T4 permitting a storage pool of hormones, which can last for many days. More than 99% of the thyroid hormones are bound to these proteins, and it is the small free unbound hormone fraction that accounts for the biological activities of the hormones. Plasma concentrations of free T3 and T4 are held at a steady state, exposing tissues to the same concentrations of free hormone. Normal thyroid function is dependent on normal function of both the thyroid and liver. Dysfunction in the liver can affect thyroid function and vice versa[27,28].

Glutathione

Intravenous infusions of glutathione are being used in therapy for chronic fatigue syndrome and fibromyalgia[29,30]. Glutathione is a tripeptide composed of the amino acids glutamate, cystine, and glycine and participates in numerous cellular reactions. It functions in many roles. As an antioxidant, it scavenges free radicals and other reactive species, removes hydrogen and lipid peroxides, and prevents oxidation of biomolecules. It acts in many metabolic activities, including storage and transport of cystine. And it serves in the regulation of signal transduction and gene expression, DNA and protein synthesis, proteolysis, cell proliferation and apoptosis, cytokine production and immune response, mitochondrial function, and more. Glutathione, most highly concentrated in the liver, is a key to the liver's ability to remove toxic substances where it is required in the process of converting fat-soluble substances into excretable water-soluble products. Liver disease can both cause and result from a glutathione deficiency.

Liver dysfunction and toxic substances appear to be involved in fibromyalgia, but what causes fibromyalgia pain and where is the pain centered? A possible answer to this question was inspired by a worsening of my own fibromyalgia pain symptoms. After quitting my job, my symptoms seemed to slowly improve. However, suddenly everything went downhill. The pain in my right leg and hip was especially bad. Lying in bed only intensified the pain and it was impossible to find a comfortable position for my right leg. After keeping the right leg straight in one position for any length of time, the slightest motion would cause the hip joint to pop accompanied by a brief, sharp, excruciating pain at the hip joint. I saw this new pain as a valuable clue for solving the mystery of fibromyalgia pain. I realized that whatever was causing this sharp hip pain had to be related to the source of my fibromyalgia pain.

It's Not the Muscle, It's the Fat

Until I experienced the sharp hip pain, I assumed that my pain was centered in the muscles. But now, this pain was specifically located in the hip joint. Joint popping results from the rubbing motion of uneven surfaces in the joint. Now if lying in bed for a time caused a slight gap between hip joint surfaces to open, inflamed and sensitive tissue in the immediate area could work its way into the gap. Then a slight leg movement would pop the joint, close the gap, and pinch the inflamed tissue causing the brief sharp pain. The question then became, just what is this inflamed tissue?

That sent me to the Internet to find information on joint anatomy and joint pain. I came across a key paper published in December 2004 that seemed to provide the answers to all of my questions, *"Adipose tissue at entheses: the rheumatologic implications of its distribution. A potential site of pain and stress dissipation?"*[31]

Fat soluble toxins and compromised liver function provide answers

Adipose tissue is fat tissue, composed of fat cells or adipocytes and is often mixed with fibrous tissue. Entheses are the attachment points on either side of a joint where muscle tendons and ligaments connect to the bone. Entheses exist everywhere joints exist, from the neck and shoulders down to the toes. The December 2004 paper is an anatomical study of entheses which found:

"Adipose tissue was present at several different sites at numerous entheses. Many tendons/ligaments lay on a bed of well vascularised, highly innervated, 'insertional angle fat.' Fat-filled meniscoid folds often protruded into joint cavities immediately adjacent to attachment sites. The adipose tissue was not simply a collection of fat cells alone but it also contained nerves and blood vessels—with the proportions varying according to site. Thus 'insertional angle fat' was generally more richly innervated than endotenon fat and some regions of fat may be more susceptible to inflammation than others by virtue of their greater blood supply."

**Insertional angle fat is found in the angle between tendon or ligament attachments to the bone.

My discovery of this paper provided a moment of great enlightenment. Inflamed, highly innervated fat tissue protruding into and being pinched by a gap in the hip joint surely caused that sharp pain I had experienced. Inflamed, highly innervated fat tissue at entheses suggests a location and cause of all fibromyalgia pain. Indeed, the locations of all my fibromyalgia pain sites centered and radiated from the vicinity of either side of the joint, exactly where entheses are located. Any motion tugging on the tendons and ligaments at those sites could irritate sensitive nerves of inflamed adipose tissue, producing pain.

I have thus concluded that fibromyalgia is not an abnormality of the brain or central nervous system. It is not an inflammation of muscle tissue. Fibromyalgia is fully explainable as an inflammation of innervated adipose tissue. And what could cause this inflammation? Fat-soluble toxic substances, possibly in the presence of an abnormally low liver production level of anti-inflammatory proteins.

Numerous potentially harmful chemicals and toxins are fat soluble and accumulate in adipose tissue where they can stay for many years or even a lifetime. Toxic, fat soluble chemicals may be inhaled, ingested, or absorbed through the skin. Such chemicals include dioxins, PCBs, pesticides, petroleum distillates, hydrocarbons, metals, chemicals used in cleaning solvents and plastics, drugs, and even personal care products. Recent research has revealed that adipose tissue functions much more than just as a storage depository for fat. Fat cells or adipocytes are now considered part of one big endocrine organ that secretes hormones and a wide range of proteins involved in inflammation and the immune system, which have been collectively named "adipokines". Taken together with the fact that nerves and blood vessels run through adipose tissue, it is not surprising that toxic substances accumulating in adipose tissue could give rise to an inflammatory response in adipocytes[32, 33, 34].

With a dysfunctional or damaged liver, as is often present in celiac disease, the limited ability of the liver to remove harmful, fat soluble substances increases the risk of accumulating toxic substances making one more susceptible to inflammation of adipose tissue and fibromyalgia. Increased intestinal permeability or leaky gut provides an additional pathway for harmful substances, undigested food proteins, and toxins to reach and accumulate in adipose tissue. Irritable bowel syndrome (IBS), which is thought to be caused by bacterial overgrowth, is common in fibromyalgia and bacterial overgrowth is a cause of leaky gut[35]. Leaky gut is also present in celiac disease. It is now clear why celiac disease may increase one's risk of developing fibromyalgia.

Women make up 80% of fibromyalgia patients. Why? The answer may lie in a relationship between estrogen, adipose tissue, and xenobiotic estrogens. Adipocytes express receptors that bind to estrogen. There are six known forms of estrogen receptors classified as ER-alpha and five forms of ER-beta1 thru ER-beta 5. Fat deposition in females differs from fat deposition in males. Research has found that the type and number of estrogen receptors expressed in adipose tissue differs at different body locations. The concentration of estrogen in conjunction with adipocyte receptor type and number seems to control where fat is deposited in the body. Estrogen treatment in males can alter male fat distribution into female fat distribution. In addition, females express a significantly greater number of adipocyte estrogen receptors than males[36, 37].

Many of the same fat soluble toxic chemicals mentioned above have properties that mimic estrogens and are called xenobiotic estrogens or xenoestrogens. These xeno-estrogens can bind to estrogen receptors and wreak havoc in the body. Exposure to xenoestrogens is believed to cause some breast cancers. Because females have a much greater number of adipocyte estrogen receptors than males, there is much more oppor-tunity for these xenoestrogens to bind with adipocytes in females than in males. Binding with xenoestrogens may cause an inflammatory response in adipocytes. Additionally, fibromyalgia is more likely to occur in women after menopause, when estrogen levels drop. The lower estrogen levels mean there are more free adipocyte estrogen recep-tors available, and less competition for them between estrogen and xenoestrogen, in-creasing the likelihood of adipose tissue inflammation and fibromyalgia in women after menopause. Thus it is the increased number of adipocyte estrogen receptors which receptors, which may account for the higher incidence of fibromyalgia in women. Also, any condition that lowers estrogen levels in women (or men) might increase the risk of fibromyalgia[38,39,40,41].

Preventing, treating, or curing fibromyalgia would seem to require stopping exposure to whatever toxic or harmful substances may be causing inflammation of the adipose tissue. This may be very difficult as identification of the substances that may be contrib-uting to the problem is a major challenge. Are the offending toxins in the air, water, or some other facet of the environment? Is it at work or at home? Are they emitted by a factory or could they be chemicals used on the job or for a hobby? Are they in a cleaning product or solvent, an adhesive, a garden product or pesticide, a personal care product, a medication, or a food? Could they come from a plastic product? Did a bac-terial or viral infection seem to trigger the fibromyalgia? Were toxins inhaled, ingested, or absorbed through the skin? Everything must be considered. For instance, one study found that reduced use of cosmetics in a group of women with fibromyalgia significantly improved their symptoms over a two year period[42].

Olestra to the Rescue?

Even if one successfully eliminates exposure to the harmful substance(s), they have already accumulated in the adipose tissue and could, depending on their properties, potentially cause inflammation for many years before eventually being eliminated by the liver. I previously mentioned that it took me four months to recover from a two week exposure to Pepto-Bismol. If the liver is damaged or dysfunctional, that time could increase even further. This explains why fibromyalgia often persists in individuals for months and years. Is there some way to "detoxify"? Is there a way to accelerate the elimination of these fat soluble substances?

There are numerous web sites promoting controversial methods of detoxification, including large doses of B vitamins, saunas, diet, herbal remedies, and chelation. Saunas, for instance, are used for "sweat" therapy. But sweating can only eliminate water soluble products and has no effect on eliminating fat soluble substances. However, there is one valid, medically proven treatment that can accelerate the removal of a number of fat-soluble toxic substances. Oddly enough, this can be achieved by eating potato chips purchased directly off the shelves of local grocery stores.

Olestra, the non-absorbable fat substitute from Procter & Gamble, has been successfully used to treat patients with excessive accumulations of dioxin and PCB. In one case, two Austrian women with record high levels of dioxin intoxication and suffering from chloracne were given Olestra, both in pure form and as Olestra contained in fat-free potato chips. This increased fecal excretion of dioxin by eight to ten fold, and reduced the normal elimination half-life of dioxin from seven years to one to two years.

In another case, a Western Australian man suffering from PCB toxicity was treated with two one-ounce servings of Pringles fat-free potato chips daily for two years. His PCB level dropped dramatically, and his chloracne vanished[43,44,45,46].

The effects of diet restriction and Olestra on the tissue distribution of a chlorinated hydrocarbon were studied in one experiment. Mice were administered hexachlorobenzene labeled with radioactive carbon-14. When diet was restricted, carbon-14 increased by 3-fold in the brain and the total amount in adipose tissue did not change. On a restricted diet combined with Olestra, there was a 30-fold increase in the rate of carbon-14 excreted in stool compared to a diet without Olestra. Dietary Olestra also reduced the carbon-14 movement into the brain resulting from a restricted diet by 50%[47].

My fibromyalgia was quite likely caused by exposure to chemicals inhaled daily at work for years. Since quitting my job, I was no longer exposed to those chemicals. For my fibromyalgia symptoms to end, I needed to eliminate those chemicals that had accumulated in my adipose tissue. If I did nothing but wait for the chemicals to be excreted over time, there was no way of knowing how long my fibromyalgia symptoms might last. There was a good chance that the chemicals to which I had been exposed were the type that Olestra can help remove, but I could not be certain. If I decided to treat myself with Olestra, there was no way to know how long it would take for me to begin to see any improvement in my fibromyalgia symptoms. But there was nothing to lose by trying.

I had a choice of fat-free Pringles or Lays Light or Ruffles Light potato chips, all made with Olestra. Pringles contain cornstarch, and I have corn sensitivity. So my choice was two daily servings of one ounce of either Lays Light Original or Ruffles Light Original potato chips. I saw no reason to alter my diet otherwise. I am already quite lean and trim, and do not need to lose weight. I planned to give it at least two months of treatment to see any improvement in symptoms, but I hoped to see at least some improvements sooner.

When I began Olestra treatment, my fibromyalgia symptoms were at their peak. My arms and shoulders ached. Reaching for anything was a dread. Walking any distance was nearly unbearable. My right leg and hip hurt and the pain was worse lying in bed. I was still experiencing that sharp hip pain when my hip joint popped. I was greatly fatigued and I could do almost no exercise or stretching. Lifting grocery bags was a trial.

After just two weeks of Olestra treatment, I was not disappointed. There was a small but very definite improvement in my symptoms. The sharp hip joint pain and popping were diminishing. There was just enough reduction in pain to begin to do some limited stretching exercises. With that ability, I could begin to monitor my symptoms on the basis of increases in ranges of motion and flexibility at joints, as well as how well I could walk.

Almost daily, there were unquestionable signs of improvement. The range of limb motion during exercise steadily increased in small, but perceptible increments. Pain levels decreased. Leg pain in bed became tolerable. I was able to add daily walks to my exercise regimen. Fatigue was decreasing. Into the 11th week of treatment all seemed to be going great. I had recovered much flexibility in my legs. My arms no longer ached and I could reach all the way across my car seat to reach the latch to unlock the passenger door without pain. I was able to do some pushups, regained some arm strength, and was able to handle grocery bags. It looked as though a full recovery might soon arrive—but then came a setback.

My left leg had been the least affected limb during my fibromyalgia. The left leg had always retained a degree of flexibility. But by the end of the 11th week of treatment, my left leg began to stiffen in pain. Fatigue increased. I had to curtail my exercise. However, despite this setback, flexibility and pain levels in my arms, shoulders, and right leg remained relatively unchanged. Overall, my condition was vastly improved over what it had been before starting Olestra treatment. I have no idea why my left leg suddenly became so affected. Perhaps it was some minor bacterial or viral infection as

I also experienced an increase in bowel discomfort at that time. All I could do was let the symptoms in the left leg run their course, and begin my exercise regimen as soon as my left leg loosened up.

As I write this, I am now into my 15th week of Olestra treatment. My left leg is just beginning to loosen up. Symptoms in my other limbs continue to be stable. In a few days, I will re-start my exercise and stretching routine, hoping to restore flexibility in my left leg. I am convinced that Olestra has played a significant role in improving my fibromyalgia symptoms.

Loose Ends

I have noticed, in addition to being very stiff in the mornings, my fibromyalgia pain seems to let up somewhat and be at its lowest level late in the evenings. The pain cycle seems to be on a 24-hour circadian clock and corresponds to levels of cortisol secreted by the adrenal glands. Cortisol, among many functions, is an anti-inflammatory. In the 24-hour cycle, cortisol secretion is at its lowest around 7:00 am, just about the time most of us need to get up in the morning. Cortisol secretion then picks up and peaks shortly after breakfast, gradually dropping off into the evening. Cortisol has the opportunity to infuse into the inflamed adipose tissue throughout the day, lowering the inflammation and providing pain relief. By late evening, the accumulation of cortisol in adipose tissue is apparently at its maximum. With little cortisol being secreted overnight the cortisol level drops off and the inflammation in the adipose tissue increases resulting in morning stiffness and pain. The relationship between cortisol secretion and fibromyalgia symptoms has been studied[48].

Exercise and stretching have been a part of my therapy. While exercise works primarily on the muscles and not adipose tissue, I have found it beneficial if not overdone. Keeping up muscle tone, strength, and flexibility improves mobility and also seems to lower the level of fibromyalgia pain. Pain, however, can severely limit one's ability to perform exercise. I usually take advantage of the reduced pain in the evening and perform my exercises then. I push myself to the threshold of pain tolerance when stretching my limbs.

Exercise has been found to have important effects on the immune system. Anti-inflammatory cytokines, such as IL-6, are released by muscle tissue during exercise[49,50,51]. Adipose tissue has also been found to secrete IL-6 during exercise under the influence of a release of epinephrine (better known as adrenaline)[52,53]. As I perform my exercise, the pain level subsides, and my range of motion increases. It seems clear that anti-inflammatories released by muscle and adipose tissue during exercise actually make it possible to do more exercise with less pain. However, this pain relief is temporary and short-lived. Not long after I complete my exercise, I begin to stiffen up.

Since liver dysfunction seems a part of fibromyalgia, can liver tests be useful? There are a number of liver function tests that can be performed which measure the blood serum levels of proteins and enzymes produced by the liver. However, these tests primarily assess liver injury rather than liver function. Abnormal test results often, but not always, indicate a liver problem and offer clues as to the nature of the problem. Normal liver function tests do not always mean the liver is normal[54]. Physicians seeing patients for fibromyalgia should consider ordering liver function lab tests. Studies of the prevalence of liver abnormalities in celiac disease rely on the results of liver function tests. Since normal test results do not rule out the possibility of liver dysfunction, the incidence of liver abnormalities in celiac disease could be much higher than reported.

Conclusion

The current prevalent medical perspective that characterizes fibromyalgia as a condition involving brain and central nervous system abnormalities does not adequately explain the symptoms of my own experience with fibromyalgia. An inflammation of highly innervated and vascularised adipose tissue in the vicinity of entheses readily offers a full explanation of the source of fibromyalgia pain. The inflammation of adipose tissue can be attributed to an accumulation of fat-soluble toxic substances within the tissue. Thus, susceptibility to fibromyalgia likely involves liver dysfunction as well as exposure to toxic substances. Liver dysfunction may decrease the liver's ability to remove fat soluble substances and production of anti-inflammatory proteins. This, too, may be a factor in the initiation of inflammation in adipose tissue. Conditions such as celiac disease have a high prevalence of liver abnormalities and a high prevalence of fibromyalgia. Increased intestinal permeability, common with bacterial overgrowth and celiac disease, provides an additional pathway for toxins, undigested proteins, and other harmful substances to overload the liver and accumulate in adipose tissue. Olestra, a non-absorbable fat substitute readily available as an additive in fat-free potato chips, holds great promise as a treatment to accelerate the removal of fat soluble toxic substances from inflamed adipose tissue offering a potential fibromyalgia cure.

Editor's note:

Abnormal insulin levels have also been connected with pro-inflammatory protein imbalances, so fasting glucose testing may also provide valuable information to those experiencing fibromyalgia.

Food Cravings, Obesity and Gluten Consumption

By Dr. Ron Hoggan, Ed. D.

Increased consumption of gluten, according to Dr. Michael Marsh, raises the risk of celiac disease symptoms[1]. Although these symptoms may not indicate celiac disease, they reflect some biological realities. Grain-based foods simply do not offer the range of nutrients necessary to human health and they damage the human body in many ways. Beginning with intestinal damage, to neurological damage, to increasing cancer risk, to directly causing cellular damage, gluten has been implicated in many non-celiac ailments and disorders. USDA and Canada Food Guides notwithstanding, if people eat grain-laden diets, they may develop symptoms of celiac disease (but in most cases, without the diagnostic intestinal lesion). The connection between eating disorders and celiac disease is well known and well documented[2,3,4,5]. Thus, the dynamics at work in celiac disease may offer insight into the broader realms of obesity and other metabolic/eating disorders, especially among those who are eating the recommended, daily quantities of grain-derived foods, while attempting to keep their weight down by eating low-fat foods.

The primary, defining characteristic of celiac disease is gluten-induced damage to the intestinal lining. Since malabsorption of vitamins and minerals is well known in the context of celiac disease, it should not be surprising that some celiac patients also demonstrate pica. (Pica is an ailment characterized by eating dirt, paint, wood, and other non-food substances.) Other celiac patients paradoxically eat excessive quantities of food, coupled with a concurrent failure to gain weight. Yet another, perhaps larger, group of celiac patients refuse to eat (One may speculate that the latter find that eating makes them feel sick so they avoid it).

Perhaps the most neglected group is that large portion of untreated celiac patients who are obese. Dr. Dickey found that obesity is more common than being underweight among those with untreated celiac disease[6]. When I ran a Medline search under the terms "obesity" and "celiac disease" 75 citations appeared. A repeated theme in the abstracts and titles was that celiac disease is usually overlooked among obese patients. While obesity in celiac disease may be common, diagnosis appears to be uncommon. Given the facts, I certainly believe that some of the North American epidemic of obesity can be explained by undiagnosed celiac disease. Although that is only a small part of the answer to our obesity puzzle, I suspect that celiac disease may offer a pattern for understanding much of the obesity that is sweeping this continent.

One example, a woman diagnosed by Dr. Joe Murray when he was at the University of Iowa, weighed 388 pounds at diagnosis[7]. Dr. Murray explained her situation as an over-compensation for her intestinal malabsorption. I want to suggest a two faceted, alternative explanation which may extend to a large and growing segment of the overweight and obese among the general population. As mentioned earlier, anyone consuming enough gluten will demonstrate some symptoms of celiac disease. If large scale gluten consumption damages the intestinal villi—but to a lesser degree than is usually required to diagnose celiac disease—fat absorption will be compromised. Deficiencies in essential fatty acids are a likely consequence.

The natural response to such deficiencies is to crave food despite adequate caloric intake. Even when caloric intake is huge, and excess calories must be stored as body fat, the need to eat continues to be driven by the body's craving for essential fats and energy. Due to gluten-induced interference with fat absorption, consumption of escalating quantities of food may be necessary for adequate essential fatty acid absorption. To further compound the problem, excessive production of insulin blocks pancreatic glucagon production. This absence of glucagon cripples the individual's ability to burn stored fats, while the cells continue to demand both essential fats and energy. We either eat, or we succumb to intense lethargy and depression.

This is what leads to the ravenous appetite associated with carbohydrate addiction. As carbohydrate consumption escalates, excess carbs are stored as fat and weight gain continues. Every dip in blood glucose incites hunger and even the smallest margin of carbohydrate excess that is beyond our immediate energy needs leads to more fat storage.

Poor medical advice also contributes to the problem. The mantra of "reduce fat intake" continues to echo in the offices of health professionals despite a growing body of converse research findings. In February of 2006, the results of a powerful, eight year study of almost 49,000 women showed little difference between the health status of women consuming low fat diets and those consuming normal diets[8]. Alarmingly, the recommendation of low fat dieting seems to have resulted in weight gain, a well recognized risk factor for a variety of diseases.

For some of us, this result was predictable. The likely consequence of a low-fat diet is an increased intake of carbohydrates while food cravings are fuelled by a deficiency of essential fatty acids and a sense of lethargy that can only be temporarily corrected by further carbohydrate consumption. If my sense of the underlying problem (caloric excess combined with essential fatty acid deficiency due to fat malabsorption) is accurate, then a low fat diet is exactly the wrong prescription. Many obese persons are condemned, by such poor medical advice, to a life of ever deepening depression, autoimmune diseases, cardiovascular disease, and increasing obesity.

At the end of the day, when these folks drop dead from heart attacks, strokes, or some similar disaster, the self-righteous bystanders will just '*know*' that the problem was a lack of willpower and eating too much fat.

I watched my mom steadily gain weight for 35 years. I watched her exercise will power beyond the capacity of most folks. Still, she could not resist her compulsive eating. I have seen her take something from the freezer and chew on it while agreeing that she had just eaten a very large meal and should feel full.

In December of 1994 I was diagnosed with celiac disease. According to the published experts in this area, my mom should also have been invited for testing. Yet, when asked for testing, her doctor refused her. Through persistence, and a pervasive faith in her son, mom finally (after months of negotiation) swayed her doctor to do the anti-gliadin antibody blood test. Despite the fact that she had been on a reduced gluten diet for the previous year, her antibody levels were slightly elevated.

She never sought a biopsy diagnosis, and the EMA and tTG were not available here in Canada at that time. However, she has been gluten-free for the past seven years or so. She dropped about 75 pounds of unwanted weight.

Her weakness was never will power. She was battling an instinct so basic that few of us could have resisted. That, I think, is the story behind much of North American obesity. The widespread, excessive consumption of gluten at every meal, in addition to the low-fat religion that has been promulgated throughout the land, is resulting in intestinal damage and a widespread deficiency in essential fats is among North Americans.

Our Adipose Prisons

By Dr. Ron Hoggan, Ed. D.

The U.S. has taken the lead of the industrialized world when it comes to weight-gain, especially obesity, and many other industrialized nations are in close pursuit. Since Ancel Keys' flawed assertion linking dietary fats and serum cholesterol with heart disease in

1951, the industrialized world has sought to reduce its consumption of fats—especially saturated fats. Thus, the last fifty years has seen a steady shift away from dietary fats. Our carbohydrate consumption, particularly in the form of grains and sugars, increased at the same time—and the obesity epidemic was begun.

A recent issue of *People Magazine* reported on a 17 year old young woman who struggled with obesity and could not halt a steady and dangerous trend of weight gain[2]. The only answer she and her parents could find was to have an adjustable band surgically placed around her stomach. This band makes it painful to eat more than very small portions. The band was loosened somewhat as she approached her target weight, but it still severely limits the quantity of food she can eat. Although she is much happier and healthier at her current size, I could not help but wonder if the surgery was a mistake. No mention was made of ruling out celiac disease before resorting to such drastic measures. It is doubtful that celiac disease was even considered. Yet Dickey and Kearney reported on an examination of data gathered on 371 newly diagnosed celiac patients. These two researchers found that 39% of these patients were overweight. One third of these people were obese, while only 5% of these celiac patients were underweight at diagnosis[3]. Further, Dr. Joseph Murray has repeatedly discussed two case histories of morbidly obese patients with occult celiac disease[4]. Tragically, the diagnosis came too late for one of these patients. She died before the gluten-free diet could reverse her obesity and the health hazards that go with it.

The information, that gluten can and does cause obesity and that a gluten-free diet can reverse it, does not seem to have reached physicians involved in general practice, those working in the field of obesity, and even, many gastroenterologists. The young woman featured in the *People* article might have been spared considerable pain and expense had she first been investigated for celiac disease and gluten sensitivity. This article also mentioned that the number of children between ages 10 and 19 who are undergoing the same gastric surgery tripled between 2000 and 2003 yet it is doubtful that celiac disease was ever considered or sought among these children. How many of them could be spared the pain and risks associated with gastric weight-loss surgery? Such experimentation with their nutrition is also suspect because their bodies are still developing and such artificial alterations may be depriving these children of important nutrients. (I have previously speculated that celiac associated obesity results from food cravings driven by specific nutrient deficiencies -see previous article.)

Given the recent report that celiac disease afflicts more than 1% of the U.S. population[5] and that gluten sensitivity has been found in 11% of those tested at a Texas shopping mall[6] and given rates of overweight and obese individuals found among newly diagnosed celiac patients, it seems likely that much of the weight-gain epidemic that is sweeping the industrialized world is being fueled by the gluten syndrome and increased grain consumption in general. I suspect that if our civilization is ever to escape this adipose prison, we must return to getting more of our calories from fats, and fewer from grains and sugars.

Editor's note:

There is a growing body of evidence that has identified vitamin D deficiency as epidemic. From bone density to the various issues discussed in the next article, vitamin D is a critical component of good health. Interaction between skin oils and sunlight can provide vitamin D, but our lifestyles may thwart this source of vitamin D. Because most of us bathe on a daily basis, our soap removes the very skin oils that are critical to this process. Many of us spend most of our waking hours sheltered from sunlight, by the buildings we work in and the vehicles in which we travel to and from work. The winter months are particularly problematic, as the sun's rays are less intense due to the tilt of the earth and the longer angle at which the sun's rays strike us. Another source of vitamin D is in the foods we consume. However, since many celiac and gluten sensitive individuals suffer from some degree of malabsorption, even on a gluten-free diet, it is not difficult to see why we should be considering vitamin D supplements. (Conversely, we might consider giving up bathing. However, this strategy might be even more socially isolating than the gluten-free diet.)

Vitamin D Deficiency May Affect Celiacs' Immune Function

By Laura Wesson

My fingernails were shredding and I was a bit out of it mentally, missing obvious things. I'd had to stop eating many foods because of intolerances to almost everything I used to eat before I went gluten-free. I wondered if I had dropped some essential nutrients when I cleared all of those foods out of my diet. So I checked my diet for nutrient deficiencies, using the USDA nutrients database at www.nal.usda.gov/fnic/foodcomp/search. I'm sure there's software that works with this database, but I wrote a little computer program to analyze my diet. I have an electronic food scale, so weighing food is easy.

The most important thing I found is that I'm low on vitamin D. You can get vitamin D from food, or from a supplement, and from the ultraviolet B in sunlight; many of us, like me, may get almost none from any of those sources. And—this is important for a lot of us—vitamin D deficiency can cause a lot of symptoms including immune system problems! I went looking on Medline and it was mentioned as having anti-inflammatory properties, and preventing cancers such as colon cancer and lymphoma; preventing infections, and helping with autoimmune diseases. Gluten intolerance is less common in the Middle East and more common in northern Europe. I've seen this explained as the result of evolution, since wheat has been used for longer in the Middle East, but I wonder if people in the north are also more likely to be gluten intolerant (an autoimmune disease) because they don't get as much vitamin D. It may also explain why people get more colds during the winter season when there's less sunlight. Vitamin D deficiency is best known for causing rickets in children and osteomalacia (softened bones, muscle weakness and pain, tender sternum) in adults. Osteomalacia is often misdiagnosed as fibromyalgia, because the symptoms are similar. Rickets is increasing in the U.S., especially among black children. Most post-menopausal bone loss in women occurs during the winter. It can take months of increased vitamin D intake to correct the health problems caused by deficiency.

There are only a few significant dietary sources of vitamin D. In the U.S., almost all milk is fortified with vitamin D to 100 IU per cup, so you should get the recommended daily intake of 400 IU if you drink 4 cups of milk per day. However, milk often doesn't have as much vitamin D as is claimed on the label. Some cereals, like Kellogg's Cornflakes, have small amounts of added vitamin D. Typically, 10 cups of fortified cereal would give you the RDI. The government encourages fortification of milk and cereal so that fewer children will develop rickets. Otherwise—you would get the RDI from nine oysters, or about 4 ounces of fatty fish like salmon or tuna, or a teaspoon of cod liver oil. Many other kinds of fish have only small amounts. You'd have to eat 2 pounds of cod to get the RDI. The only natural vegan source of vitamin D is Shiitake mushrooms. Just like people, mushrooms make vitamin D when they're exposed to ultraviolet. About 13 sun-dried shiitake mushrooms contain the RDI. And that's it. Many of us on gluten-free diets are also not eating dairy or fortified cereals, so unless we have a passionate love-affair with fish or oysters or shiitake, we would be getting almost no vitamin D from food.

You can get vitamin D the natural way, from the sun. It takes exposure to sunlight outside (not under glass) on your hands and feet for about fifteen minutes a day. I was not sure what was meant by "direct sunlight". I read someplace that ultraviolet is scattered over the whole sky. Unlike visible light, the whole sky shines with ultraviolet light. Clouds would filter out some of it. People with dark skin require more time in the sun so many black people develop a deficiency. Using even low-SPF sunscreen prevents your body from making vitamin D. The farther from the equator you live, the less UVB there is in the winter sunlight, because the sun is closer to the horizon in the winter and the sunlight filters through more atmosphere before it gets to you. At the latitude of Boston, and near sea level, there isn't enough UVB radiation between November and February for one's body to make vitamin D.

You have probably heard the public health advice to wear sunscreen—the same ultra-violet B that generates vitamin D in your body also causes skin cancer and ages skin. The small amount of exposure to sunlight required is probably only a very small cancer risk and would cause little photo-aging of the skin. Unfortunately I wasn't able to find quantitative information about how carcinogenic fifteen minutes' daily sun exposure would be. There are also vitamin D lights (see www.sperti.com/duv.htm),\ which are probably also a healthful choice.

I have severe immune system problems. I tested positive for 53 inhalant allergies—my body had developed allergies to almost all the allergens around me. I get sick for days if I eat almost any of the foods that I ate while I was eating gluten. I even get sick from a couple of foods that, so far as I can remember, I only started eating on a gluten-free diet. So I live on an exotic-foods diet. I've had a hellish time trying to get allergy shots. At a concentration of 1 part in 10 million they make me sick for a couple of days while the normal starting concentration for allergy shots is 1 in 100,000. I'm plagued by bladder infections. With cranberries being one of my intolerances, I can't even use them to help prevent the infections.

I've certainly been short of vitamin D. I live in the north, and I'm always careful to use high-SPF sunscreen when I go outdoors. I can't eat milk, fish, shellfish or mushrooms, so I can't get a significant amount of vitamin D from food. I haven't been taking any vitamin supplements, because almost all have traces of protein from some food that makes me sick. It would be lovely if vitamin D deficiency turned out to be part of the cause of my very burdensome immune problems. I'm skeptical because I was getting vitamin D from a supplement and/or from my diet up until 2 years ago, when I found I had a vast number of hidden food intolerances, and I started having reactions to vitamin pills. Fortunately there is a vitamin D supplement that I can take—vitamin D3 made by Pure Encapsulations, which I bought from www.organicpharmacy.org. The ingredients in the capsule are made from wool and pine trees. I'll find out if it helps over the next few months.

Vitamin D causes disease when taken in large amounts. If you think you are deficient, don't take too much to make up for it. Vitamin D is a hormone—it's not something to take in mega-doses, any more than, hopefully, one would take a mega-dose of estrogen or testosterone. If your doctor recommends a high dose, they should do regular blood tests to keep track of your vitamin D level. It's pretty safe to take up to 2000 IU per day on your own. Dr. Michael Holick, a vitamin D researcher at Boston University and author of The UV Advantage, believes that people need about 1000 IU per day. I asked a family doctor, who said they suggest 400-800 IU per day for middle-aged women. However, it might be a good idea for gluten intolerant people to take more, about 1000 - 2000 IU per day, since we may have difficulties absorbing vitamins and celiac disease is an autoimmune disease.

Vitamin D is very important, just as all the vitamins are. But we are conditioned by the media, and tend to think more about vitamins C and E, which get a lot of attention because they're antioxidants. Vitamin D was the absolutely last one I looked at. Then I found that it was my most serious deficiency! And nutrient deficiencies are not a trendy topic, so the possibility of developing deficiencies is something people tend to forget while trying to improve their diets. Many people who avoid gluten also have other food intolerances, or are on some other kind of special diet, and it would be an excellent idea to go to the USDA database and find out whether their new diet is giving them enough vitamins and minerals. It certainly helped me. I feel more cheerful and alert, like my mind woke up on a sunny day.

It's best to get as much as possible from one's diet, too. Whole foods have a lot in them that's good for the body that research hasn't yet identified, and if your diet gives you the RDA of all the vitamins and minerals, it will also be giving you other healthful nutrients that will do you a lot of good. This might also be true of vitamin D. Maybe it's better to get a small amount of ultraviolet, like an iguana sitting under a UV lamp, instead of taking pills. UVB might be healthy in ways we don't yet know about.

Vitamin D is a bit like stored-up sunlight. You can catch it for yourself from the sun when it's high in the sky, you can eat the sunlight the fish have gathered for you, or you can take a supplement and keep packed sunlight on your shelf.

Editor's note:

I (Ron) take 2,000 IU of vitamin D supplements every day, and I know one physician with an autoimmune disease who takes 8,000 IU each day.

CHAPTER 3:
THE BRAIN CONNECTION

Addiction to Gluten

In 1979, Christine Zioudrou and her colleagues published a startling report about the incomplete digests of wheat in _The Journal of Biological Chemistry_. They reported that morphine-like peptides (partial proteins) and other psychoactive substances are found in partly digested wheat. Zioudrou et al. named the morphine-like peptides _'exorphins'_ to reflect that they behave like endorphins, but come from outside the body. Their work was confirmed and enhanced by subsequent researchers who went on to describe the specific amino acids, and their sequences, that form at least 5 distinct exorphin peptides (Fukudome and Yoshikawa).

Zioudrou et al., in the same report, identified stimulatory materials from the partial digests of gluten as well. Thus, the digests of gluten form a kind of cocktail composed of counteracting sedating and stimulating peptides. While they do not attach to the same receptors, the stimulatory materials may offset much of the sedating impact of the exorphins, producing something of an artificial and simplistic chemical balance in most of us.

Although startling, this information was given little attention until the U. of Maryland, Baltimore group, Wang, et al., published a report in the December issue of the _Journal of Cell Science in 2000_, reporting their own new discovery. While trying to develop a cholera vaccine, they had found a protein they called zonulin. It is a protein that disrupts the protective tight junctions in the small intestine and the blood brain barrier and is excessively produced, by some individuals, in response to ingesting wheat and other grains with analogous proteins, rye and barley.

These two converging areas of research lend considerable credence to the previously marginalized perspective called 'leaky gut' and claims that partly digested proteins from gluten grains are able to bypass the intestinal barrier, into the bloodstream, and subsequently into the brain. The evidence now indicates that when susceptible individuals eat gluten, we produce excessive amounts of zonulin, which opens the barriers formed by epithelial cells, allowing exorphins to reach the bloodstream then the brain and alter brain and immune function. While there is still considerable debate about these issues, there can be little doubt that these addictive peptides are reaching the brain and, with varying degrees of impact, wreaking havoc on the consciousness of some hapless victims, while having little or no discernible impact on others. This is a puzzle that cries out to be solved and several lines of research have converged and may do just that.

We now know that, not only do these exorphins cause addiction, they also alter blood flow patterns in the brain and cause excessive stimulation, all of which are suggestive of gluten's role in a wide range of psychiatric and neurological ailments.

In the meantime, we have gone far past the stage where these highly addictive and psychoactive components of gluten can be dismissed. Thus, among the genetically susceptible, we not only have to adopt a lifestyle that excludes these hazardous grains because of their immunological impact, we must also deal with the unintended addiction and psychiatric disturbances that many of us have fallen prey to.

As many readers may know, denial is an important component of any addiction. This is no less the case in the context of gluten sensitivity and celiac disease. Thus, it is most fitting that we begin this chapter about the impact of gluten on the brain with Danna Korn's insightful and entertaining discussion of denial as it relates to breaking our addiction to gluten in the context of gluten sensitivity and celiac disease.

Dealing with Denial

By Danna Korn

You've all heard the joke proclaiming that "Denial is not a river in Egypt." No, it's not. What it *is,* though, is a very real issue for many, if not most people who have been diagnosed with celiac disease or gluten sensitivity. There are a couple of types of denial. The first type affects *us*, while the second type affects those *around* us.

When *We're* in Denial

Many people who are diagnosed—or when their kids are—go through some type of denial. It usually occurs at a few key times after diagnosis—and for a few different reasons, here are some examples:

- **Immediate denial—the diagnosis isn't right.** *Nope.* Couldn't be. I don't know anyone who has that. I don't even know what gluten is. I've never heard of celiac disease. I don't have symptoms…my symptoms are mild. It's just lactose intolerance, I'm sure. I don't have diarrhea, so I couldn't have that. I'm overweight, and all celiacs are skinny. My results were inconclusive. Someone must have made a mistake. All of these thoughts can be symptoms of denial.

- **A few weeks into the diet—I don't think that diagnosis was right.** This is when the reality of doing this *for the rest of your life* sets in. One angel (the good one, of course) sits on one shoulder whispering, "You know you need to stay gluten-free—keep it up—you can do it! Mmmm, yummy cheese on this gluten-free toast. The other shoulder is home to the Devil-in-Denial: "No *way* are you going to another happy hour and order wine and celery sticks while all the other guys are drinkin' beer and deep-fried stuff. You don't have no stinkin' intolerance. Come on—just one beer…and one piece of pizza. It won't hurtcha. No stinkin' intolerance…" This is really just a period of ambivalence, hoping beyond hope that you don't *really* have this condition, choosing to lean toward believing you don't.

- **Danger zone: I never had that.** The most dangerous type of denial occurs several months into the diet, when all of a sudden you realize you feel so good that you don't even remember the last time you felt bad. That's when people often think, "I *knew* I just needed a little bit of time to get over that bug I had! I feel *great*. I'll bet I never even had anything wrong with me."

When *Others* are in Denial

Then there's the type of denial that our family members and loved ones express. Ask anyone who is gluten intolerant or has been diagnosed with celiac disease if they have relatives who won't be tested, and chances are, you'll get a surprised look as though you just guessed what color of underwear they're wearing, and a "yeah, how did you know?" Because we *all* have them. Well, most of us do. Why is it so hard for our relatives to believe they might have this? It is, after all, one of the most common genetic diseases one can have—and it *does* run in the family. Yet we've all heard comments like:

- No, I don't have that (blunt, bold, and full-on denial).
- I don't think I need to be tested (oh, really, and that would be because….?!?)
- I was tested once, and the tests were negative (remember, once-negative does *not* mean always negative—also remember there *are* false negatives).
- I was tested, and my results were inconclusive, so I don't think I have it. ' (Inconclusive may be a euphemism for mildly positive).
- I don't have any symptoms (Oh, really? There are about 250 symptoms, and you have NONE?)

- My symptoms really aren't that severe; I can live with them (so you'll just wait till you're *really* sick and doing long-term damage to start trying to improve your health?).
- I couldn't do the diet anyway, so I'm not going to bother being tested (now there's a rational argument for you).

Bottom line is they don't *want* to have celiac disease, or they don't *want* to give up gluten. Some of your relatives may even refuse to believe *you* have it. I've met many people with celiac disease who have been accused of being hypochondriacs or neurotic.

The problem with denial is that it justifies eating gluten. When you have this epiphany "realizing" that you don't have celiac disease or don't need to be gluten-free, it's tempting to run, not walk, to the nearest Krispy Kreme outlet.

Resist the temptation. If you've been on the diet for awhile, then yes, you feel great, but it's *because* you're not eating wheat or gluten, not *in spite* of it. The danger in testing the waters is that you may not have any reaction when you do, and then you're likely to jump to the obvious (by which I mean "desired") conclusion and confirmation that you never needed to eliminate wheat or gluten in the first place.

If you still wonder whether or not you have a medical reason for cutting gluten from your diet, here are a few things you can do to help solidify things in your mind:

- Get properly tested.
- Get a second (or even a third) opinion.
- Talk to other people who have been diagnosed with the same condition about your symptoms and your feelings of denial (chances are they'll grin and say, "Yep, I felt that way at one point, too").
- Write it down: List your symptoms, the symptoms of the condition, and how you feel if you've been following the diet. Sometimes seeing it in writing is the just the proof we need.

Denial, by the way, is one of the most compelling arguments in support of proper testing and diagnosis. If you've been confirmed with a diagnosis, you may be tempted to fall into a state of denial, but it's going to seem pretty silly, even to you.

But also keep in mind that if you've been tested and your results were inconclusive or negative, you may need to consider re-testing or other alternatives. The tests have changed over the years, and maybe your tests were done long ago. There are often false negatives; *and* you can be triggered at any point in your life, so just because you were negative once doesn't mean you'll be negative again. And finally, there are people who are negative on all of the tests, yet their health improves dramatically on a gluten-free diet. Go figure.

Remember, if it looks like a duck, walks like a duck, and quacks like a duck, it's most likely a duck, even if you wish it were a pigeon.

Editor's comment

There is a great deal that we still don't know about the impact of gluten on the brain, so let's start with looking at a few things we do know and perhaps we will see where we should be looking for answers to the things we don't know. First, we know that gluten contains exorphins that can and do reach the brain in susceptible people. We also know that about 70% of untreated children with celiac disease meet all the criteria for a diagnosis of attention deficit disorder (ADD) except that they have celiac disease. We also know that the rate of ADD among these same children drops to 0% within a year of strict compliance with a gluten-free diet. Further, we know that there is a higher rate of epilepsy among people with celiac disease and that seizures become less frequent and sometimes even stop completely after removal of gluten from the diet. We also know that 56% of patients with neurological diseases of unknown origin have elevated antibodies against gluten. In other words, they are gluten sensitive.

Several studies reported in the peer reviewed medical literature claim to have investigated the link between schizophrenia and gluten without finding evidence for this connection. Yet even a cursory examination of these reports and study designs reveals deep flaws in design and implementation that absolutely predicts the outcome reported. For instance, one such study allowed patients' families to bring food to patients while on weekend visits. Other studies failed to exclude all sources of gluten.

On the other hand, two well designed single-blind cross-over studies found a clear connection between gluten/casein and some cases of schizophrenia. One of these studies was conducted by Dr. Curtis Dohan et al. Dohan ran a psychiatric ward of a VA hospital in Pennsylvania and devoted many years of study to the link between gluten and schizophrenia.

Singh and Kay conducted another very solid study with similar findings. Further, Dr. Kalle Reichelt and colleagues have reported on connections between gluten/dairy consumption and autism, depressive illness, ADHD, learning disabilities, and developmental delays.

More recently, several psychiatrists have reported individual cases where schizophrenic patients experienced near miraculous recoveries on a gluten-free diet.

I'm not suggesting that excluding gluten would help everyone with schizophrenia. I have no idea how many people with these various psychiatric afflictions are likely to benefit from a gluten-free diet. I don't know the extent to which drug therapies might be excluded in the context of a gluten-free diet. I don't even know if such patients would prefer to control their conditions with drugs or diet.

There is, however, one thing that I do know. That is that if we do not examine this possibility with an open mind, the toll of human suffering will continue unabated. Whatever the extent to which gluten is contributing to these problems is the extent to which the current degree of suffering is unnecessary and avoidable. There is inarguable evidence that gluten makes some contribution. What is needed is to determine the dimensions of this contribution.

Herbert Spencer once said:

"There is a principle which is a bar against all information, which is proof against all arguments and which cannot fail to keep a man in everlasting ignorance – that principle is contempt prior to investigation"

Thus, I would argue that the greatest gift that medical practitioners and scientific researchers can offer the gluten sensitive and celiac community is an open mind.

Eating to Learn: How Grains Impact on Our Ability to Focus, Comprehend, Remember, Predict, and Survive

By Dr. Ron Hoggan, Ed. D.

Evolution is an interactive process. Those of us who learn quickly and well are more likely to survive, thrive, and reproduce. Learning capacities then, are a factor in the survival of our genes. Research is now revealing that cereal grains, along with other allergenic and highly glycemic foods, pose a serious threat to our sustained ability to learn. These foods have been shown to interfere at almost any stage of the learning process, impeding our attempts to focus our attention, observe, ponder, remember, understand, and apply that understanding. Grains can alter learning capacities in ___at least___ four specific ways: as sequelae of untreated celiac disease; through an immune system that is sensitized to gluten; through the dietary displacement of other nutrients; and through the impact of grain on blood sugar/insulin levels.

There are many reports of learning problems in association with untreated celiac disease. A majority of children with celiac disease display the signs and symptoms of attention deficit disorder (ADD)[1,2] a range of learning difficulties[3] and developmental delays[4-6]. Many of the same problems are found more frequently among those with gluten sensitivity[7] a condition signaled by immune reactions against this most common element of the modern diet. Grain consumption can also cause specific nutrient deficiencies that are known to play an important role in learning. Grains can also cause problems with blood sugar/insulin levels resulting in reduced capacities for learning. Further, foods derived from grain are an important element in the current epidemic of hypoglycemia, obesity, and Type 2 diabetes[8-10]. Our growing understanding of the biological impact of cereal grain consumption must move educators to challenge current dietary trends.

Part of our improved understanding comes from new testing protocols which are revealing that celiac sprue afflicts close to 1% of the general population, making it the most common life-long ailment among humans, with frequencies ranging from 0.5% to more than 5% of some populations[11, 12]. It is widespread and appears to occur more frequently among populations that have experienced relatively shorter periods of exposure to these grains[13]. The importance of this newly recognized high frequency of celiac disease becomes obvious when we examine the impact it has on learning and behavior.

Research has identified ADD in 66-70% of children with untreated celiac disease, which resolves on a gluten-free diet, and returns with a gluten challenge[1, 2]. Several investigators have connected particular patterns of reduced blood flow to specific parts of the brain in ADD[13-15]. Other reports have connected untreated celiac disease with similarly abnormal blood flow patterns in the brain[16]. One might be able to dismiss such reports if viewed in isolation, but the increased rates of learning disabilities among celiac patients[3], and the increased rates of celiac disease among those with learning disabilities leave little to the imagination[17]. Further, there is one report of gluten-induced aphasia (a condition characterized by the loss of speech ability) that resolved after diagnosis and institution of a gluten-free diet[18]. Still other investigations suggest a causal link between the partial digests of gluten (opioid peptides) and a variety of problems with learning, attention, and development.

Non-celiac gluten sensitivity afflicts close to 12% of the general population[19,20]. It is characterized by a measurable immune reaction against one or more proteins in found in grains. When a person's immune system has developed antibodies against any of these proteins, undigested and partly digested food particles have been allowed entry into the bloodstream[21]. The leakage of food proteins through the intestinal wall signals a failure of the protective, mucosal lining of the gastrointestinal tract, as is consistently found in untreated celiac disease. Many of the same health and learning problems that are found in celiac disease are significantly overrepresented among those with gluten sensitivity for the very good reason that many of the same proteins are being leaked into the blood of those with gluten sensitivity.

Our cultural obeisance to grains is at odds with information drawn from the remains of ancient humans. Archaeologists have long recognized grains as a starvation food—one for which our digestive tracts are not well suited. Grains result in consistent signs of disease and malnourishment in every locale and epoch associated with human adoption of grain cultivation.

Today, grains are a poverty food. As we increase our grain consumption, we cause deficiencies in other nutrients by overwhelming the absorptive and transport mechanisms at work in our intestines. For instance, diets dominated by grains have been shown to induce iron deficiency[22]—a condition that is widely recognized as a factor in many learning dificulties[23-29]. This should not be surprising since iron is the carrier used to distribute oxygen throughout our bodies, including various regions of our brains. There is little room to dispute the hazards to learning posed by reductions in oxygen supply to the brain. Iron deficiency also reduces available iron ions which are used by the hippocampus to encode long-term memories from short term memories, revealing yet another dimension of gluten grains as mediators of learning difficulties.

There is more. The impact of grain consumption on our blood sugar levels is yet another facet of its contribution to learning problems. We evolved as hunter-gatherers, eating meats, and complex carbohydrates in the form of fruits, vegetables, and seeds. Refined sugars were a rare treat wrested from bees with some difficulty. At best, it was a rare treat for our pre-historic ancestors.

Today, with unprecedented agricultural/industrial production of refined sugars along with cultivation and milling of grain flours, these products have become very cheap and available, particularly over the last fifty years. During that time, we have added enormous quantities of grain-derived starches to the overwhelming quantities of sugar we consume. The result of this escalating dietary trend may be observed in the current epidemic rates of Type 2 diabetes, hypoglycemia, obesity, and cardiovascular disease. In the classroom, we see these trends manifest in students' mood swings, behavioral disorders (fluctuating between extreme lethargy, hyperactivity, and irrational anger), chronic depression, forgetfulness, and muddled thinking—all of which reflects the inordinate, counter evolutionary burden placed on homeostatic systems that regulate the body's blood sugar.

The pancreas has many functions. One important activity of the pancreas is to stabilize blood sugar levels. When blood sugar is not well regulated, learning is impaired[30]. The pancreas secretes carefully metered quantities of glucagon and insulin. It does so in response to the elevated presence of glucose in the bloodstream, by producing insulin. It produces glucagon in response to low blood glucose levels. The balanced presence of both of these hormones in the bloodstream is critical to learning because they regulate the transport of nutrients into cells. Too little or too much insulin can cause blood sugar levels fluctuate out of control, inducing a wide range of symptoms.

Today, when the insulin/glucagon balance goes awry, it is frequently due to insulin overproduction in response to a diet dominated by sugars and starches. The resulting elevated levels of insulin cause rapid movement of nutrients into cells, either for storage as fat, or to be burned as energy, causing increased activity levels, "hot spells", sweating, increased heart rate, etc. This energized stage requires a constant supply of sugars and starches to be maintained. Otherwise, it is soon followed by bouts of lethargy, lightheadedness, tremors, and weakness, which are all signs of low blood sugar levels.

Despite having stored much of the blood sugars as fats, we often produce insufficient glucagon to facilitate burning fats for energy, because insulin production blocks pancreatic glucagon production. As this condition progresses, and as blood sugar levels plummet, periods of irrational anger and/or confusion can result. In the context of low blood glucose, adrenaline is secreted to avoid a loss of consciousness. The next step in the progression, in the absence of appropriate nutritional intervention, is lapsing into a coma.

In the short term, the answer to these fluctuations is more frequent consumption of small amounts of sugars/starches every couple of hours. However, the long term result of such an approach is a state of insulin resistance, where more and more insulin is required to do the same task of moving glucose into cells. Then blood glucose continues to rise but the cells are starved for nutrients and they begin to die off. Once this stage is reached, the individual may be diagnosed with type 2 diabetes and it must be curtailed or a deadly state of ketoacidosis may develop. The frequency of this disease has so increased among North Americans, even among children, that an autoimmune form of diabetes, previously called 'juvenile onset', had to be renamed to "Type 1 diabetes".

By now, it will not surprise the reader to learn that Type 1 diabetes has also been shown to be significantly associated with gluten. Research reveals that there is considerable overlap between celiac disease and Type 1 diabetes. About 8% of celiacs also have Type 1 diabetes[31-33], and 5-11% of Type 1 diabetics also have celiac disease[34-38]. Further, Scott Frazer et al. have repeatedly shown, in animal studies, a causal, dose-dependent relationship between type 1 diabetes and gluten consumption[39-42].

The growing avoidance of gluten and other allergenic foods should not be confused with the several dietary fads of the 20th Century. The vegetarian perspective ignores the vitamin deficiencies that result from a strict vegetarian diet. The low-fat craze is another fad that has mesmerized the industrialized world for the last 50 years or so. Fortunately, this perspective has recently come under scrutiny. Despite having served as the driving force behind most physicians' dietary recommendations during the last several decades, the low fat dictum is overwhelmingly being discredited by research reported in peer reviewed publications.

Recognition and avoidance of allergenic and highly glycemic foods is a whole new trend that is based on scientific research and evidence. It reflects the application of an improved understanding of the function of the gastrointestinal tract, the endocrine system, particularly the pancreas, and the immune system. Past dietary fads are consistently deficient in important nutrients that are necessary to our good health and survival. Further, they frequently contain substances that are harmful to us, such as the phytates that are abundantly present in whole grain foods, and interfere with absorption of many minerals.

It is increasingly clear that grains, especially those that contain gluten, are contraindicated for human learning. The evidence is overwhelming. The mandate of eating to learn is learning to eat as our pre-agricultural ancestors did.

Editor's note:

The following personal story is very close to my heart. That's not because his first sentence promotes one of my books (although that doesn't hurt). It is because his story explores a very disturbing experience for which medical professionals failed to offer any real help, insight, or remedy. Yet, despite their own admitted ignorance, they were uniformly dismissive of the possibility that diet might underlay these serious, poten-tially devastating symptoms. They were certain that gluten could not be causing these problems. Science and its principles seem sorely lacking in this context. It is another form of denial that is especially frightening to those of us who have had to resist the certitude that often exudes from many health care professionals.

Psychiatric Symptoms and Gluten

By Jim Ford

Ron Hoggan's book <u>Dangerous Grains</u> has been an enormous help toward understand-ing something bizarre that happened to my 19 year old son, Lee, in the past year.

One day last October, Lee suddenly began exhibiting psychotic behavior, and eventu-ally had what appeared to be some kind of seizure. He lay on the couch, tensed up, and started shaking violently. His eyes were rolling back into his head and he was vocalizing loudly. After a period of time he came out of it and was somewhat lucid but seemed dazed and very confused.

We took him to the emergency room where he underwent a battery of tests that re-vealed nothing out of the ordinary. During the wait, he had two more of the seizure-like episodes. A psychiatrist was phoned and he was given neuroleptic drugs. He went to the epilepsy ward for further testing -EEG, CT scans and MRIs that did not reveal any-thing obviously wrong. Fortunately, we were able to stay with him.

On the morning of the second day he seemed better and we talked while he ate break-fast. Thirty minutes later he was having an episode- again shaking and vocalizing, and after a couple of hours started to come out of it. We noticed this pattern- eating, fol-lowed shortly afterward by seizure-like episodes and psychosis, which gradually cleared enough to converse. I started to notice what he was eating and the common denomina-tor was wheat. I gave him some rice and vegetables from home and there was no reac-tion, but bagels, bread, muffins and gravy all seemed to bring about the same violent reaction. I have food allergies and am aware that wheat is a common allergen (I learned to avoid it years ago), but I couldn't understand how he could be affected in such an extreme manner, so quickly after eating.

He was moved to a locked psychiatric ward, diagnosed with possible bipolar disorder or non-specific schizophrenia, and the neuroleptics were continued. Of course, his psychiatrist didn't want to hear about my observations regarding Lee's apparent reaction to wheat. (My wife and daughter also witnessed it on several occasions) I told the psychiatrist that Lee hadn't been having any mental changes lately but had been complaining about digestive problems and I requested a biopsy to confirm celiac disease. It was promptly denied, but I was able to get the hospital dietitian to put him on a gluten-free diet (unknown to the psychiatrist who rarely saw him, but was happy to prescribe ever increasing doses of neuroleptics). The seizures stopped the very next day-the staff no doubt assumed the drugs were having an effect in spite of my revelation about the gluten-free diet.

Over the next several weeks Lee became more psychotic and suffered terrible side-effects from the drugs. The county brought him to court and had him committed. He was ordered to continue the neuroleptics and there seemed to be little we could do. Eventually he was sent to a halfway house, but a couple of weeks after arriving he started to become catatonic. (I had told the staff about the wheat reaction but they were unable to provide a gluten-free diet). We took him to the emergency room where we learned that he was extremely dehydrated. He had lost the urge to eat or drink and was becoming very psychotic. The hospital was full, so he was sent to a sister hospital. By the time the ambulance arrived, he was completely catatonic - unable to speak and incontinent.

At the new hospital, he had a new psychiatrist. She was alarmed at the dosages of drugs he was receiving and felt he was probably experiencing the beginning of 'neuroleptic malignant syndrome,' a potentially fatal reaction to neuroleptics. The drugs were discontinued but he remained catatonic and was given Electro Convulsive Treatment several times a week. (I also spoke with the dietician when he was admitted and had Lee placed on a gluten-free diet - which was halfheartedly followed). After a few ECT treatments (and a mostly gluten-free diet) he started to come out of it.. His new doctor began to realize that he didn't seem to have any mental illness at all (now that the neuroleptics had been discontinued, the catatonia was lifting and diet was improving) and called in several specialists for a more thorough evaluation.

I told her about the reaction to wheat but she refused to believe there could be a connection. Finally, another neurologist was brought in and he had the insight to give him a gliadin antibody test and found that he was extremely reactive. He was finally "officially" put on a gluten-free diet. Before that, we had already started bringing him food from home and doing everything we could behind the scenes to keep gluten from him. He continued to improve, in spite of the side effects of the ECT.

His psychiatrist couldn't really understand what was going on with him but began to trust us enough to release him, drug-free, into our care. Three months after the ordeal began, he finally came home and is clearer now than he's been in years. He's always been kind of quiet and we realize now that gluten has probably been affecting him for years. He has done an excellent job of following the gluten-free diet, is working full time, and starts college in a few weeks.

Shortly after he came home, my mother came across Dangerous Grains and bought it for me. It all finally makes sense, and I plan to send copies to Lee's psychiatrist and neurologist. We saw countless people in the locked psychiatric wards who were suffering and, with the exception of the chemical dependencies everyone was on some type of drug or drugs. Many were receiving ECT on a routine basis. I know my son is not unique - testing and gluten-free diets could save many of these poor souls from a lifetime of drugs and suffering. I want to do everything I can to increase the knowledge of these professionals and Dangerous Grains seems the perfect vehicle.

So great thanks to Ron Hoggan (and Dr. Braly and the rest) for doing what you're doing. I know it's only a matter of time before the people who control the mental health system become enlightened enough to stop doing harm and truly begin to heal these patients. It was a close call for us and I realize Lee is a living example.

Editor's note:

What follows is an article written by a medical researcher and practitioner who is leading the way for other members of his profession. As you will see, he is well versed in the gluten issues that have caused so much frustration to those with the gluten syndrome. He is a credit to his profession and a boon to those who struggle with the health hazards posed by gluten.

Gluten Causes Brain Disease!

By Prof. Rodney Ford M.B., B.S., M.D., F.R.A.C.P.

Yes, that's what I think. Gluten-sensitivity is a disease of your brain and nerves.

The gluten puzzle

I have come to this conclusion after studying the effects of gluten on my patients for over a decade. I am a pediatric gastroenterologist and allergist. I run a busy clinic for children and their parents. I have been increasingly concerned by the large numbers of my patients who are affected by gluten I was perplexed by their wide-ranging symptoms. The puzzle was to explain how gluten could cause so much ill health to so many people in so many different ways, including celiac disease.

Faulty brain control

Eureka! The solution came when deep in discussion with my friend and colleague, Ron Harper, Professor of Neurobiology, UCLA. We were both struggling with the concept of multiple symptoms that needed to be explained. The answer appeared absurdly simple: disturbed "brain control". It suddenly seemed obvious—gluten could disturb the neural pathways of the body. Gluten was gradually damaging the brain and the nerves of susceptible people. It was the brain that was the common pathway for the manifestations of all of the gluten symptoms. So I set out to research what the world medical literature had to say.

Is gluten a neurotoxin?

I felt excited. I reviewed my patients in this new light—I began looking for a brain-grain connection. I began to see gluten as a neurotoxin—this could provide a universal model of gluten-sensitivity. This toxicity might act through inflammatory mechanisms or cross-reactivity with neurons. I began accumulating the evidence for my proposal that gluten-sensitivity is a brain and nerve disease.

"Full Of It!"

The concept of "Full of it" developed from the stories from my patients. I wrote my hypothesis down in a book now called <u>Full of it!</u> It refers to our diets being full of gluten; to the world being full of gluten-sensitive people; to the medical practitioners who are so skeptical of adverse reactions to gluten; to the enthusiasm of people who are feeling vibrant again on a gluten-free diet; and to those who are brimming with hope that the problem of gluten has now been recognized.

Food allergy skeptics

As a junior doctor I decided to formally research the food allergy phenomenon. I was awarded a research post and carried out the first comprehensive food allergy studies in New Zealand. I triumphantly demonstrated that food allergy was both a real entity and that it was common. But, to my disappointment, my colleagues were reluctant to believe me or my data. They professed a "disbelief" in food allergy. This surprised me as I had the research data.

My next step was to conduct four more years of investigation of food allergy in Australia (at the Royal Children's Hospital, Melbourne). This was a bigger and more elaborate study. My Doctoral Thesis (1982) based on this work is called: <u>Food hypersensitivity</u>

in children: diagnostic approaches to milk and egg hypersensitivity. Since then I have continued my investigations into food allergy—but still today (25 years later) medical skepticism abounds. This "disbelief" is held despite the vast body of research describing food allergy. There seems to be an underlying unwillingness for doctors to consider food allergy as a possibility. Unfortunately, this also applies to gluten reactions.

The shocking truth

The shocking truth about gluten is that gluten foods are causing tremendous damage—but currently this is going mostly unrecognized. Unfortunately, gluten grains have become our staple diet. The quantity of gluten in our food supply has been steadily increasing. Yet worse, official Health Policies endorse gluten grains as the foundation of our food pyramid.

Medics turn a blind eye

Gluten is sapping the energy and wellbeing of countless millions. To date, the medical profession has turned a blind eye to gluten's wider problems whilst focusing all of their attention on the narrow problem of celiac disease.

A typical story

Nearly every day, I receive emails like this:

"Dr Ford, I have emailed you a number of times regarding our two children.

I thought I should let you know that since going gluten free for the last three months, our son and daughter have, at last, put on some weight.

If I had kept them on a normal gluten diet (which they recommended at the hospital) we would be still be having the headaches and sore tummies as well as the bad moods, which our son would have. People just thought he was a naughty child, but now he is so different - we can talk to him without getting into any fights.

I congratulate you for all your efforts on bringing gluten intolerance to the media and medical profession. More children and their families may find long awaited help. We have had to put up with this for seven years! At long last there is light at the end of the tunnel. Kind regards, Sue and Garry."

Can gluten damage your brain?

I believe that gluten was actually causing these two children to be sick. That is the explanation for their "naughty" behavior, their moods and their headaches.

I postulate that gluten can damage your brain. I have come to this conclusion by the abundant circumstantial evidence from my observations of my patients who are gluten-sensitive. I have pondered the next questions: "Why do they have such an array of symptoms from gluten?" "Why do they recover so quickly when gluten is removed?" And "Why do they deteriorate so rapidly when only tiny amounts of gluten are eaten?" The concept of a brain/nerve disease can explain everything.

The brain/nerve hypothesis

"The symptoms from gluten occur through its action on the nervous system".

I propose that gluten-sensitivity is a **brain condition**. Each and every organ in your body has some form of brain/nerve control. I propose that gluten can injure the delicate nervous networks that control your gut's functions. A malfunction will subsequently lead to all of the gut symptoms that have so well been described. In addition, gluten can also directly affect brain function, which leads to the primary neurological symptoms that are so commonly seen with gluten-sensitivity.

What is new?

There are a number of new ideas that I put forward. These are based on circumstantial evidence. They produce a unifying theory of the symptoms that are attributed to gluten toxicity.

A brain disease

I consider that gluten-sensitivity is mostly a *neurological* problem. A major contribution to this debate is the realization that the brain has a central role in the expression of the symptoms that have, until now, been attributed to the local toxicity of gluten in the gut.

A nerve disease

I propose that gluten-sensitivity is a nerve disease. There is a gigantic network of nerves that controls every function that your gut is programmed to do. There are as many nerve cells in your gut as there are in your head! (about 25 billion nerve cells). I call it your tummy brain (or gut brain). Your tummy brain can be directly damaged by gluten reactions. This is the cause of so many sore tummies and bowel troubles.

A wide spectrum of neurological manifestations

For decades, there have been reports of unexplained brain and nerve symptoms, which are associated with celiac disease. Although these associations have been described, there has been no universal mechanism proposed. However, if gluten is seen as a *neurotoxin*, then the explanation has been found.

A very common disease

Reactions to gluten have recently been documented to be extremely common. About one-in-ten people (as ascertained by blood donor studies) have high levels of gluten antibodies in their blood. My clinical studies have arrived at this same high number of gluten-sensitive people. Others have data to show that it is even more prevalent.

Am I full if it?

You might ask, "Is he full of it?" Yes, I am full of excitement and hope for the future. So many people can now be helped, if only this information can be widely distributed. I am full of ideas and full of enthusiasm. I hope that you are full of hope for your healthy and vibrant future.

Tariq's story:

"Dear Rodney,

Thank you for your care and support of my family in regard to our allergies, gluten sensitivity and celiac disease that exists within that framework.

My son Tariq, who is nearly 12 years old, has been a patient of yours over a number of years for his multiple food allergies. Tariq also suffers from dyslexia. Over the last several years Tariq has been becoming increasingly tired, lacking in energy and motivation, struggling with school work and constantly scratching due to his eczema and rashes covering all of his body.

During this time, even though he has attended soccer training up to four times a week he somehow gained a lot of weight. Tariq was constantly grumpy and had low mood levels.

Two months ago you diagnosed Tariq with gluten-sensitivity (his tTG 4; IgG-gliadin 86; IgA-gliadin 9).

Tariq was extremely reluctant to go on a gluten free diet. But as the rest of the family had gone gluten-free—so he was forced also to become gluten-free.

The changes that a gluten-free diet has evoked in Tariq have been astounding. His energy levels have increased, his skin has vastly improved, he has lost a lot of his excess weight (even though his appetite has increased) and he has shown improvement in his dyslexia.

Tariq is not as grumpy as he was and his mood levels have improved. Tariq is now vigilant about gluten, and can see the differences it has made to his life, and the quality of it.

Also, the other soccer parents have noticed a vast improvement in Tariq's energy levels and speed. His teacher has also noticed a big difference.

Thanks again.
Regards, Rosemary"

Are you affected?

The shocking truth is that gluten can damage your brain and that so many people are being encouraged to eat gluten-foods that might be steadily eroding their health and energy. If you have any lingering doubt about your own health, then I suggest that you check out the possibility of gluten-sensitivity.

If you have any comments or questions we would love to hear from you at: http://www.drrodneyford.com/

More on Psychiatric Symptoms and Gluten

By Réjean Perron

I live near Montréal, in Québec country and I'm webmaster of a new French web site, called SOSGLUTEN.CA, devoted to gluten sensitivity. The first time I saw the word "gluten" was in year 2000. At that moment my wife, Danielle, was very sick and while she was waiting for a diagnosis from her doctor, I discovered an ailment called "celiac disease" on the Web. That was my first meeting with the word "gluten". When she went to the doctor to finally receive what is, effectively, a diagnosis of celiac disease, she had already been on a gluten free diet for three weeks, based on my own findings. After that, I continued to read, read, and read again, anything on the web concerning celiac disease and gluten sensitivity.

In 2002 when my youngest daughter, Manon, received a diagnosis of anxiety and depression, I requested a blood screening for celiac disease. As you may have expected, the doctor initially refused. It was only after my insistence that he finally ran these tests. From this, Manon received a diagnosis of celiac disease and she stopped having to take Paxil after six gluten-free months.

In 2003, I helped a sister of my wife, Suzanne, to understand that gluten might be behind her skin disease and other health problems. She finally received a diagnosis of dermatitis herpetiformis and celiac disease after seeking a second medical opinion. In 2004, I also helped another sister of my wife, Noelline, to understand that gluten might also be behind her bone pain, joint pain and many other health problems. Despite two negative blood tests and two negative biopsies, she started a gluten free diet and it turned out to be the best decision of her life.

More recently, in 2005, I requested, for me and my son Eric, the opinion of Dr. Kenneth Fine via Enterolab. My son, an engineer at 25 years old, had finger joint pain and he was always a little inclined to depression. I frequently had esophageal reflux, indigestion with chest pain, and insomnia since I was three or four years old (I'm now 53). The diagnosis from Dr. Fine was a diagnosis of gluten sensitivity for my son Eric with a copy of HLA DQ2 gene (from his mother) and for me a diagnosis of gluten sensitivity with only gluten sensitive genes. Today, we are all on a gluten free diet and have been since Christmas 2005, and all symptoms have disappeared for Eric and me.

As you can understand, avoiding gluten is in the center of our lives, and that is the reason I have decided to create a French web site devoted to celiac disease and gluten intolerance. I now have personal proof that gluten intolerance is not limited to celiac disease.

To conclude, the main goal of this article is to share my family's experiences with you, and to ask you to visit my web site at: http://www.sosgluten.ca Naturally, if you consider that this young and new site is worthy to figure among your web links, it would be appreciated.

Teach Your Children Well

By Dr. Ron Hoggan, Ed. D.

Virtually every parent and professional person who works with children wants them to learn, grow, and achieve their greatest potential. The vast majority of these caregivers know that nutrition plays an enormous role in each child's life-quest. Unfortunately, that is where broad agreement ends. There are almost as many perspectives on what constitutes a healthy diet as there are people on this planet. Some claim that the healthiest diet is that of a vegetarian which almost invariably leads to a heavy reliance on grains and which is devoid of vitamin B_{12}. Others assert, based on cardiovascular disease being our number one killer that the best diet includes the smallest amount of fats. They believe that fat consumption is related to blood cholesterol levels. They also believe that blood cholesterol levels are the best predictor of heart attacks. Yet there is little solid evidence to support these beliefs, while low cholesterol has been linked to increased cancer risk. Still others argue for the health benefits conferred by a high protein diet. They point out the importance of proteins in providing the building blocks for immune system function and the body's maintenance and repair at the cellular level. A small but growing faction points to the health benefits of a diet dominated by fats with little or no carbohydrate content. Other diets target refined sugars and flours as problematic. Added to this diversity, there is a plethora of dietary perspectives that advocate rigid proportions of fat, protein, and carbohydrates. The proportions of each component vary according to the data that is given the most credence by the creators and advocates of each diet. Many dietary rituals have grown up around cancer avoidance or therapy, weight loss strategies, treatments for cardiovascular disease or its avoidance, and autoimmune diseases. Book, video tape, audio tape, menu guides, and other media sales are just a starting point. Some advocates of specific dietary strategies are even selling special foods that comply with their recommendations. The profit motive can be a powerful factor in creating bias. Then there are the government sponsored healthy eating guides. Of course, each paradigm assumes that one diet can be recommended for all people. The USDA has recently devised recommendations that do make a few concessions to gender and stage-of-life, with separate recommendations for children, adults, and seniors.

However, even with these changes, the USDA provides a clear message advocating plenty of grains and little fat. It is difficult to determine just how much these recommendations have been influenced by special interest lobbies. Agricultural and food production corporations have made astronomical investments in current dietary practices and shaping new dietary trends. Is it reasonable to expect them to be responsive to evolving research findings that might compromise their investments?

Those of us who have experienced illness and were sometimes deathly ill from grain proteins that come highly recommended by government food guides, have had to revise our views of healthy eating and reject such dangerously flawed guidance. Gluten sensitivity and celiac disease often crop up in the context of what many health care professionals tout as a healthy diet. Prior to my own diagnosis of celiac disease, I remember one physician recommending that I eat bran every morning to reverse some of the gastrointestinal problems I was having. He would not believe that eating bran made me vomit and left me feeling ill for some time.

There is a persistent sense that we should all know what constitutes a good diet. Almost every one of us who have to avoid gluten knows that it is an unhealthy choice for us, irrespective of government or private sector recommendations for healthy eating. We have learned not to trust these prescriptions filled with certitude and rigidity. We experienced some degree of return of our health through adopting eating habits that are diametrically opposed to those recommendations.

Thus, many of us will have a very different view of conventional dietary wisdom. For instance, Dr. Eve Roberts, a scientist at Toronto's Hospital for Sick Children, was quoted on Monday, September 24th in the Victoria Times Colonist as saying: "I do not want children to grow up with liver disease because we forgot to tell them how to eat"[1]. I'm sure that same attitude abounds throughout the medical profession. Unfortunately, despite the overwhelming consensus that children should not suffer such diet-induced illnesses, there is little agreement on exactly what we should be telling children (or adults for that matter) to help them avoid fatty liver disease.

In fact, dietary contradictions abound throughout the medical literature. So how are we to choose a healthy diet? What can we teach our children about eating well? For those of us who are gluten sensitive or have celiac disease, gluten avoidance is a given. For our children, the answer may be less clear. They will be at greater risk of having celiac disease or gluten sensitivity, but what should we teach them about these grains? Should they avoid gluten entirely? Should they eat normally until they become ill—perhaps risking permanent neurological damage or a deadly cancer as their first sign of the gluten syndrome? Should they be constantly vigilant with regular blood tests, endoscopies, or IgG allergy testing?

Many of us have been told to "just eat a balanced diet". It sounds appealing, but it is so vague as to provide little meaningful direction. What is a balanced diet and how do we judge if any special interest group is more interested in health than profits? Just how much can we trust information that has a price tag attached to it? Somebody is profiting. Can they really provide objective guidance? These questions should form part of our search for information. There is nothing wrong with making a profit or earning a living from providing dietary advice. However, it is important to be aware of any possible conflicts of interest or vested interests that might shape that advice.

For these reasons, I have developed my own strategy for determining what advice and guidance I can provide to my children and grandchildren. I acknowledge that this approach is limited by my own biases, my finite capacity for assimilating and synthesizing information, my incomplete familiarity with nutritional research, and my own personal experiences. On the other hand, I don't have to worry about being directly influenced by profiteering or lobby groups diverting me from my primary purpose.

On that basis, I have proceeded to explore my own dietary program. I have conducted some trial-and-error experiments on myself, and I have read as extensively as my part-time avocation of dietary investigation permits. From this, I have learned to trust my own gut. If something doesn't feel right in my stomach, I avoid it. I have also learned to trust my sense of smell. If a food does not smell appetizing to me, I don't eat it. I suspect that this is a tool that evolution has provided us with to determine what is and is not safe to eat. Those without a smell-induced aversion to unhealthy substances probably stopped contributing to the human gene pool.

I have also learned that IgG allergy testing is an effective tool with which I can reduce the lengthy trial-and-error process necessary for identifying the majority of my delayed food sensitivities. I realize that this testing has its weaknesses, but so does almost every other form of medical testing. I have come to accept that as long as human beings are involved, we will have imperfect testing regardless of claims to the contrary. Finally I try to read critically. I read medical and scientific research reports to stay abreast of new findings and gain a better understanding of this complex field. And I try to "catch" any sign of design flaws that will pre-determine the outcome of studies that are presented as unbiased.

The tentative conclusions I have reached, pending new information, are as follows:

1. Gluten grains probably aren't very good for people. They are highly allergenic affecting at least 10% of the general population, and perhaps as much as 40% of the population. And our gastrointestinal tracts are much shorter and have fewer stomach chambers than animals that evolved eating grains.
2. These grains also contain opioids, which are morphine-like substances that can be highly addictive and have a deleterious effect on our ability to resist cancer and other ailments from which natural killer cells usually protect us. They also contain large quantities of starch that is converted very rapidly into sugars.
3. The evidence suggests that refined sugars and starchy foods cause many of our problems with obesity, vision problems due to growth related distortions of the eyeball, type II diabetes, and hypoglycemia.
4. Dairy products probably aren't very good for most people either. They are also highly allergenic and contain opioids similar to those found in gluten. Further,

about two thirds of the world's adult populations are lactose intolerant. They don't retain enzymes for digesting milk sugars after childhood.

5. I think it is wise to avoid processed foods where possible. The more they've been processed, the further they are from the state in which our pre-historic ancestors ate them.

6. I believe it is a good idea to avoid eating soy because it has been linked to neurological diseases and other health problems that I don't want to develop.

7. I avoid foods to which IgG testing of my blood has shown an immune reaction against.

8. I try to avoid juices, as these are mostly sugar.

Those are the things I try to avoid. On a more positive note, there are several specific strategies that I try to follow:

1. I take supplements of vitamins and minerals which evidence has shown that I either absorb poorly or have been depleted from the soils in which my food is grown.

2. I try to eat whole fruits and vegetables.

3. I try to eat when I am hungry—not according somebody else's idea of appropriate mealtimes.

4. If I am ever diagnosed with cancer, I will follow a ketogenic diet. That is a diet that is dominated by fats, includes about 30% protein, and excludes all carbohydrates. I have tried this diet for about a month. I can't say that I enjoy it very much, but I'd be happy to forego the pleasure of carbohydrates if my life is at stake.

5. I'm very grateful to my wife who works very hard at finding tasty treats so I don't have to feel isolated or deprived in social situations where food is consumed.

6. I'm convinced that even a little exercise is a critical feature of a well balanced diet. I'm not advocating work-outs suitable for professional athletes, but I do try to walk regularly.

I realize that these strategies are often impractical and I don't pretend to live up to all of them all of the time (except for gluten and dairy protein avoidance). I also suspect that I would be better off if I ate organic fruits and vegetables along with range fed meat. I should probably avoid any genetically modified food as well. We really don't know what's in that stuff! However, I haven't reached the point yet where I am sufficiently motivated to change my diet to that extent, although I do realize that it would probably be a good idea. I am convinced that Dr. Barry Sears is onto something when he advocates specific proportions of each food type for optimal health and performance. Unfortunately, my diet is already complex enough that without some specific and highly motivating reason, I'm just too busy or lazy to be bothered with measuring such things. I just let my taste buds and availability (my wife only cooks one cake at a time) determine my portion sizes.

This is the balanced diet I recommend. I sorely doubt that my children or my grand-children will follow my advice, except when they visit during mealtimes. However I am confident that such a diet, should they choose to accept it, will not cause them to self-destruct due to dietary disease.

CHAPTER 4:
DIFFERENTIATING/IDENTIFYING CELIAC DISEASE AND GLUTEN SENSITIVITY

Editor's comment:

The next article is an attempt to equip readers with tools for enhancing their collaborative relationship with medical practitioners in the shared search for a diagnosis. The bias expressed arises both out of my own experiences with challenging relationships with physicians and other health care workers, as well as my discussions with many celiac patients who waited a very long time for an accurate diagnosis, then struggled to get appropriate follow-up testing and treatment.

MOM, F.R.C.M. (Fellow of the Royal College of Mothers)

By Dr. Ron Hoggan, Ed. D.

My doctor is a nice guy. He is also very bright and has an impressive memory for many complex terms as well as the details of various biochemical reactions. He couldn't have gotten through medical school—*he couldn't even have gotten acceptance into medical school* - without being pretty bright and very capable.

But he hasn't lived inside my skin. He can't know as much about me as I do. Neither has he observed my children for as long or with as much love and concern as I have. If we are ever to achieve balanced relationships with physicians, we must all acknowledge each others' areas of expertise. The history of the discovery of the gluten-free diet is really a story that should improve doctor-patient collaboration if the facts ever become widely known.

Not long ago I listened to a conference speaker, once again, crediting World War II grain shortages in The Netherlands for Dr. Dicke's discovery of the gluten-free diet as the treatment of choice for patients with celiac disease. This is a myth that has been perpetuated for far too long. This faulty tale sullies the memory of a great scientist, Dr. Willem Karel Dicke, and robs a concerned mother of the credit she richly deserves. The facts are available in Dr. Dicke's Ph. D. thesis. Dr. Chris Mulder has generously provided an English translation of Dr. Dicke's thesis, which is available at http://members.shaw.ca/dicke/index.htm

In his thesis, Dr. Dicke clearly states that he was treating celiac patients with a wheat-free diet by November of 1937. See case history of GH, page 28 and following. The insight came from a 1932 meeting with two colleagues: "The basis of this therapy stemmed from an observation by M.E. van Dusseldorp and H.A. Stheeman while he was treating a young celiac patient....."

This was long before World War II even began, and the grain shortages actually occurred late in the war.

Further, in the follow-up commentary at the end of the translation, Dr. Mulder reveals that the idea, which led to these 1932 insights, originated with a concerned mother's observations of her own child, and her comments to Dicke's colleagues. Please stop for a moment and consider this issue. Who is more likely to notice worsening symptoms following specific dietary intake - a busy physician spending a few minutes with a child, or a concerned mom?

The myth about World War II grain shortages simply does not jibe with the facts. It seems far more likely that a concerned mom, not a busy pediatrician, would notice what a child ate and how that affected his bowel movements. To my ears, this explanation has the ring of truth.

The question of who deserves the credit for this pivotal insight may not appear very important at first blush. However, our increasingly specialized society presses us to place more and more trust in the specialist, whether lawyer, physician, or auto mechanic. When we are placing our own and our child's health and safety in the hands of another person, we may reasonably expect these specialists get their facts straight on simple historical issues that can be easily investigated.

Dr. Dicke's important role, as a physician and a man of science, was to investigate this concerned mother's hypothesis. His memory is enhanced by the recognition that he freely rendered to the originators of the idea. We not only violate Dicke's memory, we insult his stature as a scientific investigator, when we perpetuate the false claim that the chance occurrence of WW II grain shortages led to the discovery of the treatment value of a gluten-free diet.

He deserves credit for having been open to other peoples' insights and for having tested and harnessed these ideas for the betterment of human health.

This issue also speaks to the importance of trusting ourselves, our own observations, and our own assessments—our own guts, if you will, in our quest for health. Dr. Dicke's work was extremely important and it constituted a huge contribution to Humanity. His research has already saved countless thousands of lives and will continue to do so. It may even result in a significant shift in worldwide nutritional trends. But we need to remember that the original insight that identified the trigger for celiac disease came from an observant, concerned mother. In remembering this, many of us will feel empowered to collaborate with our physicians rather than blindly accepting yet another prescription for yet another chemical agent. And that is the pivotal importance of publicly recognizing where the idea of a gluten-free diet originated.

We need to recognize that the physician's expertise is only one important element in the diagnostic and treatment process. We may often defer to physicians' superior knowledge of medical issues. However, our own expertise as the occupants of our bodies and/or as parents must also contribute to this process of diagnosis and subsequent healing. We need to trust our own observations and judgment. Dismissal or denigration of our unique expertise bespeaks a competitive spirit; not a collaborative one. Such a competitive attitude will weaken the diagnostic process and/or hinder our recovery.

Editor's note:
The next essay explores the developing field of blood tests for finding and diagnosing celiac disease. Dr. Kumar has worked for many years in this area, spearheading research that has helped make diagnostic blood tests for celiac disease a reality. Please bear in mind however, that his focus is on testing for celiac disease only.

How Effective are the Serological Methods of Diagnosing Celiac Disease?

By Vijay Kumar, M.D.

Celiac disease is an autoimmune disorder that may occur in genetically susceptible individuals. It is initiated by ingestion of gluten present in cereals, primarily wheat and to a much lesser extent other cereal proteins such as prolamines of barley and rye. Celiac disease is characterized by malabsorption resulting from inflammatory injury to the small intestinal mucosa. The classical symptoms of celiac disease include diarrhea, weight loss and malnutrition, however, only a small percentage of patients with celiac disease present with classical symptoms. Such patients represent the tip of the iceberg of gluten sensitivity. Many patients with celiac disease may present with short stature, iron and folate deficiency, anemia, bone loss, aphthous stomatitis, arthralgia, and dental enamel defects. Because of the varying and mild clinical presentations, celiac disease is often diagnosed when the patient has grown to adulthood rather than as a child. Adults may present with iron deficiency, anemia, macrocytic anemia and hypocalcemia (*see Table 1 below*).

Table 1:

Clinical Presentations of Celiac Disease	
Classical	**Features Atypical**
Chronic Diarrhea	Iron-deficiency anemia
Failure to thrive	Dental enamel defects
Abdominal distension	Short stature
	Osteoporosis/osteopenia
	Coexistence with other autoimmune disorders

Diagnosis based solely on clinical criteria can be misleading and may lead to improper diagnosis and treatment as a result of the variety of clinical presentations often seen in other conditions. Problems with diagnosis have a serious impact on the patient. Delays in diagnosis commonly extend 10-13 years from the first presentation of clinical symptoms, leaving the patient subject to chronic symptoms while searching for proper diagnosis. Failure to diagnose this condition in the short term may predispose an individual to long term complications such as splenic atrophy and intestinal lymphoma. On the other hand, attempts to diagnosis a patient based primarily on clinical criteria may unnecessarily place the individuals on lifelong gluten-free diet as several transient conditions may mimic Celiac disease clinically (*see Table 2 below*).

Table 2:

Cancer Morbidity on Normal, Reduced-Gluten and Gluten-Free Diet in celiac disease					
Diet Group	Number	Observed Malignancies	Expected Malignancies	Observed/ Expected	Excess Morbidity Rate
Normal	46	7	0.19	36.8	10.7
Reduced Gluten	56	5	0.12	41.7	5.0
Gluten-free	108	3	0.46	6.5	1.2

(Howelle PD, Is Coeliac Disease a Pre-Malignant Condition? Gastrointestinal Immunology and Gluten-Sensitive Disease, 1994. p.185)

The true prevalence of celiac disease is difficult to ascertain. However, with the advent of serum antibody methods, incidences as high as one in 300 have been described in the general population [editor's note: As of 2010 this number is now recognized to be at least 1 in 133], both in Western Europe and in the U.S. Celiac disease is prevalent worldwide, but may be rare in individuals of Chinese and Japanese descent (*see Table 3 below*).

Historically, the diagnosis of celiac disease was based primarily on histological studies of the jejunal biopsy characterized by villous atrophy, crypt hyperplasia, and lymphocytic and plasma cell infiltrate in the lamina propria. Histological examination of the small intestinal biopsy remains the gold standard for diagnosing celiac disease, but has its limitations. Many patients with celiac disease are small children and histological studies may be viewed by many, especially a child's parents, as a great discomfort. There may also be problems with accuracy. Occasionally, a biopsy with abnormally high density of intraepithelial lymphocytes with a normal villous architecture may be reported as normal. It has also been reported that some patients with latent or even active celiac disease show normal histopathology (Gastroenterology 104:1263-72, 1993). Celiac disease might also be confused with other disorders when diagnosed histologically. Parasitic infections (giardia lamblia) and malabsorption syndrome, for example, may mimic celiac disease histology.

Table 3:

Prevalence of Celiac Disease		
Country	Prevalence based upon Clinical	Prevalence based upon Laboratory
Finland	1:1000	1:330
Italy	1:1000	1:184
Germany	1:2300	1:500
Netherlands	1:4500	1:250
Denmark	1:10,000	1:330
USA	1:10,000	1:250

Guandalini S & Gupta P Clin appl Immun Rev 2:293-305, 2002

As these limitations have been recognized, serum antibody tests have gained acceptance in screening for celiac disease and in follow-up of patients with celiac disease to determine their compliance to a gluten-free diet. The various serological tests employed in the work-up of patients suspected to have celiac disease include anti-gliadin antibody

(AGA), anti-endomysial antibody (EMA), anti-reticulin antibody (ARA) and anti-tissue transglutaminase (tTG) antibody tests. Antibodies to gliadin and tTG are detected by ELISA, whereas endomysium and reticulin antibodies are detected by indirect immunofluorescence. Of the serum antibody tests, EMA and tTG antibody primarily detects antibodies of IgA immunoglobulin isotype, whereas the AGA test detects both IgG and IgA isotypes. No IgM class antibodies to these antigens are detected in patients with celiac disease. Hence there is no need to test for IgM class antibodies in the work-up of patients with celiac disease.

Of these tests, AGA was the first to be described in the literature and has been evaluated most extensively. IgG class AGA antibodies are more sensitive but less specific then IgA-AGA. The major utility of IgG-AGA is in celiac disease patients who are IgA deficient. In a study conducted recently in our laboratory, all of the 15 IgA-deficient celiac disease patients tested positive for IgG-AGA and negative for IgA-AGA and other autoantibodies (Celiac Disease and IgA deficiency: How effective are the serological methods of diagnosis? *Clinical diagnostic lab Immunology 9:1295-1300, 2002*).

EMA and ARA are very specific indicators of celiac disease. These assays are immunohistochemical methods and require experience in reading immunofluorescence reactions. Some investigators suggest that they are less sensitive. However, in all the studies conducted since our laboratory first described EMA back in 1983, we find the EMA assay to be 100% specific and sensitive for celiac disease. Other investigators may find EMA to be less sensitive due to the selection of the substrate, fixation of tissue sections, specificity of conjugate employed or serum screening dilution. Internally, we find that testing for EMA at dilutions of 1:2.5 or 1:5 yield 5% of patients positive for EMA yet negative at 1:10 or 1:20. It could be that some of the investigators who have reported low sensitivity might be screening the patients at high serum dilutions.

Since the identification of tTG as the endomyisal antigen, ELISA methods have been described for detecting antibodies in the sera of patients with celiac disease. The advantage of the anti-tTG antibody assay is that it is an automatable assay that is less subjective than EMA and it is more sensitive and specific than AGA. For these reasons, many laboratories have opted to use the tTG antibody method as the screening method. In these laboratories, it may be the only assay used for detection of celiac disease cases. In the majority of studies of the tTG antibody method, the specificity and sensitivity were found to be between 90-95%. (*Table 4 below*) summarizes the specificity of the AGA, EMA and tTG antibody methods most commonly employed by laboratories performing tests for celiac disease.

Table 4:

Diagnostic Specificity of Serological Markers for Celiac Disease		
Assay	Specificity	Sensitivity
Anti-gliadin Antibody IgG	78%	88%
Anti-gliadin Antibody IgA	86%	52%
Anti-endomysial Antibody	100%	100%
Anti-tissue transglutaminase	98%	90-95%

If the prevalence of undiagnosed celiac disease is 4.8 per thousand as reported by Lagerqvist et al (J Intern Med 250:241-48, 2001) then of all the serological methods, EMA is the only method that provides 100% positive and negative predictive value for celiac disease. This raises the question of the optimum method of screening for celiac disease. The answer will vary according to the likelihood of celiac disease in the population studied and upon the experience of the laboratory performing the test. Some investigators may use the AGA or tTG antibody methods for screening and, if positive, confirm using the EMA test. We recommend this approach as it also helps to identify all celiac disease patients, whether IgA-deficient or not (see Table 5, below).

Celiac disease patients are prescribed a gluten free diet for life. Serological tests are useful in monitoring a patient's response and adherence to the gluten free diet. The levels of the various antibodies (AGA, EMA, ARA and tTG) decrease and eventually disappear in the majority of the patients on a complete gluten free diet. Similarly, these antibodies either appear or rise in level when the patient is on a gluten containing diet. Serological methods, therefore, play a significant role in both diagnosis and follow-up of celiac disease patients.

Celiac disease has been associated with many other autoimmune disorders such as type 1 diabetes, thyroid autoimmunity and other autoimmune disorders. Approximately five percent of patients with type 1 diabetes have celiac disease. Similarly, a slightly larger percentage of celiac disease patients also have type 1diabetes. It has been proposed that early detection of celiac disease may be beneficial in such cases as it is believed that

Table 5:

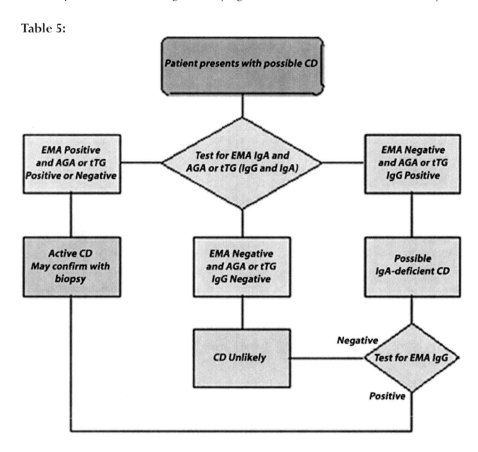

adherence to a gluten-free diet may delay the onset of diabetes. If true, this further emphasizes the utility of and need for serum antibody tests in the screening of population genetically susceptible for celiac disease.

In conclusion, clinical symptoms of celiac disease are variable and often mild, resulting in significant delays in diagnosis. The use of serological tests has improved the ease of detection, monitoring, and hence—the continuing care of celiac disease patients.

Challenging the Gluten Challenge

By Ron Hoggan, Ed. D.

There is an abundance of stories about people who begin a gluten-free diet, find that they feel better then decide they want a firm diagnosis of celiac disease. They are facing several problems. First, they may be gluten sensitive without the intestinal lesion of celiac disease. This is very likely since about twelve percent of the population is gluten sensitive, but only a little more than one percent of the general population has celiac disease. Another problem faced by gluten-free individuals who want a diagnosis is that it can take years after returning to a regular gluten-containing diet before the characteristic damage of celiac disease can be seen on a biopsy[1]. Simply put, after beginning a gluten-free diet, only a positive biopsy is meaningful. A negative biopsy does not rule out celiac disease.

A variety of opinions have been offered regarding how much gluten, for how long, should result in a definitive biopsy. The reality is that no such recommendation is consistent with the medical literature[1-4]. Some people with celiac disease will experience a return of intestinal damage within a few weeks of consuming relatively small amounts of gluten. Such brief challenges are valuable for these individuals. However, many people with celiac disease or dermatitis herpetiformis will require much larger doses of gluten, over much longer periods, to induce characteristic lesions on the intestinal wall. Unfortunately for these latter individuals, a negative biopsy after a brief gluten challenge can, and often is, misinterpreted as having ruled out celiac disease. Blood tests can compound this problem. If, as seems likely, celiac patients who are slow to relapse are also the ones who develop milder intestinal lesions, they are the very celiac patients for whom blood tests are very unreliable[5]. Claims to have ruled out celiac disease based on brief challenges with small quantities of gluten are mistaken and they can lead to serious, even deadly, consequences.

We may forget that gluten consumption by a person with celiac disease can lead to deadly cancers and a variety of debilitating autoimmune diseases. Any recommendation of a gluten challenge should be accompanied by a clear warning that the process may overlook many cases of celiac disease. The absence of such warnings is inexcusable.

And what about non-celiac gluten sensitivity? The absence of an intestinal lesion does not rule out gluten-induced damage to other tissues, organs, and systems. Evidence and research-based information in this area is sadly lacking but we do know that undigested or partly digested gliadin can damage a wide range of human cells[6] and we also know that gluten sensitivity is associated with elevated mortality and cancer rates. Thus, one need only be consuming gluten and experience increased intestinal permeability for gluten-induced damage to be a factor in an astonishing number of ailments.

There are several partial answers to this problem. One, which I've raised before, is to employ Dr. Michael N. Marsh's rectal challenge for the diagnosis of celiac disease, particularly when the individual has already begun a gluten-free diet. This test permits a definitive diagnosis of celiac disease for up to six months after beginning a gluten-free diet. That would catch a great number of celiac patients who have found relief through a gluten-free diet and now want a diagnosis. Another piece of this puzzle is to test for IgG anti-gliadin antibodies. Although these antibodies are considered "non-specific," they inarguably identify an immune response to one of the most common foods in a regular North American diet. Although these individuals may experience improved wellness on a gluten-free diet, we just don't know enough about non-celiac gluten sensitivity to do more than recommend that they continue on this diet since it makes them feel better and it may well stave off autoimmune disease[7].

Editor's note:

What follows is another perspective that can be seen as complimenting the approach advocated by Dr. Kumar above. Although there are some areas of disagreement, these two paradigms need not be mutually exclusive.

Associated ailments can signal gluten sensitivity or celiac disease even in the absence of better recognized symptoms. From a wide range of psychiatric and neurological symptoms (as explained in the last chapter) to autoimmunity, bone disease, endocrine disease, muscle and nerve ailments, reproductive problems, several types of cancers, cardiovascular diseases, lung diseases, kidney diseases, liver diseases and a host of deficiency conditions and ailments, gluten can be a factor that contributes to, or is a sole cause of many of these symptoms and illnesses. In your quest for wellness, try to resist the corrosive dismissals and derision that may sometimes arise in the context of that quest. Try to have confidence in your own sense of what is wrong. Most serological and endoscopic testing is currently aimed at finding celiac disease, and all of these tests have shortcomings in that regard. You need not have celiac disease for gluten to be contributing to your problems. Each year the research literature continues to unearth more and more conditions in which gluten is a contributing or causal factor. Thus, the gluten-free diet seems a very reasonable course of action, even in the absence of celiac disease, when anti-gliadin antibodies are found.

Early Diagnosis of Gluten Sensitivity: Before the Villi are Gone

By Kenneth Fine, M.D.

Transcript of a talk given by Kenneth Fine, M.D. to the Greater Louisville Celiac Sprue Support Group—transcribed by Marge Johannemann; Edited by Kelly Vogt

Gluten sensitivity is the process by which the immune system reacts to gluten contained in wheat, barley, rye, and oats. The reaction begins in the intestine because that is where the inciting antigen, gluten, is present (from food). When this immunologic reaction damages the finger-like surface projections, the villi, in the small intestine (a process called villous atrophy) it is called celiac disease (or sometimes celiac sprue or gluten-sensitive enteropathy). The clinical focus of gluten-induced disease has always been on the intestine because that is the only way the syndrome was recognized before screening tests were developed.

The intestinal syndrome consists mainly of diarrhea, gas, bloating and nausea, vomiting, fat in the stool, nutrient malabsorption, and even constipation. Although the small intestine is always the portal of the immune response to dietary gluten, it is not always affected in a way that results in villous atrophy. Even though recent research has shown that celiac disease is much more common than previously suspected, affecting 1 in 100-200 Americans and Europeans, past and emerging evidence indicates that it accounts for only a small portion of the broader gluten sensitive clinical spectrum (often referred to as the "Tip of the Gluten Sensitive Iceberg").

With better understanding of how gluten triggers immune and autoimmune reactions in the body, under the control of various genes, and advancing techniques for detecting these reactions, it is becoming apparent that the majority of the gluten sensitive population (the submerged "mass of the iceberg") do not manifest villous atrophy in its classic, complete form and therefore do not have celiac disease.

In these non-celiac, gluten sensitive individuals, the brunt of the immune reaction either affects the function of the intestine, causing symptoms without structural damage, affects other tissues of the body (and virtually all tissues have been affected in different individuals) or both. This is important because the commonly used diagnostic tests of clinically important gluten sensitivity (blood tests for certain antibodies and intestinal biopsies) are only positive when villous atrophy of the small intestine is present. But if only a small minority of gluten sensitive individuals actually develop celiac disease, the majority, who have not yet or may never develop villous atrophy, with or without symptoms, can remain undiagnosed and untreated for years. This can result in significant immune and nutritional consequences, many of which are irreversible even after treatment with a gluten-free diet. Some of these disorders include loss of hormone secretion by glands (hypothyroidism, diabetes, pancreatic insufficiency, etc), osteoporosis, short stature, cognitive impairment, and other inflammatory bowel, liver, and skin diseases, among others. Only with early diagnosis, can these problems be prevented or reversed.

I am here to report on a scientific paradigm shift regarding early diagnosis of gluten sensitivity based on about 30 years of medical research by myself and others. My message is that earlier and more inclusive diagnosis of gluten sensitivity than has been allowed by blood tests and intestinal biopsies must be developed to prevent the nutritional and immune consequences of long-standing gluten sensitivity.

Imagine going to a cardiologist because your blood pressure is high or you're having chest pain, and the doctor says he is going to do a biopsy of your heart to see what is wrong. If it 'looks' O.K., you are told you have no problem and no treatment is prescribed because you have not yet had a heart attack showing on the biopsy. You would not think very highly of the doctor utilizing this approach because, after all, isn't it damage to the heart that you would want to prevent?

But for the intestine and gluten sensitivity, current practice embraces this fallacious idea that until an intestinal biopsy shows structural damage, no diagnosis or therapeutic intervention is offered. This has to change now because with newly developed diagnostic tests, we can diagnose the problem before the end stage tissue damage has occurred; that is, "before the villi are gone," with the idea of preventing all the nutritional and immune consequences that go with it.

There are many misconceptions regarding the clinical presentation of gluten sensitivity or celiac disease: For example, that you cannot be gluten sensitive if you have not lost weight, are obese, have no intestinal symptoms, or are an adult or elderly. However, the most widely held and clinically troublesome misconception is that a negative screening blood test, or one only showing antigliadin antibodies, (without the autoimmune anti-endomysial or anti-tissue transglutaminase antibody) rules out any problem caused by gluten at that time or permanently.

For some reason, the high "specificity" of these blood tests has been tightly embraced. Specificity means if the test is positive, you surely have the disease being tested for with little chance that the positive is a "false positive." But sadly, a negative test does not mean you do not have the problem. This is the biggest pitfall of all because the only thing a very specific test, like blood testing for celiac disease, can do is "rule in" the disease; it can not "rule it out."

If you've got very far advanced and/or long-standing celiac disease, it is likely that the test will be positive. However, several studies have now revealed that it is only those with significant villous atrophy of the small intestine who regularly show a positive antiendomysial or anti-tissue transglutaminase antibody, the specific tests relied upon most heavily for diagnosis of gluten-induced disease. When there was only partial villous atrophy, only 30% had a positive test. More disturbing perhaps, were the results with respect to screening first degree relatives of celiacs with blood tests. Despite some biopsy-proven early inflammatory changes in the small intestine, but without damage to the villi, all blood tests were negative.

For some reason, it's been perfectly acceptable to celiac diagnosticians that a patient must have far advanced intestinal gluten sensitivity, i.e., villous atrophy, to be diagnosed and a candidate for treatment with a gluten-free diet. That means from the specific testing standpoint, there's never (or rarely) a false positive. But what about the larger majority of gluten-affected people who do not presently have or may never get this end stage, villous atrophic presentation? They are out of luck as far as blood testing is concerned. So we have erroneously relied on specificity (always picks up gluten sensitivity after it has caused villous atrophy, never having a false positive) instead of sensitivity (doesn't miss gluten sensitive people even though they might be picked up early, even before full-blown celiac disease develops). Would a test relying on specificity rather than sensitivity be good enough for you, or your children? Consider the risk of not getting an early diagnosis versus going on a gluten free diet a few months or years prematurely. While I do not recommend anyone to have a biopsy (especially children) for diagnosis because of the shortcomings and invasive nature of this technique, I particularly do not want someone to have a biopsy showing villous atrophy, since by that time, associated bone, brain, growth, and/or gland problems are all but guaranteed.

And here is another related problem: You have a positive blood test but, if a small bowel biopsy comes back normal or nearly normal, you are told that the blood test must have been a "false positive" and that gluten is not your problem. Would you believe that, especially in light of the fact that most such people would have gotten the blood test in the first place because of a specific symptom or problem? Let's hope not. A positive blood test, negative biopsy means only that the gluten sensitivity, as evidenced by antibodies to gliadin in the blood, has not yet damaged your intestines severely.

Evidence of this comes from a study that I performed. We tested 227 normal volunteers with blood tests for celiac disease. Twenty-five of these people (11%) had either antigliadin IgG or IgA in their blood versus only one (0.4%) that had antiendomysial, anti-tissue transglutaminase, and antigliadin IgA in the blood. So for every one person in a population that has the antibodies that have 100% specificity for celiac disease of the intestine (antiendomysial and anti-tissue transglutaminase), there are 24 that have antibodies to gliadin that may not have celiac disease. So what is going on with the 11% with antigliadin antibodies in blood? Are these false positives (rhetorically)? You're telling me that there is a disease called celiac disease and it is associated with antibodies to gliadin in the blood and sometimes it damages the intestine? But people with antigliadin antibody in their blood but no other antibodies do not have a clinically significant immunologic reaction to gluten? Do you see the problem? How can 11% be false positives? What about the 89% with none of these antibodies? You cannot equate having no antibodies at all (a negative test) with having antigliadin antibodies alone. If you have antibodies to gliadin, something is going on here. Where there's smoke there's fire. The purpose of this study was to test this hypothesis: That an antigliadin antibody alone does indicate the presence of an immune reaction to gluten that may be clinically important. Using tests for intestinal malabsorption and abnormal permeability (i.e., tests of small bowel function, unlike a biopsy which says nothing about function), we found that 45% of people with only an antigliadin IgG or IgA antibody in blood (without either antiendomysial or anti-tissue transglutaminase antibody) already had measurable intestinal dysfunction, compared to only 5% of people with no antibodies to gliadin in their blood. When we did biopsies of these people's intestines, none had villous atrophy with only a few showing some early inflammation. Thus, having an antigliadin antibody in your blood does mean something: That there is nearly a 1 in 2 chance that functional intestinal damage is already present even though it may not be visible structurally at the resolution attained by a light microscope assessment of a biopsy.

As mentioned at the outset, not all gluten sensitive individuals develop villous atrophy. Evidence for this has been around for a long time. In 1980, a medical publication titled "Gluten-Sensitive Diarrhea" reported that eight people with chronic diarrhea, sometimes for as long as 20 years, that resolved completely when treated with a gluten-free diet, had mild small bowel inflammation but no villous atrophy. In 1996 in a paper called "Gluten Sensitivity with Mild Enteropathy," ten patients, who were thought to have celiac disease because of a positive antiendomysial antibody blood test, had small bowel biopsies showing no villous atrophy. But amazingly, these biopsies were shown to react to gluten when put in a Petri dish, proving the tissue immunologically reacted to gluten (which was likely anyway from their positive blood tests).

Two other reports from Europe published in 2001 showed gluten sensitivity without villous atrophy, and hence without celiac disease. In one of these studies, 30% of patients with abdominal symptoms suggestive of irritable bowel syndrome having the celiac-like HLA-DQ2 gene but no antibodies to gliadin in their blood, had these antibodies detected in intestinal fluid (obtained by placing a tube down into the small intestine). Thus, in these people with intestinal symptoms, but normal blood tests and biopsies, the antigliadin antibodies were only inside the intestine (where they belong if you consider that the immune stimulating gluten also is inside the intestine), not in the blood. This is the theme we have followed in my research, as we are about to see.

More proof that patients in these studies were gluten sensitive came from the fact that they all got better on a gluten-free diet, and developed recurrent symptoms when "challenged" with gluten. Although the gluten-sensitive patients in these studies did not have the villous atrophy that would yield a diagnosis of celiac disease, small bowel biopsies in many of them showed some, albeit minimal, inflammatory abnormalities. Yet, when a symptomatic patient in clinical practice is biopsied and found to have only minimal abnormalities on small bowel biopsy, clinicians do not put any stock in the possibility of their having gluten sensitivity. As much as I would like to take credit for the concept, you can see from these studies that I did not invent the idea that not all gluten sensitive patients have villous atrophy. It has been around for at least 23 years, and reported from different parts of the world.

For many years there has also been proof that the intestine is not the only tissue targeted by the immune reaction to gluten. The prime example of this is a disease called dermatitis herpetiformis where the gluten sensitivity manifests primarily in skin, with only mild or no intestinal involvement. Now from more recent research it seems that the almost endless number of autoimmune diseases of various tissues of the body also may have the immune response to dietary gluten and its consequent autoimmune reaction to tissue transglutaminase as the main immunologic cause. A study from Italy showed that the longer gluten sensitive people eat gluten, the more likely they are to develop autoimmune diseases. They found that in childhood celiacs, the prevalence of autoimmune disease rose from a baseline of 5% at age two to almost 35% by age 20. This is a big deal if you think of how much more complicated one's life is when one is both gluten sensitive AND has an additional autoimmune disease.

So preventing autoimmune disease is one very important reason why early diagnosis and treatment of gluten sensitivity is important. Early diagnosis before celiac disease develops also holds the potential of preventing other clinical problems such as malnutrition, osteoporosis, infertility, neurologic and psychiatric disorders, neurotube defects (like spina bifida) in children, and various forms of gastrointestinal cancer. Another reason for early diagnosis and treatment is very straightforward and that is because many gluten sensitive individuals, even if they have not yet developed celiac disease (villous atrophy), have symptoms that abate when gluten is removed from their diet. Furthermore, from a study done in Finland, a gluten sensitive individual who reports no symptoms at the time of diagnosis can improve both psychological and physical well-being after treatment for one year with a gluten-free diet.

Despite the common sense and research evidence that early diagnosis of gluten sensitivity offers many health advantages over a diagnostic scheme that can only detect the minority and end-stage patients, the limitation, until now, lay in the tests being employed. As mentioned above, the main tests used for primary(before symptoms develop) and secondary (after symptoms develop) screening for celiac disease, blood tests for antigliadin and antiendomysial/anti-tissue transglutaminase antibodies, are only routinely positive after extensive damage to intestinal villi. As shown in a 1990 publication, this is because unless you have full blown, untreated celiac disease, the IgA antibodies to gliadin are only INSIDE the intestine not in the blood. Measuring antigliadin antibodies in blood and intestinal fluid (obtained by the laborious technique of having research subjects swallow a long tube that migrates into the upper small intestine), researchers found that in untreated celiacs, antigliadin antibody was present in the blood and inside the intestine, whereas after villous atrophy healed following a year on a gluten-free diet, the antigliadin antibody was no longer in the blood but was still measurable inside the intestine in those with ongoing mild inflammation.

An important conclusion can be drawn from these results, as these researchers and myself have done: Gluten sensitive individuals who do not have villous atrophy (the mass of the iceberg), will only have evidence of their immunologic reaction to gluten by a test that assesses for antigliadin IgA antibodies where that foodstuff is located, inside the intestinal tract, not the blood. This makes sense anyway, because the immune system of the intestine, when fighting an antigen or infection inside the intestine, wages the fight right in that location in an attempt to neutralize the invading antigen, thereby preventing its penetration into the body. It does this with T cells on the surface of the epithelium, the intraepithelial lymphocytes, and with secretory IgA made with a special component called secretory piece that allows its secretion into the intestine.

The excellent English researchers that made the discovery that they could detect the immunologic reaction to gluten inside the intestine before it was evident on blood tests or biopsies knew it was a breakthrough, testing it many times over, in different ways, and further extending the clinical spectrum of gluten-induced disease to include a phase before the villi are damaged—so called "latent celiac sprue". Furthermore, they developed this technique of assessing the intestinal contents for antigliadin antibodies into what they viewed as a "noninvasive screening test for early or latent celiac sprue" (what others and I would simply call *"gluten sensitivity"*). However, this was not exactly a noninvasive test. Nor was it simple. The procedure required the patient to swallow a tube, followed by a complete lavage of all their gastrointestinal contents with many gallons of nonabsorbable fluid that had to be passed by rectum and collected into a large vat to be analyzed for the presence of antigliadin antibodies.

While this was indeed a conceptual breakthrough, it practically went unnoticed by the medical community because the cumbersome procedure of washing out the intestine just could not be done in a normal clinical setting. To this day, I am not sure how many people even know that it was not me, but rather this well known celiac research group, led by the late Dr. Anne Ferguson, who pioneered the assessment of the intestinal contents as a viable and more sensitive source of testing material for the early reactions of the immune system to gluten. What we did in my research was to refine and simplify the method of collecting and measuring these intestinal IgA antigliadin antibodies before they can be detected in blood. That is, instead of washing out the antibodies from the intestine, we allow them to be excreted naturally in the stool (feces). And so with that idea, and our ability to measure these antibodies in stool, as others before us had done for fecal IgE antibodies directed to food antigens, our new gluten (and other food) sensitivity stool testing method was born.

My research of microscopic colitis actually led me to discover that stool analysis was the best way of assessing for gluten sensitivity before celiac disease develops. Microscopic colitis is a very common chronic diarrhea syndrome, accounting for 10% of all causes of chronic diarrhea in all patients, and is the most common cause of ongoing chronic diarrhea in a treated celiac, affecting 4% of all celiac patients. However, from my published research, despite the presence of the celiac HLA-DQ2 gene in 64% of patients with microscopic colitis, very few get positive blood tests or biopsies consistent with celiac disease.

Yet, small bowel biopsies revealed some degree of inflammation sometimes with mild villous blunting in 70% of cases. According to the facts and previously discussed shortcomings of celiac blood tests, antibodies to gliadin are unlikely to be detected in the blood in these patients because they lack villous atrophy.

So negative blood tests for antigliadin antibodies per se did not, in my mind, rule out the possibility that these patients with microscopic colitis, a disease that under the microscope looks like celiac disease (but of the colon), and that affects many celiac patients, were not gluten sensitive themselves. But as Dr. Ferguson's research revealed, these antibodies might be detectable inside the intestine. And since we surely were not going to perform that cumbersome intestinal lavage test in my patients, we decided to see if we could find these antibodies in the stool as a reflection of what is coming through the intestine.

Here's the first set of data that we found showing the superior sensitivity of stool testing versus blood tests for antigliadin IgA antibodies. In untreated celiac disease patients, we found 100% positivity in the stool versus only 76% in blood. In hundreds of micro-scopic colitis patients since tested, only 9% have antigliadin antibody in blood but 76% have it in stool. And the same is true of 79% of family members of patients with celiac disease; 77% of patients with any autoimmune disease; 57% of people with irritable bowel syndrome-like abdominal symptoms; and 50% of people with chronic diarrhea of unknown origin, all of whom have only about a 10-12% positivity rate for blood tests (like normal volunteers). Thus, when you go to the source of production of these antibodies for testing - the intestine - the percentage of any population at a higher than normal genetic and/or clinical risk of gluten sensitivity showing a positive anti-gliadin stool test is 5 to 7.5 times higher than would be detected with blood tests.

In normal people without specific symptoms or syndromes, the stool test is just under 3 times more likely to be positive than blood (29% vs. 11%, respectively). That's a lot more people reacting to gluten than 1 in 150 who have celiac disease. 29% of the nor-mal population of this country, almost all of whom eat gluten, showing an intestinal im-munologic reaction to the most immune-stimulating of dietary proteins really is not so high or far-fetched a percentage, especially in light of the fact that 11% of them display this reaction in blood, and 42% carry the HLA-DQ2 or DQ8 celiac genes.

Why is this so important? Because some people with microscopic colitis never get bet-ter when they're treated, and most autoimmune syndromes only progress with time, requiring harsh and sometimes dangerous immuno-suppressive drugs just for disease control. If the immune reaction to gluten is in any way at the cause of these diseases, as research suggests, and if we had at our disposal a sensitive test that can diagnose this gluten sensitivity without having to wait for the intestinal villi to be damaged, then treatment with a gluten free diet might allow the affected tissues to return to normal or at least prevent progression. *We now have that test in fecal antigliadin antibody.* Just a few weeks ago we completed the first follow-up phase of our study: What happens when a gluten sensitive person without villous atrophy goes on a gluten-free diet for one or two years?

While I am still gathering and analyzing the data, most of the subjects reported substantial improvement in clinical status (using an objective measure of symptoms and well being). Not everybody gets well because, sadly, not everyone stays on a gluten-free diet—as they sometimes admit on the surveys. Some people have the misconception that if they don't have celiac disease, but "I just have gluten sensitivity" then maybe they do not have to be strict with their gluten elimination diet. I do not think that is the case. Although a gluten free diet is like anything: Less gluten is not as damaging as more gluten, but certainly no gluten is optimal if a gluten sensitive person desires optimal health.

Of the first 25 people with refractory or relapsing microscopic colitis treated with a gluten-free diet, 19 had their diarrhea resolve completely, and another five were notably improved. Thus, a gluten-free diet helped these patients with a chronic immune disease of a tissue other than small bowel (in this case the colon). They have also been shown to be gluten sensitive by a positive stool test in my lab. The same may be true of patients with chronic autoimmune diseases of any other tissue, but who do not have full-blown celiac disease. Gluten-free dietary treatment, sometimes combined with dairy-free diet as well, has been shown to help diabetes, psoriasis, inflammatory bowel disease, eczema, autism, and others.

Thus, my approach, and the one I believe to be most sensitive and complete for screening for early diagnosis and preventive diagnosis for clinically important gluten sensitivity, is a stool test for antigliadin and anti-tissue transglutaminase IgA antibodies (IgG is not detectable in the intestine) and a malabsorption test. The malabsorption test we developed is special, because you no longer have to collect your stool for three days; we can find the same information with just one stool specimen. Stool testing in combination with HLA gene testing, which we do with a cotton-tipped swab rubbed inside the mouth, is the best diagnostic approach available for gluten sensitivity.

Who should be screened for gluten sensitivity? Certainly family members of celiacs or gluten sensitive people are at the highest genetic risk. For the most part, all of the following patient groups have been shown to be at higher risk than normal for gluten sensitivity: Chronic diarrhea; microscopic colitis; dermatitis herpetiformis; diabetes mellitus; any autoimmune syndrome (of which there is an almost end-less number like rheumatoid arthritis, multiple sclerosis, lupus, dermatomyositis, psoriasis, thyroiditis, alopecia areata, hepatitis, etc.); Hepatitis C; asthma; chronic liver disease; osteoporosis; iron deficiency anemia; short stature in children; Down's syndrome; female infertility; peripheral neuropathy, seizures, and other neurologic syndromes; depression and other psychiatric syndromes; irritable bowel syndrome; Crohn's Disease; and people with severe gastroesophageal reflux (GERD).

Autism and possibly the attention deficit disorders are emerging as syndromes that may improve with a gluten- free (and additionally casein-free) diet. A diagnosed celiac might be interested in our testing to know (after some treatment period no shorter than a year) that there is no on-going damage from malabsorption, for which we have a test. If a celiac is having ongoing symptoms or other problems, a follow-up test should be done just to be sure there's no hidden gluten in the diet, or something else that could be present, like pancreatic enzyme deficiency which often accompanies celiac disease, especially in its early stages of treatment.

Historically, with respect to diagnostic methods for celiac disease, from 100 A.D., when celiac disease was first described as an emaciating, incapacitating, intestinal symptom-causing syndrome, to 1950, we had just one diagnostic test: Clinical observation for development of the end stage of the disease. Between 1940 and 1960, when the discovery of gluten as the cause of celiac disease occurred, the best diagnostic test was removing gluten from the diet and watching for clinical improvement. It was during this period that the 72-hour fecal fat and D-xylose absorption tests were developed as measures of gluten-induced intestinal dysfunction/damage.

In the mid- to late 1950's, researchers pioneered various intestinal biopsy methods that showed total villous atrophy as the diagnostic hallmark of celiac disease. You've heard the intestinal biopsy called the "gold standard"? Well, as you can see, it is a 50 year-old test, and thus, the "old" standard. It was not until the 1970's and 80's, with improvements in the 1990's, that blood tests for antigliadin and antiendomysial/anti-tissue transglutaminase were developed But these tests, like all methods before, can reliably reveal only the "heart attack" equivalent of the intestinal celiac syndrome: Significant villous atrophy or bad celiac disease.

We are in a new century, a new millennium, and I have built upon what my research predecessors have started; mostly on the work of researchers who laboriously put down tubes and sucked out intestinal fluid for testing for antigliadin antibody when it was not present in blood. We now know that a stool test for antigliadin antibody is just as good and much simpler. The wide-reaching ramifications of knowing that so many more people and patients are gluten sensitive than has ever been previously known has led me to assume a professional life of medical public service. To do so, I started a 501(c) not-for-profit institute called the Intestinal Health Institute, have brought these new diagnostic tests to the public on the Internet (at http://www.enterolab.com), and volunteer my time helping people with health problems by email and by lecturing. With greater awareness and education of both the public and medical community, more early diagnosis of gluten sensitivity can be achieved before the villi are gone, more of the gluten sensitivity iceberg will be uncovered and treated early, leading to a reduction in gluten-related symptoms and diseases, and saving lives.

Gluten, Lung Function and Zonulin

By Dr. Ron Hoggan, Ed.D.

Melissa Jones pointed out that I missed an important element of the topic when I discussed the discovery of zonulin and the therapeutic promise offered by this discovery. Melissa's complaint was that I should have included a discussion of the connection with lung disease. I agree. After some reflection, I think that there is a good deal more that should be said about this recently discovered protein, including its connection with lung disease. Excessive amounts of zonulin are produced by those who have intestinal diseases and/or autoimmune diseases. These particularly include people with celiac disease and type 1 diabetes. Zonulin is a likely factor in autoimmune thyroiditis, systemic lupus erythematosus, Sjogren's syndrome, scleroderma, and at least sub-groups of multiple sclerosis patients and many patients with rheumatoid arthritis. Zonulin may also be a major factor in the development and maintenance of many learning disorders and psychiatric illnesses. Current research has shown that zonulin weakens protective barriers throughout the body, in the intestines, lungs, blood vessels, skin, and perhaps, the brain. Research has also connected increased zonulin production to gluten consumption, but there may be additional factors that can trigger production and the resulting compromise to the various protective barriers this protein regulates. Lung disease is only one facet of this complex issue.

The range and rate of lung diseases among celiac patients is broad and elevated, so Melissa's concerns are well grounded. Some researchers report a greater frequency of many lung diseases including bird fancier's lung, farmer's lung, Idiopathic pulmonary hemosiderosis, lymphocytic bronchoalveolitis, pulmonary sarcoidosis, cavities in the lung walls, fibrosing alveolitis, and while there is some disagreement in the literature, there may also be higher rates and greater severity of asthma among celiac patients. Nonetheless, it should not be surprising that we experience an increased risk of lung disease since there is considerable similarity between the barrier functions of the mucosa of the lungs and that of the intestines. Thus, the search for a drug that can help us maintain the integrity of this barrier could protect against lung disease and provide important benefits for gluten sensitive individuals who are at greater risk of developing breathing problems along with the host of other ailments that involve compromised protective barrier function.

For instance, investigations of zonulin have the potential to help people with autoimmune diseases. This research may even offer a new, proactive therapy for workers in the baking and milling industries, for severe burn victims who will predictably develop intestinal distress, and for cancer patients who are undergoing radiation treatments. Even patients with skin diseases may be helped. The therapeutic promise of the gluten-free diet for improving various psychiatric diseases, learning disabilities, and behavior problems might also be realized, at long last. The potential therapeutic implications of zonulin research, for a wide range of patients, are startlingly broad.

I attended Blake Patterson's presentation at the 12th International Celiac Disease Symposium on Saturday, November 11, 2006 in New York City. Alba Therapeutics, with Blake Patterson at the helm, was then developing a drug aimed at delivering Larazotide with meals. This substance blocks zonulin action by cloning the receptors which bind to zonulin but do not relax the tight junctions and are subsequently wasted in feces. This would decrease the compromising impact of zonulin by reducing permeability at tight junctions between cells of the protective tissues of the intestine, lungs, blood vessels, and perhaps, the blood barrier. This blockage, if it is achieved, may provide a means of regulating the tight epithelial junctions that create the various protective barriers mentioned earlier. Although he was extremely conservative when discussing the potential benefits of the drug Alba is developing, there can be little doubt that he has considered many more potential applications than I can think to list.

The short-range objective, and the intended market of this drug, is to provide a more rapid and complete disease remission. Although it may ultimately allow a celiac patient to eat a normal diet, this is not the only objective of their development work. I have little personal interest in eating gluten again, but it would be nice not to have to worry about accidental and trace sources of gluten if that is part of what the drug offers. Research has already shown that a gluten-free diet can prevent type I diabetes from developing in two genetically susceptible people. One was at high risk of developing diabetes while the other already had it. This confirms the many animal studies that have shown, among the genetically susceptible, a dose-dependent relationship between gluten ingestion and the development of type 1 diabetes. It is a small leap to infer that if Larazotide restores the barrier function in the intestinal wall of diabetic patients, as a gluten-free diet does, it should also stop the autoimmune attack on islet cells, which make insulin in the pancreas.

The current belief is that when gluten is leaking into the bloodstream and genetically susceptible people mount an immune response against that gluten, the antibodies identify certain sequences of amino acids in the protein structure. These sequences are similar to those found in islet cells, so the antibodies will also attack and destroy these insulin producing cells of the pancreas. By tightening the junctions of the protective barrier in the intestinal wall, thus stopping the leakage of gluten into the bloodstream of genetically susceptible individuals, Larazotide should also stop the autoimmune result of this process frequently referred to as molecular mimicry. Larazotide could be used not only to protect surviving islet cells in the type 1 diabetic who still has some production capacity, it can also aid the long-term survival of transplanted islet cells. These transplants are somewhat limited, in current circumstances, because the transplanted cells are destined to be destroyed by the same autoimmune process that destroyed the individual's original islet cells.

Thus, the therapeutic implications for this drug go far beyond Alba's short term objectives. Many celiac patients, myself included, experience significant lung disease. I am well aware that my history of smoking cigarettes, now fifteen years in the past, contributed to my lung disease. On the other hand, I'm also aware that when I visit rural locations where there is little air pollution, my lung function improves dramatically.

My own lung problem results, in part, from extensive scarring on the walls of my lungs. This scar tissue impedes the normal exchange of oxygen and carbon dioxide across the lung wall, to and from the blood. This component of the problem probably won't get much better. There is also an allergy-driven asthma component to my difficulties. This facet of my lung problems, as shown by my improved lung function when away from urban air pollution, could be helped dramatically by a drug that tightens the barriers in the lining of my lungs and protects me from the absorption of these airborne particles of pollution.

Zonulin and Larazotide research is so new that it is difficult to predict where it might go, or the medicinal purposes it might serve. At the time I am writing this, the FDA has approved Larazotide for testing in other autoimmune disorders. Those of us who have been frustrated by watching the medical community overlook the scope and severity of gluten-induced illness may well be vindicated by this work. I had the privilege of speaking to a support group at the University of Arizona Medical School in Tucson last year. At that time I stated that the discovery of zonulin should lead to the Nobel Prize for Fasano, et al. because of the enormous implications of their discovery. The more important outgrowth of this research is that many millions of sick and/or vulnerable people may benefit enormously from Larazotide If it can successfully and effectively regulate the impact of zonulin in humans, Larazotide will save and enhance the quality of many lives.

So Why Do Celiacs Still Need a Biopsy?

By William Dickey, Ph.D., M.D., F.A.C.G.

For many years, biopsy of the small bowel demonstrating villous atrophy has been fundamental to the diagnosis of celiac disease. Older celiacs will remember, fondly or otherwise, the Crosby suction biopsy device which was swallowed attached to a long tube and made its way down to the small bowel where, position confirmed by x-rays, it guillotined a small portion of tissue. The procedure was tedious and technical failures common—only identified when the device was hauled up after several hours. Later it became clear that biopsies from the duodenum obtained during endoscopy were just as good, and the biopsy process became a five minute job with no need for X-rays. Nevertheless, many celiacs are reluctant to undergo biopsy and its necessity is increasingly questioned, particularly now that blood tests for celiac-related antibodies are highly sensitive and specific. There are a number of reasons why, in my own practice, biopsies continue to be helpful in celiacs diagnosed in adulthood:

1. Biopsies are necessary when blood tests are negative. While endomysial (EmA) and tissue transglutaminase (TTGA) antibodies are detectable in most cases where villous atrophy is present, 5-10% of patients lack these antibodies[1]. In this situation, where the story is suggestive of celiac, perhaps with a family history or strongly suggestive symptoms, biopsy is the only way to make the diagnosis. Increasingly, physicians recognize that many patients with gluten sensitivity do not have villous atrophy (Grade III of the Marsh classification) of "classic" celiac disease, but have milder abnormalities such as crypt hyperplasia (Marsh II) or an excess of the inflammatory cells called lymphocytes (Marsh I). Patients in these categories are less likely to have positive serology[2].

2. Biopsies are necessary where false positive blood tests may occur. TTGA, particularly where levels are low, may be associated with diseases other than celiac: ulcerative colitis, Crohn's disease, arthritis and liver diseases without any evidence of celiac disease have been linked[3]. Newer TTGA tests have steadily improved in

this regard but I still would be reluctant to diagnose celiac on a TTGA test alone. "False positive" EmA is a different issue, which I will return to.

3. Biopsies give a baseline for comparison. Suppose a patient starts a gluten-free diet without biopsy—we don't know whether she or he had Marsh I, II or III or even normal histology. A year later, same patient develops new symptoms of diarrhea, weight loss, whatever. We'll get a duodenal biopsy as part of the workup, but it's going to be difficult to interpret without knowing what things were like before going gluten-free. Specifically, a baseline to look back at tells us whether the small bowel is better, worse or no different, and helps us decide whether we need to focus on celiac disease as the most likely cause of new problems or explore other possibilities involving the rest of the gut. The biggest diagnostic disaster of all, of course, is the gluten-free diet started without any sort of baseline investigation including antibodies, raising the specter of the infamous gluten challenge if a definitive diagnosis is needed.

4. Biopsies provide a "gold standard" assessment of the state of the bowel. There has been much excitement recently about capsule endoscopy, a wireless device the size of a large pill (not to be confused with the Crosby capsule!) which makes its own way down the small bowel taking pictures as it goes. Characteristic abnormalities can be seen in celiac disease, raising the possibility that this device might be useful in diagnosis. If experience with conventional endoscopes is any guide, however, these abnormalities are missing in a sizeable minority of celiacs particularly with mild disease[4] (Capsule endoscopy, in its present state of development, can not take biopsies). Certainly the capsule allows assessment of the bowel beyond the reach of conventional "anaconda-style" endoscopes, but I am not convinced at present that it can replace biopsy.

5. A follow-up biopsy gives an indicator of progress. I offer my patients a repeat biopsy after two years gluten-free and, perhaps surprisingly, most take up the offer and are keen to hear how things have improved. I've increased the biopsy interval from one to two years because only 40% of people had complete recovery after 12 months gluten-free[5]. EmA and TTGA disappearance is only a marker of how successful gluten exclusion has been and is not a reliable indicator of bowel recovery. Does persisting villous atrophy matter if the patient is doing well on a gluten-free diet? Intuitively, one might like to keep a closer eye on the patient with persistently flat biopsies, who could be at greater risk of complications in the future[6].

6. The endoscopy not only allows examination and biopsy of the duodenum but also a look at the esophagus and stomach. Sad fact of the ageing process is that you start to collect diseases like trading cards, and just because you're celiac doesn't mean

you can't have something else. It's important to have a good look for bleeding lesions in the upper gut even if the blood work for a seventy year old with anemia says celiac (and check out the colon too, but that's a topic for another day).

On the other hand, we recognize that biopsies are not always the final arbiter in diagnosis. While the jury is still out on what a TTGA positive, biopsy negative result means with regard to gluten sensitivity, there is plenty of evidence that a positive EmA generally does mean that biopsy abnormalities will follow: My own follow-up of EmA positive, biopsy negative patients indicates that they will develop abnormal histology if not treated[7]. So it makes sense to start EmA positive people on gluten-free without waiting for significant bowel damage—and as already stated, even a normal baseline biopsy will provide a reference for any problems that might arise in the future.

Sometimes I meet a patient with bad gut symptoms but completely normal blood work up and biopsies and when all else fails I will run a trial of gluten-free. It often works, particularly if there is a family history of celiac. But then again, if it doesn't, we have a baseline normal biopsy to say there is no need to persevere.

I guess in the future diagnosis of gluten sensitivity will rely on totting up various factors, none individually essential: blood tests, biopsies, family history, genetic testing for the HLA celiac genes. Some researchers are making a case for dropping the biopsy requirement if the antibody blood work checks out in children[8], for whom (and for the parents) endoscopy and biopsy is a major issue. In adults however it is quick, straightforward and safe and will remain a key part of my celiac workup.

The Gluten Spectrum—Why does this Grain Protein Make So Many People So Sick?

By Prof. Rodney Ford M.B., B.S., M.D., F.R.A.C.P.

Gluten has puzzled me for a long time. Why does this grain-protein, gluten, make so many people so sick? I am a professor in pediatrics. I run the Children's Gastroenterology and Allergy Clinic in New Zealand. For over thirty years I have been investigating and looking after children (and their families) who have reactions to food—in other words those with food allergies and food intolerances. Their symptoms are often due to gluten. I see a lot of families with celiac disease and gluten-sensitivity.

Gluten and Cow's Milk

The puzzle was this. Gluten, that sticky protein that makes wheat-flour so wonderfully chewy is well known to make people sick. But, conventionally, it has been only been implicated as causing celiac disease (that is gut damage of the small bowel caused by gluten). Consequently, the bunch of symptoms that celiac sufferers experience has been directly attributed to this gut damage (and also to the subsequent nutritional deficiencies). However, I think that this explanation is too simplistic.

By contrast, in the area of cow's milk allergy and intolerance, medics recognize that the cow milk proteins can cause a multitude of different problems, such as diarrhea, vomiting, gastric reflux, colitis, constipation, enteropathy, migraine, rashes, eczema, urticaria and poor growth. These complaints are instigated by a number of different immunological mechanisms.

My point is this: if cow's milk can cause a host of different problems, surely gluten can behave in a similar manner.

Gluten—the Culprit

It is my observation that gluten is the culprit for setting off most of the celiac type symptoms. It does not seem plausible that all of the symptoms experienced by celiac sufferers are caused through a nutritional deficiency or from the damaged gut. Clearly, with extensive gut damage, there will be significant malabsorption of foods and nutrients with subsequent diarrhea and poor nutrition. But these are the more extreme cases. My theory is that gluten harms the nerve network that controls a person's gut—this brings about gut malfunction, which in turn sets off many symptoms.

The symptoms reported in association with celiac disease vary widely. Some celiacs, even some with severe gut damage, have few symptoms. While others, even with their gut fully healed (because they have been on a gluten-free diet), experience extreme symptoms from exposure to small traces of gluten. Surely, this can only be explained by people having different degrees of sensitivity to gluten, rather than by the extent of their gut damage.

Medical evidence is accumulating that confirms this picture. To illustrate this, I would like to tell you about the last ten of my gluten patients who I saw this week. Their names, ages and problems are listed below (see **Table 1**).

Table 1:

Name	Age (years)	Symptoms	Diagnosis
Jemma	1	Eczema	Gluten-sensitive
Emily	2	Eczema, diarrhea	Gluten-sensitive
Hamish	2	Gastric reflux	Gluten-sensitive
Emma	3	Vomiting	Celiac
Lilly	5	Abdo pain, diarrhea	Celiac
Rose-Anne	5	Abdo pain, slow growth	Celiac
Connor	6	Eczema, tricky behavior	Gluten-sensitive
Jack	7	Abdo pain, Gastric reflux	Gluten-sensitive
Edward	10	Abdo pain, Gastric reflux	Gluten-sensitive
David	16	Abdo pain	Gluten-sensitive

All of these ten children have had a small-bowel biopsy by endoscopy: only three showed the typical celiac gut damage. All ten children had high IgG-gliadin antibody levels. All ten children recovered on a gluten-free diet. In this group, they were all very sensitive to gluten: that is they all get their symptoms back again when they eat even tiny amounts of gluten.

The things we can learn from these children are:

- Only three have celiac disease. Most, the other seven, can be called "non-celiac gluten-sensitive".
- Gastric reflux is a common symptom of gluten-sensitivity.
- Eczema can be driven by gluten.
- Gluten causes a wide spectrum of symptoms, including celiac disease.
- We need to actively look and test for gluten sensitivity to ever make the diagnosis.
- They were diagnosed by finding a high gluten antibody level in their blood (elevated IgG-gliadin).
- They improved within weeks of going gluten free.
- They found going on the gluten-free diet is quite easy with a little bit of help.
- The children with eczema and reflux can usually come off their medications once they are established on their gluten-free diet.

Gluten—the Diagnosis

I have now diagnosed many hundreds of children and adults with celiac disease and thousands of people with gluten-sensitivity. After seeing all of these patients, I now realize that I cannot clinically distinguish between those with celiac disease and those without. Therefore, I test everyone! My mantra is "Test—don't guess". I test both for celiac disease and gluten-sensitivity.

Celiac Disease versus Gluten-sensitivity

Celiac disease: The story of celiac disease began over a hundred years ago with Samuel Gee describing the "Coeliac Affliction". Fifty years later, in 1950, Dr W Dicke first reported gluten toxicity. Gluten was subsequently linked to the gut damage a few years later. With the clinical picture now described, a small bowel biopsy became, within a few years, a mandatory test for the diagnosis of celiac disease. Nowadays, celiac disease is still considered to be a gut disease which is confirmed by finding the classic microscopic tissue damage called "villous atrophy". Over the last eight years the 'gut damage blood test' called tTG (tissue TransGlutaminase) has helped make celiac much easier to detect. About one in a hundred people have celiac disease. But doctors seem to still be looking for the classic celiac: sick people with bloated tummies and diarrhea. However, most people who are getting sick from gluten have subtle symptoms.

Gluten-sensitivity: The recognition of adverse reactions to grains also has a long history. However, blood tests for gluten antibodies have been only available over the last fifteen years. This has radically changed our understanding of gluten-sensitivity. Population tests have shown that at least ten percent of the population has elevated levels of gluten antibodies. (That is the IgG-gliadin antibodies, also called Anti-Gliadin Antibodies.) "Non-celiac gluten-sensitivity" is now the term used to describe these people who have the clinical manifestations of celiac disease but who have a normal endoscopy and who recover on a gluten-free diet. Studies are finding that at least one in ten people are gluten-sensitive.

Glutened for 30 Years

Sylvia is 60 years old. I saw her last week and she told me: "I never realized how bad I was until now that I feel so good! Yes! Now I actually realize how bad I was!"

Next, Sylvia said a sad thing: "I didn't know that I could get a test! I have been having trouble with my gut for about 30 years and have been suspicious about wheat but I didn't know I could be tested. I get symptoms of tummy bloating, headaches, abdominal pains, extreme tiredness, and sometimes I just feel dreadful. People think that I am a hypochondriac or something because I am so often unwell."

"It is such a relief at last to be recognized as having gluten sensitivity. I have been off gluten for the last six weeks. I am feeling great for the first time ever! It's wonderful!"

What a story! After 30 years of being unwell, Sylvia has discovered that gluten was the cause of it all. She has non-celiac gluten sensitivity. The tTG is normal but she has high gluten antibodies.

How do you know if you are being Damaged by Gluten?

Simply, if you or your child have any ongoing symptoms, then you should arrange to get your blood tests. Why? Because both celiac disease and gluten-sensitivity exhibit a very wide range of symptoms. You can't tell if you don't test. Check my website for my recommendations for blood tests.

How Early Can Celiac Disease Be Diagnosed?

By Prof. Rodney Ford M.B., B.S., M.D., F.R.A.C.P.

This question, "how early can you diagnose celiac disease?" is a major concern for both parents and pediatricians. This is because, like many diseases, celiac disease comes on slowly. This means that it can take a long time to make the diagnosis.

Celiac disease can develop slowly

Yes, celiac disease can develop very slowly. The symptoms can be subtle. It is a progressive disease. When you are first born, you cannot have celiac disease as you have never been exposed to gluten. However, if you have the right genetic make up, that is, if you have the celiac gene and foster the right environmental circumstances, such as eating gluten and getting gut inflammation, then celiac disease can develop.

Finding tissue damage

Celiac disease is a condition that is recognized when you get damage to your small bowel tissue. This damage is triggered by gluten.

The standard way to detect this tissue damage is by taking a gut biopsy of the small bowel skin also called the mucosa. This is done by the technique of upper endoscopy whilst under an anesthetic. Tiny fragments of gut tissue are snipped off with a pair of forceps. This tissue is then sent to a pathology lab. The lab people, called histologists, look down their microscopes at this tissue sample. They are looking for the gut damage called villous atrophy, which is characteristic of disease.

Early antibody changes – IgG-gliadin

Importantly, long before the tissue becomes obviously damaged by gluten, your body can begin to react to the gluten in your diet.

An early sign of a gluten immune reaction is that your body produces antibodies to the gluten in your diet. This can be seen in a blood test that looks for an antibody called the **IgG-gliadin antibody** (also known as anti-gliadin-antibody). Also the IgA-gliadin antibody can develop at this time.

Even in these early stages of gluten reactions (before the development of any gut damage of celiac disease), you or your child can be feeling unwell. Many of the symptoms of celiac disease can be recognized in these early stages. This is *before* the tissue damage can be seen by the histologist.

The blood test to look for tissue damage is called the **tissue transglutaminase antibody** (abbreviated as tTG).

Early bowel damage cannot be seen

The next thing to happen is that the tissue in the small bowel gets slightly injured but not enough to be identified by the histologist. However, such damage can be shown by an electron microscope. This early damage can also be detected by the presence of the tTG antibody.

Usually, when the tTG blood test goes up, this is an indication to do the endoscopy and look for any tissue damage. However, early in the progression of celiac disease, this damage may not show up by conventional methods. This means that the small bowel biopsy and the histology results are good for confirming celiac disease, but they cannot rule it out.

To act or to wait?

In my experience, I have seen a number of children develop celiac disease whilst I have watched and waited. While we doctors wait and see if the gut will become progressively damaged, these children will continue to experience their gut symptoms and they may not be growing so well. We doctors are waiting to make a certain diagnosis of celiac disease. We want to repeat their blood tests and do another endoscopy.

Is this reasonable? Experience has changed my mind. I have come to the conclusion that this is not an appropriate way to deal with these children. Currently, most medical specialists are adamant. They will not make a diagnosis of celiac disease until the histologist can confirm the typical tissue damage.

How long can you wait?

I have given up the "wait and see" approach. I act. I carefully scrutinize the symptoms and the blood test results - the gluten antibodies (IgG-gliadin) and tissue damage antibody (tTG) levels. I may organize an endoscopy test. If these findings suggest the development of celiac disease, then I make a pre-emptive diagnosis of "early celiac disease", often *before* the gut gets badly damaged. I give these children a trial of a gluten-free diet – I see what their clinical response is. Pleasingly, most get completely better! If they get better, then they want to stay gluten-free.

The problem is that the diagnosis of celiac disease currently hinges on the abnormal appearance of the small bowel. This damage can take years to develop.

The main argument against my approach is that if you do not have a "definite" diagnosis of celiac disease, then you cannot advise a gluten-free diet for life. In my opinion, the decision to go on a gluten-free diet is not a black and white choice. For children, I give them the option of a gluten-free diet early in their disease. Let them feel well. Let them grow properly. Later, as an adult, they can challenge their diagnosis and have a formal gluten challenge when they understand the issues.

Conclusion – my approach

As you can see, it is difficult to say how early you can diagnose celiac disease. It is my practice to carefully assess children regarding their symptoms, their antibody levels, their genetic status and their endoscopy results (if appropriate).

I do not think it is logical to leave children with significant symptoms waiting for the small bowel damage to eventually occur. Indeed, I think that these long delays in treatment are inhumane. Postponing a gluten-free diet will cause these children to suffer ongoing symptoms. Worse, they can have growth failure, from which they may not recover.

My approach is to put these children on a gluten-free diet *early*. I watch and see if they have a clinical response—if they get better. The evidence shows that you cannot rely entirely on the small bowel biopsy for your diagnosis of celiac disease. These children can have a gluten challenge later in their lives.

The onset of celiac disease is progressive. Why wait until the bitter end before going gluten-free? The onset of celiac disease is progressive. Why wait until the bitter end before going gluten-free? You can find out a lot more from my webpage: www.doctor-gluten.com

Endoscopy in Celiac Disease

By Dr. Scot Lewey

When undergoing an evaluation for possible Celiac disease or gluten sensitive enteropathy doctors usually recommend an upper endoscopy with small intestinal biopsy. What that is and why it is recommended may not be clear to many people who are facing the decision of whether to undergo the procedure themselves or whether to subject their child to this exam.

What is it and how is it done?

During upper endoscopy a thin flexible tube, about the diameter of a fat pencil, is passed in the mouth down the upper gastrointestinal tract. This tube has a video chip on its tip. From the mouth it is advanced down the esophagus, or inside a feeding tube, into the stomach. It is then advanced into the first part of the small intestine known as the duodenum. Thus, upper endoscopy is also known as esophagogastroduodenoscopy or EGD for short. The scope has internal channels for flushing water, suctioning secretions and passing instruments that can obtain pinch biopsy samples of tissue for microscopic examination. The scope dials control internal cables that allow the tube to be turned up/down and right/left at the tip.

Do you feel it or remember it?

Typically, people undergoing the exam in the U.S. are sedated with medication. These medications are similar to Valium. They have a good amnesia and relaxing effect and are called *midazolam* or versed and are usually combined with a narcotic pain medication like *meperidine (Demerol)* or *Fentanyl*. The result is a sort of drowsy twilight amnesia. Lately, a very short-acting intravenous sedative, called *propofol (diprovan)* is increasingly being used for deeper sedation or general anesthesia. Occasionally, usually in very young children or people with severe lung problems, general anesthesia is required. The exam is usually not felt or remembered because of the medications.

What is examined and how well the lining is seen?

Celiac disease affects the upper portion of the small intestine, in the two sections known as the duodenum and jejunum. The examination of the small intestine is usually limited to the first section, termed the duodenum, though occasionally the second section known as the jejunum may be reached especially when a longer endoscope is used. The video images are very high resolution with the latest endoscopes and may have a magnification and color contrast mode to detect very subtle signs of damage of the small intestine.

What are the typical endoscopy findings?

The characteristic appearance of the surface of the small intestine in celiac disease includes superficial ulcerations that are commonly linear, flattening of the folds, notching or scalloping of the folds and a mosaic-like pattern. However, the surface may appear normal and only under microscopic examination of samples will the lining show signs of gluten-induced injury.

What are intestinal biopsies? What are their limitations? What can be missed?

Samples of small intestine are obtained with biopsy forceps that consist of tiny jaws with cups that permit pinching off samples of the intestinal lining. This is painless and very safe. The samples are placed in a preservative solution and sent to a pathology lab. The tissue is then processed, embedded in paraffin wax, cut into thin slices and mounted on a microscope slide. The slides are stained before being examined under the microscope by a pathologist. Small intestine injury from gluten may be patchy. Therefore, several samples are recommended. A minimum of 4 pieces and preferably 8 to 12 samples should be obtained to avoid missing microscopic signs of Celiac disease.

What does the pathologist look for on the slides to determine if there is Celiac disease or gluten injury?

The pathologist examines the slide for evidence of damage or injury characteristic of gluten sensitivity. Occasionally special stains are required to see signs of irritation known as inflammation. Inflammation in the gut is characterized by an increased number of a type of white blood cells. For Celiac disease the characteristic white blood cell involved in gluten-induced intestinal injury are called lymphocytes. In early celiac and gluten sensitivity without celiac disease, the biopsy may be normal and the diagnosis may not be established by intestinal biopsy without special stains or, in the research setting, by electron microscopy.

Summary

The procedure of endoscopy is safe, painless, and very helpful for confirming the diagnosis of celiac disease while excluding other upper intestinal disorders. However, the main drawback of endoscopy is that nearly everyone must have sedation to tolerate the exam and it can be expensive if not fully covered by the patient's insurance. Furthermore the biopsies may not confirm the diagnosis. If the biopsy is normal, misread as normal, or is borderline, the diagnosis of celiac disease is neither confirmed nor excluded.

Sometimes, celiac disease is diagnosed by endoscopic biopsy in people who either have normal blood tests or as an incidental finding in those undergoing endoscopy for other reasons. When the biopsy is abnormally classic for Celiac disease and the blood tests are negative but the patient responds to a gluten-free diet, the term seronegative (blood test negative) celiac disease is often used. Fear or confusion about endoscopy should not prevent anyone who is suspected of having celiac or gluten sensitivity from undergoing endoscopy.

Editor's comment:

There are many conditions and symptoms that are suggestive of celiac disease. Iron deficiency and short stature are two of the more common ones. Not everyone with iron deficiency or short stature has celiac disease. Similarly, everyone with celiac disease does not have iron deficiency or short stature. Nonetheless, there is enough overlap in these conditions to warrant testing for celiac disease in the context of either of these conditions. The following article explores short stature as it relates to celiac disease.

Screening Children of Short Stature for Celiac Disease

By Kathleen LaPoint

Celiac disease is under-diagnosed because many celiac disease patients do not show classic gastrointestinal symptoms. Highly sensitive and specific serological tests have led to the diagnosis of celiac disease in patients for whom short stature may be the only obvious symptom. Researchers from Brazil and Italy have previously reported that celiac disease accounts for 1-5% of short stature in children.

Prevalence of celiac disease varies widely according to geographic location. Although epidemiological studies are lacking in India, celiac disease reporting has increased exponentially due to targeted screening and better serological tests. To better understand the relationship between short stature and celiac disease, researchers from the Endocrine Clinic of the Postgraduate Institute of Medical Education and Research in Chandigarh studied children referred for a work-up of short stature from January 2005 to December 2006.

Researchers enrolled 176 patients, half male and half female, who fit the criteria for short stature: height $\geq$ 2.5 standard deviations below the mean for chronological age, growth rate below the fifth percentile for chronological age, and height $\geq$ 2 standard deviations below mean for chronological age when corrected for mid-parental height. Most patients were 10-15 years old (mean age of 14.5).

Researchers took detailed histories and carried out clinical evaluations and screening tests. If they could find no endocrine cause for short stature or if diarrhea had been present for more than 3 months, researchers estimated IgA anti-tissue transglutaminase antibodies (anti-tTG) and performed an endoscopic biopsy.

Celiac disease was found in 27 (15.3%) of the patients, making it the single most common cause of short stature. 25 children had pituitary disorder (14%), 24 had hypothyroidism (14%) and constitutional delay of growth and puberty or familial short stature accounted for 18 (11%). Other less common causes of short stature were metabolic bone disease, Turner syndrome, adrenal disorders, diabetes mellitus, and nutritional deficiency. All celiac disease patients were positive for tTG antibodies and had a duo-denal biopsy suggestive of celiac disease. All celiac disease patients were symptomatic; the most common symptoms after growth retardation were anemia (88%), weight loss (80%), diarrhea (69%), and delayed puberty (54%).

The average time to diagnosis for these patients was 5.5 years (95% cI: = 2.5 to 8.5 years). The celiac disease patients were treated with a gluten-free diet, calcium (500 mg/day), vitamin D (300,000 U cholecalciferol once every 3 months), and iron and multivitamin supplementation including folic acid and vitamin B12. During the 6-9 month follow-up period, growth rate velocity increased significantly from 2.9 cm/year (95% cI = 2.41 to 3.39 cm/year) to 8.9 cm/year (95% cI = 6.7 to 11.1 cm/year).

Celiac disease can lead to short stature by causing autoimmune hypothydroidism, resistance to growth hormones, and malabsorption of protein, calcium and vitamin D. Additionally, celiac disease can lead to hypogonadism which inhibits the pubertal growth spurt. Researchers recommend that all short children be screened for celiac disease.

Editor's note:

A new test for celiac disease is on the horizon. The company that is currently selling these tests in Canada and negotiating with the U.S. government to do the same in the United States has provided the following information:

Home Celiac Test Kit

By Vanessa Maltin

The Biocard Celiac Test Kit is an at-home test that measures (anti-tTG) IgA antibodies from a fingertip blood sample. It works by taking a small blood sample from pricking your finger, mixing the blood with a buffer and applying the mixture onto a test card. The test can be administered from the comfort of your own home and you'll get results in just 10 minutes. The Biocard Celiac Test is positive if you have two red lines on the test card. One red line appears in the control field, which indicates that you have done the test correctly. The second red line will only appear if you are having an immune system response to the gluten protein. If the test comes out positive for celiac disease, the makers of the test recommend consulting with a doctor to confirm the diagnosis with an intestinal biopsy.

According to the marketers of the test kit at 2G Pharma Inc., the test is as accurate as a tissue transglutaminase (tTG) laboratory test that your doctor would request. Additionally, a study published in the British Medical Journal found that the simple rapid antibody test allowed nurses working in primary care medical offices to detect celiac disease in patients who were not picked up during routine clinical care. The study evaluated 2,690 children around six years old and 120 nurses. The study found 31 newly diagnosed celiac patients. The rapid test accurately detected celiac disease in 30 of the 31 patients. The Biocard Celiac Test is approved by Health Canada and is under-going review by the US FDA with an anticipated approval in 2010.

The Biocard Celiac Test is a landmark development for the entire celiac community. It is the first time that patients will have immediate access to find out if they have the autoimmune disorder. It makes celiac disease as easy to diagnose as strep throat! It will also allow for simple screening, especially amongst family members of those already diagnosed and high risk groups such as those with unexplained infertility, unexplained iron deficiency anemia or Type I Diabetes.

This company may be contacted at: www.celiachometest.com

CHAPTER 5:
IMPORTANT FACETS OF CELIAC DISEASE AND GLUTEN SENSITIVITY

Gluten's Connection with Infertility, Problem Pregnancy, and Miscarriage

By Dr. Ron Hoggan, Ed. D.

A friend traveling in Columbia recently contacted me to ask if celiac disease is associated with hypogonadism (small testicles) or male infertility. It seems that she and her husband had become friends with a couple who could not have children. They had identified the husband as the cause of their infertility and believed that it was due to his condition of hypogonadism. My friend wrote to ask if this could be associated with celiac disease.

While I was aware that male infertility can be associated with gluten sensitivity, I was not aware that stunted testicles were also found in the context of celiac disease. After a brief sojourn through the medical literature I quickly discovered that this is, indeed the case.

I wrote back to my friend to affirm the connection and provide the citations from PubMed so they could explore the literature themselves. I also pointed out something that is well known in the celiac community; that female infertility has long been recognized as a problem associated with celiac disease. In many cases, pregnancy quickly follows institution of a gluten free diet.

Similarly, miscarriage is about seven times more common in the context of untreated celiac disease while celiac disease is about ten times more common among women who have experienced spontaneous abortion. It seems that researchers have found that untreated celiac disease can impact the entire cycle of female fertility, from delaying puberty, to causing irregular periods or cessation of periods for one or more cycles, to causing early menopause. Premature births and having babies with below normal birth weights are also twice as common among mothers with celiac disease who are eating gluten.

Most of these problems with fertility and pregnancy diminish to normal or near normal levels after following a strict gluten-free diet for a period of six months or more. Thus, the good fortune that Danna Korn discusses in the next article may be of particular relevance to those struggling with infertility.

Diagnosed with Celiac Disease? How Lucky You Are!

By Danna Korn

At first, a diagnosis of celiac disease can be daunting, to say the least, and for some people, even devastating. It means giving up some of your favorite foods—pastas, breads, pizzas, cakes, cookies, and pretzels—at least as you used to know them. So why should you consider yourself lucky if you've been diagnosed with celiac disease? Because you've been given the *key* to better health.

Okay, so I've never been good at saving the punch line for the end. It's true though, you DO have the key to better health: A gluten-free diet.

Still not feeling like you just won the lottery? Well, consider this: Celiac disease is the most common genetic disease of humankind—yet for every person diagnosed with celiac disease, 140 go undiagnosed. *They* may still suffer from gastrointestinal distress, headaches, depression, joint pain, or other symptoms. Many are told they have "irritable bowel syndrome," fibromyalgia, or chronic fatigue syndrome—and that there's nothing that can be done for them. "Go forth and live your life in misery," is, in essence, their lifetime sentence. You, however, know that simply a dietary modification (no, I didn't say a "simple dietary modification," and you're probably acutely aware of the difference) is the key to better health.

The gluten-free diet is a medical necessity for our family, but it is also a *healthy* way of life. Sometimes I used to think, "If only I could not have to worry about making tonight's meal gluten-free, I'd make…" What? What *would* I make?!? Would I make macaroni and cheese from a box? Ick! Would I make spaghetti? So what! The gluten-free stuff is just as good these days. Would I make a quick trip to Kentucky Fried Chicken or a pizza place? Oh, now *there's* a healthy meal (well okay, every now and then maybe!).

People often tell me they find the cost of the gluten-free diet to be prohibitive. True, the cost of a loaf of gluten-free bread could buy you an entire meal in some restaurants…but think of this: What if your condition required prescription medication? The cost of even some of the cheapest medications could buy (at least) a loaf of gluten-free bread each day.

We are fortunate to live in a time when celiac awareness is at an all-time high. Gluten-free foods are delicious and readily available (even the "PollyDanna" in me couldn't have said that with so much conviction 13 years ago when we first began this lifestyle!). These days, customer service reps on the other end of the toll-free lines at food companies actually know what we're talking about when we ask if their products are gluten-free. Excellent cookbooks and resource books abound, as do support groups and seminars.

Yes, if you've been diagnosed with celiac disease, you can consider yourself lucky for a number of reasons. If you've read my books or heard me speak, you know my mantra, so sing it with me now: "Deal with it…don't dwell on it!" Before long, you too will realize how very lucky you are.

Editor's note:

For more than two decades, Dr. Martin Kagnoff has been suggesting that certain viral infections may contribute to our susceptibility to celiac disease.

Magnesium Helps Rebuild Bones in Celiac Disease

By Dr. Ron Hoggan, Ed. D.

Five years ago I became concerned about weakness in my bones after a couple of surprising fractures. At one point, I broke a rib while shingling a storage-shed roof. I leaned across the peak of the roof's ridge to pick up a shingle. I never expected such light pressure to cause a problem. However, I felt a sudden, sharp pain, and heard an odd sound. This, along with a couple of less dramatic, but similar injuries, caused me enough concern to begin looking into the question of celiac disease and bone strength.

My explorations taught me that calcium absorption probably is not our main problem. People with celiac disease seem to be able to absorb adequate calcium[1], but the primary problem appears to come from excreting too much of it, thus causing us to lose more calcium than we are absorbing. I also learned that research shows little or no benefit from calcium supplementation for celiac patients, while magnesium supplementation alone results in significant improvements[2]. The explanation for this may be that some of the antibodies caused by active celiac disease attack the parathyroid gland[3]. This organ is an important player in regulating calcium metabolism. Magnesium is necessary for the body to repair the parathyroid and to maintain its continued good function.

Being convinced by this research, I began to take magnesium supplements without any calcium. I found that I had to be careful. Too much had me visiting the washroom frequently, and I was afraid that too little would fail to provide me the benefits I was seeking.

At the same time, I also requested a bone density test. I wanted objective information that would allow me to evaluate the progress I hoped to make. The first test was conducted in March of 1997. The results (called "T scores") are reported based on comparison with the density of bones found in young adults. For instance, a score of 0 indicates that the bone density is about the same as would be found in an average young adult. A score in the minus range indicates a bone that has less mineral and more pores than is found in the same young adult. Thus, a score of –1.0 to –2.5 indicates mild to moderate mineral losses, while a score of –2.5 or lower indicates osteoporosis.

My test results were not as bad as I had feared. The mineral density in my lower back was normal for my age, at –0.23. However, my upper leg, where it fits into my hip, was reported as –2.02, and my forearm was slightly stronger than that of a normal young adult at +0.19.

As I saw it, there were only two causes for concern. First, at the tender age of 50, my hips were very close to osteoporotic, and certainly at a substantially increased risk of fracture. Such fractures can be very serious. Secondly, since only three skeletal areas had been tested for mineral density—and since there was such a wide range of density variation reported for each of these areas, it seemed impossible to estimate the density of the rest of the bones in my body.

About three years after my first bone density test, some Calgary-based research made me suspect that the amount of vitamin D supplements I was taking might be too low[4]. I increased my intake to 1,000 IU daily.

By the fall of 2001, I began to wonder if I was being foolish by avoiding calcium supplements based on the reports I had read. I therefore began to supplement 350 mg of calcium each day.

In July of 2002, I underwent a second bone scan. They did not test my forearm this time, but the other two areas appear to have improved substantially. The T score for my lower back was now at + 0.06, and the T score for my hip had improved to –0.72.

I realize that what I am reporting is just one person's experience. It is what the medical professionals call "anecdotal," and does not usually carry much weight. However, my experience does support the only published research of the impact of mineral supplements on bone density in celiac patients that I can find. Based on my own experience, and the relevant research, I am now convinced that magnesium is the most important supplement to consider in the context of celiac disease. I was thrilled to read my latest bone density report. Vitamin D may also be an important factor, but limitations of time and space force me to leave this topic for another day.

Editor's note:

In the next article calcium, vitamin D, and exercise are asserted to be the answer for those with celiac disease. I'm hoping that readers will err on the side of caution and follow both sets of recommendations. Magnesium, calcium, vitamin D, and exercise are all healthful. One of the great things about these two minerals is that if we get too much of either, our bodies won't even absorb them through the intestinal wall.

Bone Up on Calcium and Vitamin D

By Shelley Case, B.Sc.

Getting enough calcium in the diet is essential for people of all ages, as this mineral performs many important functions in the body. In addition to bone health, calcium is required for muscle contractions, nerve impulses, normal blood clotting and regulating blood pressure. It may also offer protection from colon cancer.

Children and adults with celiac disease need to pay particular attention to calcium and other nutrients as many already have or will develop early bone disease such as osteopenia or osteoporosis. Osteopenia is low bone mineral density and osteoporosis is characterized by a significant decrease in bone mass resulting in brittle, easily broken bones. The hip, spine and wrist are most susceptible to fracture. Early diagnosis and treatment of celiac disease is critical for the prevention of bone disease. To maintain good bone health it is important that all people with celiac disease have routine bone density tests done to assess their overall bone health, and to follow the tips outlined below.

- **Follow a strict gluten-free diet.** Healthy villi will result in normal absorption of nutrients.
- **Meet your daily calcium requirements.** See Table 1 for the Dietary Reference Intake (DRI) for calcium.

Table 1: Dietary Reference Intake for Calcium	
Age	**Calcium (mg/day)**
Infants 0- 6 months 7-12 months	 210 270
Children 1-3 years 4-8 years	 500 800
Females and Males 9-13 14-18 19-30 31-50 51-70 71 +	 1300 1300 1000 1000 1200 1200

Choose calcium-rich foods. See Table 2 for a list of gluten-free foods. Remember that not all calcium sources are created equal. Milk (fluid, powdered or evaporated) and milk products such as cheese and yogurt contain the most readily available source of calcium. Other foods such as salmon, and sardines with the bones, calcium-fortified beverages (soy, rice and orange juice), tofu made with calcium sulfate and vegetables (broccoli, collards, kale, mustard greens, turnip greens and bok choy) also contain calcium that is easily absorbed by the body. However, the calcium found in almonds, sesame seeds, dried beans and spinach are absorbed less efficiently because these foods contain calcium-binding substances called oxalates. Although the calcium content of these foods should not be counted as part of your daily calcium intake; they do provide many other nutrients important for good health.

- **Consider calcium supplements.** If you are unable to consume enough dietary calcium you may need a gluten-free calcium supplement. Look for the amount of "elemental calcium" on the label. Your body can only absorb 500 mg at one time therefore it is best to divide your dose throughout the day. Calcium carbonate is more slowly absorbed and should be consumed with meals. Calcium citrate is well absorbed with meals or an empty stomach. Bone meal or dolomite calcium supplements are not recommended as some products have been found to contain lead and mercury.
- **Limit caffeine intake.** Studies have shown that caffeine increases calcium loss through the urine. Most experts agree that 2-3 cups of coffee/day is probably not harmful provided that calcium intake is adequate, so limit your coffee and cola intake.
- **Limit sodium intake.** Sodium also has been shown to increase the loss of calcium through the urine. Therefore it is advisable to limit your intake of processed foods, table salt and salt in cooking.
- **Get enough Vitamin D.** Vitamin D helps the body use the calcium in food. It can increase calcium absorption by as much as 30-80 %. See Table 3 for the Dietary Reference Intake for vitamin D. The easiest way to get vitamin D is from exposure to sunlight, which causes the body to make its own vitamin D. All you need is 15 minutes per day; however, aging significantly decreases 1) the ability of the skin to produce vitamin D and 2) kidney function that is involved in converting the inactive to active form of vitamin D. Also, sunscreen blocks the production of vitamin D in the skin. Another concern is that between the months of October and March in Canada and the northern USA, vitamin D synthesis in the skin is very limited. To make up for the lack of sunlight look for other sources of vitamin D listed in Table 4, and remember the points below.

Table 2 Calcium Content of Gluten-Free Dairy Foods		
Food	Serving	Calcium (mg)
Buttermilk	1 cup (250 ml)	303
Cheddar cheese	2 oz. (50 g)	350
Cottage cheese, creamed	½ cup (125 ml)	76
Feta cheese	2 oz (50 g)	255
Ice cream	½ cup (125 ml)	90
Milk (whole, 2%, 1%, skim)	1 cup (250 ml)	315
Milk (chocolate)	1 cup (250 ml)	301
Milk, powder, dry	3 Tbsp. (45 ml)	308
Mozzarella cheese	2 oz (50 g)	287
Parmesan cheese, grated	3 Tbsp. (45 ml)	261
Processed cheese slices	2 regular (62 g)	384
Swiss cheese	2 oz (50 g)	480
Yogurt, fruit-flavored	¾ cup (175 g)	240
Yogurt, plain	¾ cup (175 g)	296
Almonds	½ cup (125 ml)	200*
Baked beans	1 cup (250 ml)	163*
Bok choy, cooked	½ cup (125 ml)	84
Broccoli, cooked	½ cup (125 ml)	38
Collards, cooked	½ cup (125 ml)	81
Orange juice, calcium fortified	1 cup (250 ml)	300-350
Salmon, sockeye, canned with bones	Half a 7.5 oz (213 g) can	243
Sardines, canned with bones	6 medium (72 g)	275
Sesame seeds	½ cup (125 ml)	89*
Soybeans, cooked	½ cup(125 ml)	93
Soy beverage, fortified	1 cup (250 ml)	312
Tofu, regular, processed with calcium sulfate**	1/3 cup (100 g)	150

* The calcium from these sources is absorbed less efficiently by the body.

** The calcium content of tofu is an approximation based on products available on the market. Calcium content can vary greatly from one brand to another and can be low. Tofu processed with magnesium chloride also contains less calcium.

-Milk is fortified with vitamin D but most other dairy products such as cheese, yogurt and ice cream are not fortified. Recently some companies have been adding vitamin D to other dairy products so be sure to read the ingredient label and nutrition panel.

-Fatty fish (sardines, salmon and herring) and cod liver oil and halibut liver oil are high in vitamin D.

-Many soy and rice beverages are fortified with vitamin D. Check the ingredient list carefully as some products may contain barley malt extract/flavoring and must be avoided.

-Nut beverages (e.g. Blue Diamond Almond Breeze) and potato beverages (e.g. Vances DariFree) are fortified with vitamin D.

-Multivitamin supplements usually contain 200-400 IU of vitamin D.

-Some calcium supplements may contain vitamin D. Amounts vary so check the label.

Table 3: Dietary Reference Intake for Vitamin D	
Age	**Vitamin D (IU)**
Birth – 50 years	200
51- 70 years	400
Over 70 years	600

- **Don't just sit there...get moving!** Regular weight bearing exercises such as walking, stair climbing, dancing, and tennis and muscle-strengthening exercises can reduce the risks of falls and fractures. Consult your doctor before beginning a vigorous exercise program. So remember the ABC's: All Bones need Calcium, vitamin D and Exercise!

Table 4: Sources of Vitamin D		
Food	Serving Size	Vitamin D (IU)
Cod liver oil	1 tsp. (5 ml)	450
Cod liver oil capsule	1 capsule	100
Halibut liver oil capsule	1 capsule	400
Sardines, canned	3.5 oz (100 g.)	300
Salmon, canned, with bones	3.5 oz (100 g.)	500
Egg	1 medium	25
Milk	1 cup (250 ml)	90
Soy Beverage (fortified)	1 cup (250 ml)	90

Editor's note:

Many people with celiac disease seem to react to milk proteins, in addition to gluten. Thus, reliance on dairy products as a source for calcium may not be a good idea for some gluten sensitive individuals. Lactose intolerance is another digestive problem that should suggest caution with respect to consuming dairy products. More than two-thirds of the world's adult population is lactose intolerant, so lactose tolerance may more legitimately be seen as an abnormal condition.

Lactose Intolerance

By Shelley Case, B.Sc.

Milk and milk products contain a natural sugar called lactose (see table below). People who are lactose intolerant or, more precisely, who are lactose maldigesters, lack enough of the enzyme lactase needed to completely digest the lactose into its simple sugars, glucose and galactose. Lactase is produced in the villi of the small intestine. Symptoms of lactose intolerance may include some or all of the following: cramping, bloating, nausea, headache and diarrhea. Symptoms can occur 15-30 minutes after digestion of lactose or as long as several hours later.

Lactose intolerance and celiac disease

Many people with celiac disease, especially those who are newly diagnosed, may also develop secondary lactose intolerance. This is a temporary condition in which the level of lactase has fallen as a result of injury to the gastrointestinal tract. Once on a gluten-free diet, the villi begin to heal and the level of lactase increases back to normal levels. This process may take several weeks to months. For some, a temporary lactose-free diet may also be necessary, in addition to a life-long gluten-free diet, to control symptoms. There are a variety of products specially developed to help in the management of lactose intolerance:

- **Lactose-Reduced Milk and Ice Cream.** The lactase enzyme has been added to regular milk and 99% of the naturally occurring lactose has been converted to simple, easily digested sugars. This milk tastes slightly sweeter than regular milk, but has the same nutritional value. Ice cream made with lactose-reduced milk is also available.
- **Lactase Enzyme Drops.** These contain the lactase enzyme that can be added to liquid dairy products making them more easily digestible. Approximately 70-99% of the lactose is broken down based on the number of drops used.
- **Lactase Enzyme Tablet and Caplets.** They are available in regular strength, extra-strength and ultra-strength and should be taken just before a meal or snack that contains lactose.
- **Non-Dairy Beverages.** There is a variety of soy, rice, nut or potato-based beverages that can be substituted for regular milk. Be aware that some products may contain barley malt extract/flavoring so read labels carefully. Choose gluten-free beverages that are enriched with calcium and vitamin D.

Diabetes Mellitus: More than a complication of celiac disease

By Dr. Ron Hoggan, Ed. D.

First reported in 1925, the coexistence of diabetes mellitus and celiac disease is not a new phenomenon. However, as late as 1984, the connection was still viewed with skepticism. Prior to the use of intestinal biopsies, some researchers reported an increase of diabetes mellitus among family members of celiac patients, while others reported contradictory findings.

After development of techniques for taking jejunal biopsies, modestly increased rates of diabetes were reported. These numbers were usually close to 1% of the celiac patients who were reported as having both diseases. When faced with these increased numbers of diabetes mellitus among celiac families and celiac patients, many asserted that certain genetically determined features of the immune system (HLA) were common among people with either condition. Such genetic factors, they argued, might predispose to autoimmune diseases in general, and would therefore be likely to increase the frequency of both conditions within the same families, and sometimes, within the same individual. The issue was further confounded by the overlap between classical symptoms of celiac disease and diabetes mellitus. Thus, a second diagnosis was often overlooked because all symptoms were considered to result from the first condition diagnosed. The reported rates of coexistence thus underrepresented the true overlap.

It was only through systematic research among large numbers of diabetic patients who were biopsied, along with the development and use of serological testing for celiac disease, that the increased coexistence of these diseases gained recognition during the mid to late 1980s. Still, the dominant view ascribed a common origin for both autoimmune conditions. Thus, when other autoimmune diseases were recognized as overly common among celiac patients, little thought was given to the notion that gluten might trigger more than celiac disease.

Several startling research findings threatened this perspective and offered a new window through which to view celiac disease and autoimmunity in general. Although this work was initially given little attention, each of several distinct areas of research were building toward a critical mass.

Exploration of intestinal permeability, and its relationship to celiac disease, was investigated throughout the 1990s and has continued through the first decade of the Twenty-First Century. This work not only provided convincing evidence for the use of sugar absorption tests to screen for celiac disease in developing nations, it also established that intestinal leakage of food proteins is a consistent feature of active celiac disease.

One spin-off result of this work was to increase the credibility of molecular mimicry as a viable theory to explain autoimmunity through the leakage of food proteins into the bloodstream. These foreign proteins were shown to cause immune system reactions that damaged both the foreign proteins, self-tissues with similar protein structures, and complexes formed by attachment of these foreign proteins to self-tissues.

Meanwhile, another area of research was increasing the use of serum antibody testing, called celiac panels, which soon revealed that celiac disease was dramatically more common than previously suspected. These tests also established that the coexistence of celiac disease and diabetes mellitus is also quite common. When diabetic patients were tested, about 5% were shown to have celiac disease. When celiac patients were tested, up to 10% were found to have diabetes mellitus.

Developments in similar serum antibody testing, related other autoimmune diseases, also revealed that compliance with a gluten-free diet, following diagnosis of celiac disease, actually resulted in reductions of these other antibodies. These studies suggested that gluten might actually play a causal role, not only in diabetes, but in a wide range of autoimmune diseases that were previously considered to be coincidentally associated with celiac disease. Hope dawned for many who suffered from a wide range of autoimmune diseases. Simple dietary changes might aid new treatments and bring relief to these many sufferers of autoimmunity. Even in cases where gluten is not the underlying cause, we are gaining understanding of the dynamics by which autoimmunity develops.

The crowning moment, with respect to Type 1 diabetes, came in January of 2003 when A.J. MacFarlane, et al. published their findings in the _Journal of Biological Chemistry_. Their work demonstrated that wheat proteins might be a major causal factor in at least some cases of diabetes mellitus. Rooted in prior animal research that was largely spearheaded by Fraser Scott, this most recent research identified immune reactions, in diabetic humans, against wheat proteins, which were also closely linked with the attack on the islet cells of the pancreas. This is an exciting moment for those with type 1 diabetes. Many of them may be aided in the maintenance of islet cell transplants (another new development) through following a gluten-free diet.

This work also provides a potential turning point for everyone who suffers from autoimmunity. Thanks to the recent establishment of celiac disease as very common in North America, we now know that about 1 in 133 Americans have celiac disease. We also know that this common condition is triggered by gluten. This family of grain proteins also appears to cause some, perhaps many, cases of diabetes mellitus.

The evidence against gluten is also growing in the investigation of other autoimmune conditions. It appears that celiac disease will soon be the window through which we will gain a better understanding of autoimmunity, and the gluten-free diet may be the cornerstone of the treatment of many cases of autoimmune diseases.

Understanding the Genetics of Gluten Sensitivity

By Dr. Scot Lewey

All of us have patterns of proteins on the surface of our white blood cells. These proteins are known as human leukocyte antigens (HLA), one of which is DQ. Celiac disease and non-celiac gluten sensitivity (NCGS), and several autoimmune conditions occur more frequently with certain HLA DQ types. DQ gene testing is performed by analyzing cells from a blood sample or from a Q-tip swab of the mouth. HLA types have a naming system that can be confusing even to scientists and physicians but here is my explanation of the testing, the results, and what they may mean to you and your family.

Each of us has two copies of HLA DQ. Because there are 9 serotypes of DQ we are all DQx/DQx where x is a number between 1 & 9. For example, I am DQ2/DQ7. I received the DQ2 from one of my parents and the DQ7 from the other. Because we get one DQ type from each of our parents and give one to each of our children it is easy to see how the DQ genes pass through a family. This is important because two DQ types, DQ2 and DQ8, are estimated to be present in over 98% of all people who have celiac disease, the most severe form of gluten sensitivity.

Rarely, true celiac disease or dermatitis herpetiformis, the skin disease equivalent of celiac, have been reported to occur in people who do not have DQ2 and/or DQ8. However, according to unpublished data from Dr. Ken Fine of Enterolab, the other six types, except DQ4, are associated with risk for elevated stool antibodies to gliadin, the toxic fraction of gluten, and/or tissue transglutaminase (tTG) an enzyme. Both of these antibodies are usually elevated in the blood of individuals with celiac disease though they may be normal in the blood of individuals who are gluten sensitive and have a normal small intestine biopsy but respond favorably to a gluten-free diet.

Fine has publicly reported that elevated stool antibodies to gliadin and/or tTG have been detected in all of the untreated celiacs tested in his lab and 60% of non-celiacs who have symptoms consistent with gluten sensitivity but in none of the controls tested including cow manure. Follow up surveys of those individuals with elevated stool antibodies who initiated a gluten-free diet compared with those with elevated antibodies who did not reportedly showed significantly improved quality of life and improved symptoms in the gluten-free group.

He also reported DQ2 and DQ8 positive individuals have had, as a rule, the highest elevations of stool gliadin antibody followed by those who are DQ7 positive. Only those who are doubly positive for DQ4 have not been found to have significantly elevated antibodies that indicate gluten sensitivity. This is consistent with the differences in prevalence rates of celiac disease seen in various parts of the world since DQ4 is not generally found in Caucasians of Northern European ancestry where celiac incidence is highest but in those from Asia or Southern Africa where there is a very low incidence of celiac disease and gluten intolerance.

DQ2 & DQ8, the two major types present in 90-99% of people who have celiac disease, are present in approximately 35-45% of people in the U.S., especially those of Caucasian race of Northern European ancestry, with highest risk of celiac disease but the prevalence in U.S. of celiac disease is 1%. Though a prevalence of 1 in 100 is very common and much higher than had been believed for years, only a fraction of the genetically at risk are confirmed to have celiac disease by abnormal blood tests and small intestine biopsies. However, the number of people who report a positive response to gluten-free diet is much higher.

The stool antibody tests results would support this and the concept of a spectrum of gluten sensitivity that is much broader and in need of better diagnostic definitions. I am an example of someone who is DQ2/DQ7 who has normal blood tests for celiac disease but abnormal stool antibody tests and symptoms that responded to gluten-free diet. The strict criteria for diagnosing celiac disease, which is abnormal blood tests and a characteristic small intestine biopsy showing classic damage from gluten, is much narrower than what is being seen clinically.

It is becoming obvious to many of us who have personal and professional medical experience with gluten intolerance and celiac disease that the problem of gluten sensitivity is much greater and extends beyond the high risk celiac genes DQ2 and DQ8. Traditionally it is reported and believed by many that if you are DQ2 and DQ8 negative you are unlikely to have celiac disease or ever develop it, though this cannot be said with 100% certainty especially since there are documented cases of celiac disease and the skin equivalent of celiac disease, known as dermatitis herpetiformis (DH) in individuals who are DQ2 and DQ8 negative.

Therefore, knowing your DQ specific serotype pattern may be helpful for several reasons. For example, if you have more than one copy of DQ2 or DQ8, you carry two of the major genes. For example, if you are DQ2/DQ2, DQ2/DQ8, or DQ8/DQ8, a term Scott Adams of www.celiac.com has dubbed a "super celiac" you may be at much higher risk for celiac disease and have more severe gluten sensitivity. Certainly if you are DQ2 and/or DQ8 positive you are at increased risk for celiac disease. After a single copy of DQ2 or DQ8, it appears that DQ7/DQ7 might be next highest risk. Dr. Fine has also noted some other associations of the DQ patterns with microscopic or collagenous colitis, neurologic manifestations of gluten sensitivity and dermatitis herpetiformis, which has been one of the gluten sensitive conditions noted to be, at times, occurring in DQ2, DQ8 negative individuals.

Why some people get celiac disease or become gluten sensitive is not well understood. However, contributing factors are thought to include puberty, pregnancy, stress, trauma/injury, surgery, viral or bacterial infections -including those of the gut, medication induced gut injury or toxicity, e.g., non-steroidal anti-inflammatory medications such as aspirin, ibuprofen, etc., immune suppression or autoimmune diseases - especially since several of those factors are associated with onset or unmasking of gluten sensitivity in someone who is at risk or not previously manifesting any recognizable symptoms.

There is also well known group of individuals who are termed "latent" celiacs. They are at high risk because they have close relatives who have celiac disease with whom they share one or more of the celiac genes DQ2 and/or DQ8 though they usually have few or no symptoms but sometimes have abnormal blood tests and/or biopsies indicating possible or definite celiac disease. Others have negative blood tests and normal biopsies but symptoms that respond to a gluten-free diet.

The severity of the sensitivity to gluten appears to be related to the DQ type, family history (highest risk is in the non affected identical twin of a celiac), pre-existing intestinal injury, degree of exposure to gluten (how frequent and large a gluten load an individual has consumed) and immune status. Once initiated, gluten sensitivity tends to be lifelong. True celiac disease requires life-long complete gluten avoidance to reduce the increased risk of serious complications of undiagnosed and untreated celiac such as severe malabsorption, cancers, especially of the GI tract and lymphoma, other autoimmune diseases and premature death due to these complications.

Again, DQ testing can be done with cells from blood or by a swab of the inside of the mouth but not all labs test for or report the full DQ typing but only the presence or absence of DQ2 and DQ8. The lab that performs DQ testing is usually determined by the insurance company on the basis of contracts with specific commercial labs. However, if your insurance contracts with Quest Labs or the Laboratory at Bonfils (Denver, CO) full DQ can be done if ordered and authorized by the insurance company.

For those willing to pay out of pocket, Bonfils performs full DQ testing for Enterolab (www.enterolab.com) on a sample obtained by a Q tip swab of the mouth. Since it is painless and non-invasive it is well tolerated especially by young children. Also because the testing can be ordered without a physician and the sample obtained in their home using a kit obtained from Enterolab it is convenient. The kit is returned by overnight delivery by to Enterolab who forwards the test onto Bonfils. The cost is $149 for the genetic testing alone and has to be paid for in advance by credit card or money order and is generally not reimbursed by insurance.

Enterolab also provides the stool testing for gliadin and tissue transglutaminase antibodies to determine if gluten sensitivity is evident. The gliadin antibody alone is $99 or the full panel includes genetic typing, stool testing for gluten and cow's milk protein antibodies, and a test for evidence of malabsorption is $349.

Again, the advantages of full DQ testing is determining if someone has more than one copy of DQ2 or DQ8 or carry both and therefore have a higher risk for celiac disease or more severe gluten intolerance. If you are DQ2 or DQ8 negative then your risk of celiac disease is low, though not non-existent. If you are not DQ4/DQ4 then you do have risk for gluten sensitivity. If you determine all DQ types within enough family members you can piece together a very accurate history of the origin of celiac and gluten sensitivity within a family and make some very accurate predictions of risk to other family members.

Though the lay public and many clinicians are finding the genetic tests helpful, many, including most physicians, do not understand the genetics of gluten sensitivity. We are awaiting Dr. Fine's published data on the significance of stool antibody tests and their association to the other DQ types as his lab is the only lab offering the stool antibody tests in the U.S. Other celiac researchers in U.S. have failed to reproduce his assay but scattered reports in the literature are appearing including a recent article in the British Medical Journal indicating stool antibody testing is feasible, non-invasive, and using their protocol, highly specific but not sensitive for celiac disease in children. In the meantime, many patients are faced with the uncertainty and added cost of full DQ testing and stool testing due to the failure of traditional blood tests, small bowel biopsies, and the presence or absence of DQ2 and DQ8 to diagnose or exclude gluten sensitivity. Physicians unfamiliar with this testing are increasingly presented with the results and confused or skeptical pending published reports. The medical community continues to lack a consensus regarding the definitions of non-celiac gluten sensitivity and what tests justify recommendations for gluten-free diet. It is clear that gluten sensitivity, by any criteria, is much more common than ever thought and a hidden epidemic exists.

Your DNA Results Indicate: Super Celiac!

By Scott Adams

I recently decided to have my DNA and that of my son screened for the genetic markers, also known as HLA alleles, which make celiac disease possible. Both my mother and I have long since been diagnosed with the disease, so I naturally worry that my son, Spencer, may also end up with it at some point in his life. Even though he has been mostly symptom-free for all three and a half years of his life, last year I subjected him to serological screening after he had a several week bout with diarrhea. We were happy to discover that he did not have it, but I still knew that such tests could not rule the disease out of his future. Even so, it was nice to learn that he did not have the active disease, although a blood draw at two years of age was not exactly a pleasant experience for him—or for his parents! I swore then that I would try to avoid any unnecessary blood draws in the future, even though I knew that it might still be necessary from time to time—unless he somehow did not inherit the genetic markers for it. That idea led to my decision to have Spencer's DNA screened for celiac disease.

After mentioning my plans for the DNA screening at a family dinner, my brother also grew interested, as he too has had unexplained symptoms and a recent negative celiac disease antibody panel and biopsy. He, too, felt that it would be nice to find out once and for all if this was something that he was going to have to worry about in the future. He also pointed out to me that genetic screening had the potential to save him money over the long haul, since the test is only necessary once in a lifetime. Periodic antibody screening for the disease can prove to be quite expensive, and a negative DNA test would effectively rule out the necessity of any future testing. After we finished our dinner that evening, I sat down with my brother and we reviewed several offerings on the Internet by companies who provide genetic services for celiac disease. We were particularly impressed by Kimball Genetics, located in Denver, Colorado, as their DNA collection method did not require a blood draw and instead employed a simple and painless cheek cell collection using a swab.

The next day I telephoned Kimball Genetics and was connected with a very knowledgeable genetic counselor. After a discussion with her about my family's history I decided to order three celiac disease genetic tests, one each for my son, my brother, and myself. I requested three cheek cell collection kits to be sent to my home, where the samples would be collected and sent back to Kimball Genetics for testing. For individuals, the cost of a kit is 10% off of $325, or $292.50 per test, with a 20% family discount for testing additional family members, which brings the per test price down to $260.

Kimball Genetics also offers assistance with billing your health insurance company, which can often result in the recovery of all or part of the costs incurred for the tests. This includes detailed help with the forms, insurance CPT codes for the procedure, as well as obtaining the ICD9 codes, which are the diagnostic and symptom codes that come from your doctor. At this point I realized that to get reimbursed for the tests a person should first make an appointment with their doctor. Ideally this appointment should take place before actually ordering a test kit. This will ensure that you and your doctor are on the same page regarding the importance and necessity of the genetic tests.

The cheek cell collection kits arrived in the mail within a couple of days, and I phoned my brother to arrange a "DNA collection party" at my house. On collection day we opened the kits to find enclosed two brushes for sample collection, a Test Request Form, a consent form, medical literature regarding Kimball Genetics DNA screening test for celiac disease, and detailed instructions that outlined how to properly collect and mail the samples. The kits also included a stamped return envelope that was pre-addressed to their laboratory. The Test Request Form included an area where one could enter their credit card information, and this form along with the consent form and a check or card information were required to be sent along with the sample in the return envelope.

The medical literature included with the kits comprised of a three page document titled "Celiac Disease DNA Test." The following two sections, which I found to be particularly helpful, are reproduced below from this document, which is also available on their Web site www.kimballgenetics.com:

Indications for Celiac Disease DNA Testing

- Clinical diagnosis of celiac disease.
- Negative or equivocal antibody results (antiendomysial, tissue transglutaminase, or antigliadin) or intestinal biopsy results in an individual with symptoms of celiac disease.
- Relatives of individuals with celiac disease.

- Individuals with iron-deficient anemia.
- Individuals with dermatitis herpetiformis.
- Adults with diarrhea, abdominal pain and distention, recurrent aphthous stomatitis (canker sores), osteoporosis, infertility, multiple miscarriages, anxiety, and/or depression.
- Children with abdominal pain, diarrhea, abdominal distention, failure to thrive, short stature, delayed puberty, irritability, attention-deficit disorder and/or poor school performance.
- Children with Type I diabetes.

Our Celiac Disease DNA Test Service Provides:
- PCR analysis for DQ2 alleles (DQA1*0501, DQA1*0505, and DQB1*0201/*0202) and DQ8 allele (DQB1*0302).
- Detailed reports with genetic interpretation, recommendations, and education.
- Free genetic counseling for physicians, patients, and families.
- Free shipping.

The sample collection went very smoothly for each of us, and Spencer found it to be slightly more annoying than having to brush his teeth. We each rinsed our mouths out with water beforehand, and then rolled one brush at a time 20 times over the entire inside surface area of one check, and then did the same on the other cheek with the second brush. We let the samples dry for 30 minutes, and then put everything in their respective packages and envelopes along with the filled out paper work. Our final step was to put them out for the Mail Carrier to pick up. Their literature promised a 3-4 day turn around, and sure enough, both my brother and I got a call from someone at Kimball Genetics several days later. They needed our doctors' fax numbers, which we had forgotten to include on the paperwork. Once they had this information, a call to our doctors was all that was necessary to have our doctors forward the results directly to us by fax, and we also received the original reports by mail. Amazingly the Celiac Disease DNA Test at Kimball Genetics takes just one business day from the day the lab receives the sample (if it arrives by noon) to reporting of results.

I have to admit that besides hoping that my son did not inherit the genetic makeup that makes celiac disease possible—as the results were printing out from my fax machine—I still held out the very slight hope that they had not found the markers in my genetic sample, and that my whole diagnosis was some sort of big mistake. This hope was quickly crushed as the report indicated that I was in fact part of an elite genetic group—one that carries *both* markers for celiac disease: DQ2 *and* DQ8—which I later discovered meant that I inherited genetic traits for celiac disease from *both* of my parents, rather than just from my mother, which was my original assumption. My father is no longer alive, but after discussing his results with my mother we decided that it is possible that he also had undiagnosed celiac disease, and it is interesting to note that he had diabetes.

I couldn't help but think that my results make me something like a "Super Celiac," although the genetic counselor at Kimball Genetics reassured me that having both markers for it doesn't necessarily mean that the disease will present itself any differently. Spencer turned out to be positive for DQ2, and my brother found out that he too tested positive for both DQ2 and DQ8. On the down side their results indicate that they will need to watch out for any future signs of the disease for the rest of their lives, and probably get screened for it from time to time. On the up side there is still only a small chance that either will ever develop the disease, and at least we will know to watch for its symptoms in the future, which likely would lead to a quick diagnosis and treatment should one of them ever get it.

Ultimately anyone who decides to undergo genetic screening must be comfortable with the results—positive or negative. I advocate testing because I believe in the saying that *knowledge is power*, and that it is better to know than not to know—especially when it comes to your health. Unlike other testing methods, genetic screening for celiac disease has the amazing potential to reveal whether someone has been misdiagnosed with the disease, even though the odds for such a scenario are small. It also can confirm a diagnosis, or let relatives of celiacs know that they do or don't need to worry about it in the future. My mother felt vindicated by our results, as they indicated that she wasn't the only person who passed celiac genes to her children—my father did too. Who knows, your genetic results may even have the potential to elevate your celiac status, as it did in my case, to that of—*Super Celiac!*

Additional Food Allergies - Incomplete Recovery or Refractory Sprue?

By Dr. Ron Hoggan, Ed. D.

It is not much of a reach to suspect additional food sensitivities in the context of celiac disease or gluten sensitivity. After all, celiac disease causes increased intestinal permeability[1] otherwise known as "leaky gut." Since large, undigested gluten proteins can sometimes pass into the bloodstream, other food proteins are also likely to reach the circulation. The immune system reacts against such foreign proteins in an attempt to protect us. The presence of non-self proteins causes an immune system reaction just as if they were infectious microbes. And herein lies one answer to some, perhaps many, cases of incomplete recovery and refractory sprue. These conditions may sometimes be relatively easy to correct through the detection and avoidance of additional food sensitivities.

Adult-diagnosed celiac patients have usually experienced many years of a leaky gut, with or without symptoms and ill health. Even after diagnosis and strict adherence to a gluten free diet, intestinal recovery is usually incomplete[2]. Admittedly, these signs and symptoms can result from a variety of causes including nutritional deficiencies due to malabsorption, abnormal immune responses, damaged protective mucosa of the intestinal wall resulting in a leaky gut, additional autoimmune conditions, and opportunistic infections. It sometimes seems that celiac disease just rolls out the red carpet for a host of additional ailments. Increased intestinal permeability, resulting in additional food allergies, is just one of the many contributors to this witches' brew of additional ills that arise in untreated celiac disease and may continue despite careful avoidance of gluten.

Considerable evidence has long pointed toward additional food allergies. Unfortunately, this information has largely been ignored. But recent developments in serological testing are now making it feasible, economical, and convenient, to identify and correct such food allergies. One article appeared almost thirty years ago in the peer reviewed literature reporting complete resolution of what was previously diagnosed as refractory sprue following removal of additional allergenic foods from the diet[3]. Another such publication documented the progress of one celiac patient who was thought to have refractory sprue. This individual recovered with the additional dietary exclusion of egg, chicken, and tuna[4]. This patient became *very* ill before the possibility of immune reactions to other dietary proteins was considered.

More recent reports of the success of elemental diets in reversing refractory sprue further support this perspective[5]. Another group has indicated that 36% to 48% of celiac patients demonstrate antibody reactions to milk proteins[5]. Although there are some reports that the frequency of such sensitivities reduce with treatment time on a gluten-free diet[7,8], they also report a higher initial frequency of reactions to milk proteins.

I have not heard of any new evidence suggesting that the injury to the intestinal mucosa caused by gluten can now be distinguished from similar injuries caused by milk protein allergies. Thus, any of a variety of food allergies might be contributing to such damage to the mucosa.

The peer-reviewed reports cited above, along with the many posts to the Celiac Listserv indicating that additional food sensitivities are a factor in individual cases of celiac disease, suggest the need for vigilance among celiac patients, particularly those who are experiencing incomplete recovery on a strict gluten-free diet.

Before leaping to the use of steroids, further antibody testing seems prudent. There are a number of commercial laboratories in the United States and at least one in the United Kingdom that offer IgG testing for delayed-type allergies to common foods. Although such tests are not perfect, they can provide valuable information for those who have not experienced a full recovery on a gluten-free diet, or some individuals who have been diagnosed with refractory sprue. The therapeutic use of systemic steroids can produce some very dangerous side effects. IgG blood testing and dietary exclusion of identified allergens, on the other hand, involves a simple, convenient test followed by the kind of dietary inconvenience that most of us are already well versed in.

If possible, ELISA or similar testing ought to be done *prior* to beginning steroids, as such drugs may be unnecessary, or they may compromise the accuracy of the blood test.

Other Food Intolerances

By Laura Wesson

According to *Dangerous Grains* by Dr. Ron Hoggan and James Braly, M.D., intolerances to foods other than gluten are the most common reason that people continue to have health problems after they've gone on a gluten-free diet. Yet, from the hundreds of emails I've gotten from people on the celiac email list, and from online forums, I've found that many people don't investigate other food intolerances, even though they suffer from health problems they could likely cure by eliminating problem foods.

I was sick for five months solid in the summer of 2004, after I'd adopted a gluten-free diet. I would get up in the morning feeling half well; I'd get my shopping done first thing in the morning. Then I'd go home and lapse into a semi-stuporous state. I would sit in a chair for the rest of the day, my mind slogging slowly through a swamp. I thought at the time it was hay fever from my 53 inhalant allergies, but I was taking six different allergy medicines, to no avail.

I later found that I actually had intolerances to about 90% of the foods I'd been eating. What had really been happening, it seemed, was that I felt somewhat better after fasting overnight. Then I would eat something containing an allergen for breakfast. I'd get my shopping done then I'd start to feel sick from my breakfast. My inhalant allergies were actually only a small part of the problem. After going on an exotic foods diet, I became much healthier. In the summer of 2005, I went running every day and my mind was much clearer. My 53 inhaled allergies no longer bothered me as much.

This is typical for people with multiple food intolerances. They can be hidden just like gluten intolerance. If you're like me, your body probably didn't like gluten long before you were aware of it. It's not like a peanut allergy. If you were allergic to peanuts, you'd probably know it. Your body isn't able to suppress that allergic reaction. But if you're gluten intolerant, you can eat gluten every day and never know what's making you so sick. Your body hides its reaction, so you don't notice feeling worse after eating gluten. Wheat might even have been one of your favorite foods.

After you stop eating gluten, your body no longer has to work so hard to suppress food intolerance reactions. So if you have other food intolerances, after a few months or so you may start to feel obviously worse after eating those foods. This is an excellent reason for sticking strictly to a gluten-free diet - it will help you find any other food intolerances you may have, and thus speed your recovery. If you don't do a careful elimination diet, you may be in for a long, agonizing process of eliminating the foods you're intolerant to, one by one, feeling sick perhaps for years after starting a gluten-free diet.

Food intolerance can cause many other problems. Joint pain and stiffness is a common symptom. Just before I found out about my gluten intolerance, both my elbows and knees were hurting, and the tendons in my forearm and hand hurt so much I couldn't lift a cast iron pan with one hand. After I eliminated the many foods I'm intolerant to, in addition to gluten, I was able to run without pain. I've also noticed that my old joint injuries often stiffen after food challenges. Joint inflammation and stiffening are thought to accelerate joint destruction in osteoarthritis, the wear-and-tear arthritis that many people suffer from as they get older.

Many diseases are partly caused by chronic inflammation. Inflammation contributes to the onset and progression of tumors, and is involved in atherosclerosis. Hidden food intolerances can cause chronic inflammation and irritation in many areas of the body, so finding your food intolerances could help with any problem that involves irritation or inflammation. I think that when food intolerances are hidden, the body compensates somewhat for their pro-inflammatory effects, because my C-reactive protein and sedimentation rate, measures of inflammation, were high at a time when my food intolerances were in the process of being unmasked - but my C-reactive protein was actually lower than normal when I was still eating tiny amounts of some foods that I later found I had hidden intolerances to. However, the body doesn't seem to be able to compensate completely for the pro-inflammatory effects of food intolerances.

A gluten-containing diet raises the risk of some GI tract cancers in celiacs. Perhaps other food intolerances also cause GI tract cancer - a scary possibility!

I had a hard time with carbohydrates for more than twenty years. When I tried highly glycemic carbs, I would feel jittery, hungry, irritable, and tense. My carbohydrate reactions went away after I found my non-gluten food intolerances. I can eat almost any amount of tapioca starch mixed with maple syrup—an enjoyable, sticky goo with a very high glycemic index - and all that happens is that I get high and happy and I feel like going out and exercising.

My jittery, anxious food reactions weren't simply reactions of intolerance. For example, I have intolerances to foods like peanuts. A tiny trace of peanut oil made me sick for days, but peanuts had never made me feel jittery or anxious when I ate them before I found my hidden food intolerances. Rather, it seems that having hidden food intolerances caused my body to release a lot of adrenaline after I ate carbohydrates, or else it made my body more sensitive to adrenaline. A study of people with suspected reactive hypoglycemia showed that they were hypersensitive to adrenaline.

If you have emotional or psychiatric problems, it's also worth looking for hidden food intolerances, although according to Brostoff and Gamlin's book _Food Allergies and Food Intolerance_, people who have psychological problems from food intolerance usually have physical health problems as well.

Some other problems that are possibly related to food intolerance are asthma, fatigue, rashes, irritable bowel syndrome, migraines, sinusitis, recurring urinary tract infections, and light and/or noise sensitivity.

If you have food reactions that you might attribute to accidentally being exposed to gluten, but you can't verify that you actually had gluten, you might actually be reacting to other foods.

The gold standard for finding food intolerances is to do an elimination diet for a week or two and then to try foods one by one, and see if they have some kind of bad effect. If you think you have a food reaction that's delayed for days, it would be a good idea to try the food again to see if the same reaction happens again. Here's another caution:

once or twice, I've thought I'd reacted to a food challenge, when actually I had a bladder infection.

If you do the elimination diet perfectly, you can probably find all of your food intolerances at once, which would save many people from many years of sickness. However, this is very difficult, because doing an elimination diet correctly means eliminating all common food allergens – that is, all foods that you normally eat fairly often, as well as all foods that might cross-react with those foods. Brostoff and Gamlin's book has a lot of information on food intolerance cross-reactions that very accurately reflects my experience. Ideally, you should also quit taking any medications or supplements that you normally take, or get your medications made by a compounding pharmacy without fillers, because most medications have many allergenic non-medical ingredients such as corn starch. Even your toothpaste could be causing a reaction. After I found my intolerance to birch, I kept on using toothpaste that was sweetened with birch xylitol, washing my mouth carefully with water after brushing my teeth. Once, though, I forgot to wash my mouth out, so a little toothpaste went down my throat, and I got sick for four days. You can brush your teeth with baking soda, which you won't have an intolerance to, since it's not made from anything organic.

It's also very difficult to do an elimination diet because people are often addicted to foods they're intolerant to. On one elimination diet I did, I was unable to stop using fructose made from corn. Later, I painfully, slowly, quit using fructose over many months. When I finally eliminated all corn products from my diet, I found that my body had been masking about 30 or 50 other food intolerances, as a side effect of masking my corn intolerance. After I eliminated corn, I suddenly started getting sick after eating many of the foods I'd been eating all along.

Elimination diets and food challenges can be done in an in-patient setting, which might be the only way to completely adhere to the diet. If you have an IgE mediated food allergy, food challenges should only be done with medical supervision. Brostoff and Gamlin's book has a number of elimination diets of varying degrees of strictness.

Some people rely instead on IgG ELISA blood testing for food intolerances. The idea behind the test is that a higher than normal level of IgG antibodies to a food might mean that one has an intolerance to it. The body normally makes IgG antibodies to foods. One research study showed that eliminating foods based on IgG ELISA testing helped many people with irritable bowel syndrome. Otherwise the tests haven't been validated by research. Investigators have also tried sending several blood samples obtained from the same person at the same time to different labs, or more than one blood sample to the same lab, and found the test results were very inconsistent.

Finding your hidden food intolerances is often a long, painful process that is full of errors and guesses. It's also very important to do if you are not completely healthy on a gluten free diet.

Immunoglobulin Deficiency and Celiac Disease

By Vijay Kumar, Ph.D., FACB

Celiac disease is an autoimmune gastrointestinal disorder that may occur in genetically susceptible individuals triggered by the ingestion of gluten-containing grains such as wheat, barley and rye. Of the many autoimmune disorders, celiac disease represents one of the few where the etiological agent is known and the disease subsides and goes in remission once the etiological agent is withdrawn from the diet.

Celiac disease is characterized by malabsorption resulting from inflammatory injury to the small intestinal mucosa, which, when prolonged, can cause malnutrition. The classic symptoms of celiac disease include diarrhea, weight loss and malnutrition. However, only a small percentage of patients with celiac disease present with the classic symptoms. Consequently, the clinical spectrum of celiac disease has grown much broader to include patients without classic symptoms. It is not uncommon for the initial symptoms to be non-gastrointestinal or for gastrointestinal symptoms, if present, to be mild or intermittent. Some of the common non-gastrointestinal manifestations include short stature, iron and folate deficiency, anemia, bone loss, aphthous stomatitis, arthralgia, dental enamel defects, etc. The inclusion of a wider range of clinical presentation has led to greater numbers of individuals diagnosed with celiac disease later in life than ever before. Adults may present with iron deficiency, macrocytic anemia and hypocalcaemia.

Studies have found the prevalence of celiac disease to be highly variable from population to population[1] and the true prevalence has been difficult to ascertain. The disparate criteria used in the diagnosis of celiac disease are often the cause. If only the clinical criteria are used in determining prevalence, the incidence of celiac disease is much lower as compared with incidence established by serological methods[2]. Using serological methods of diagnosis, the incidence of celiac disease in the general population is approximately one in 200 [editor's note: As of 2010 this number is now recognized to be at least 1 in 133].

Diagnosis of celiac disease based on clinical criteria can therefore be misleading and may lead to serious delays in proper diagnosis. Frequently, delays in diagnosis extend 10-13 years from the first clinical presentation of symptoms. Failure to diagnose celiac disease early on may predispose an individual to long-term complications such as splenic atrophy and intestinal lymphoma. The incidence of lymphoma arising in the context of celiac disease is difficult to ascertain. One study has shown incidence of lymphoma involving the gastrointestinal tract in patients with celiac disease to range from 3.6 percent to 40 percent[3]. In another recent study, celiac disease was found to be associated with significantly elevated risk for intestinal lymphoma, especially for non-Hodgkin's[4]. A gluten-free diet normalizes the mucosa and helps reduce the malignant potential.

Histological examination of the small intestinal biopsy is considered to be the gold standard for diagnosing celiac disease, but it has its own limitations. Certain studies have shown some patients with latent or even active celiac disease that may have normal histopathology[5].

Serological Methods of Detecting Celiac Disease

The revised European Society of Pediatric Gastroenterology and Nutrition (ESPGAN) criteria for diagnosis of celiac disease include only a single biopsy with clear-cut remission of clinical symptoms on a gluten-free diet[6]. Positive serology at the time of diagnosis with a decline in antibody levels on a gluten-free diet contributes to the diagnosis. The various serological tests employed in the work-up of patients suspected to have celiac disease include anti-gliadin antibody (AGA), anti-endomysial antibody (EMA), anti-reticulin antibody (ARA) and anti-tissue transglutaminase (tTG) antibody tests. Antibodies to gliadin and tTG are detected by the ELISA method, whereas endomysial and reticulin antibodies are detected by indirect immunofluorescence. EMA are very specific indicators of celiac disease. One study[7] concludes that "EmA-IgA is 100 percent sensitive and specific in active, untreated IgA-sufficient celiac disease patients when performed by an established laboratory."

tTG has been identified as the endomysial antigen. This discovery has enabled development of automatable ELISA methods for detecting antibodies in the sera of patients with celiac disease. Many laboratories have opted to use the tTG antibody method in screening for celiac disease. In these laboratories, it may be the only assay used for detection of celiac disease cases. Various studies on the efficacy of the tTG antibody method for screening have found the specificity and sensitivity of this method to range from 90 percent to 95 percent[8]. Assays using human tTG have been described to improve the sensitivity of detection of tTG antibodies. Surprisingly, in a recent report by the Medicines and Healthcare Products Regulatory Agency (MHRAM) on various anti-tTG IgA isotype assays the specificities were found to be good but assay sensitivity was often poor, indicating considerable variation in reliability of detection.

One limitation of existing serological methods is that, with the exception of IgG–gliadin, they detect only the IgA isotype of the antibodies; hence, IgA deficient celiac disease patients may yield false negative serology[9]. This may compromise the utility of the serum antibody methods in detecting all celiac disease cases[10].

What is IgA deficiency?

In the blood there are proteins called immunoglobulins that generally provide immuno-logical protection. There are five types of immunoglobulins, known as IgG, IgA, IgM, IgE, and IgD. IgG and IgM provide protection in the circulatory system whereas IgA is transported to the surface of mucosal linings such as in the gastrointestinal tract and oral mucosa, safeguarding these mucosal surfaces from infection. Certain individuals that fail to produce the IgA immunoglobulin are referred to have selective IgA deficiency. The cause of this selective IgA deficiency is not known.

What is known is that patients with selective IgA deficiency have a defect in differ-entiating B cells (one of the white cell types) into cells that manufacture immuno-globulins called plasma cells. The concentration of IgA in the plasma of normal in-dividuals is about 300 mg/dl. In individuals with selective IgA deficiency the IgA levels are less than 0.05 mg/dl. IgA deficiency is one of the most common immu-nodeficiencies, found in one in 500-700 healthy blood donors[11]. In most situations, these IgA deficient individuals are healthy. Those who develop symptoms suffer from sino-pulmonary infections, allergies, and autoimmune disorders, especially celiac disease[12].

The incidence of IgA deficiency in celiac disease patients is between 2-3%, representing a 10-15 fold increase over the general population. Familial inheritance of IgA defi-ciency occurs in 20% of cases. While the selective defect of B cells limits the number of IgA secreting plasma cells, IgA deficient individuals have normal function of IgG and other immunoglobulin secreting plasma cells. Celiac disease patients with IgA defi-ciency produce IgG immunoglobulin normally, and the antibodies to EMA, tTG and gliadin are of the IgG isotype rather than IgA. To prevent false negative results in IgA deficient cases of celiac disease, it is necessary to include serological methods that can detect antibodies of IgG isotype.

How can we detect Celiac Disease in patients with IgA deficiency?

In patients with known selective IgA deficiency, the IgG antibody levels for EMA, tTG and gliadin can be measured and are very effective in identifying patients with celiac disease. However, one generally does not know if the individual is IgA deficient. Until specific tests for IgA levels are performed, the IgA status of an individual may never be known. As IgA deficiency is more prevalent in the celiac population than the general population, it has been proposed that all patients who are considered for celiac disease be tested for IgA levels to identify cases of IgA deficiency. Checking all routine samples referred to a laboratory for celiac disease testing, Lock and Unsworth found that testing for IgA levels in identifying IgA deficient celiac disease patients is excessive and more likely to identify non-celiac disease cases[13]. They concluded that testing of IgA levels is not cost effective. Testing for IgG antibodies to EMA, tTG or AGA, however, is cost effective. Detection of these antibodies either individually or in combination helps to identify all cases of IgA deficient celiac disease on normal diets. Using this method, we reported the first IgA deficient celiac disease case in 1989. Since then, others have reported on large populations of IgA deficient celiac disease and non-celiac disease cases and found the serological methods to be effective (see table on pg. 17). The levels of these antibodies are also of interest, as antibody level tends to correlate with the severity of the disease. When a patient is on a gluten free diet, the levels of these antibodies will decrease and eventually disappear, suggesting that the patient is in remission. Thereafter, tests for antibody levels could be checked annually or bi-annually to ensure the individual's dietary compliance. Intake of gluten in individuals who are in remission will result in the re-appearance or increase of these antibodies in the serum (see figure at right).

Recognizing Celiac Disease Down the Endoscope

By William Dickey Ph.D. MD FACG

Among the many symptoms associated with celiac disease, some of the commonest fall into the broad category of "dyspepsia". These are symptoms more usually attributed to acid reflux from the stomach into the esophagus (heartburn, regurgitation, even difficulty swallowing a.k.a. dysphagia) or to peptic ulcer disease (upper abdominal pain, indigestion, fullness). While we are not entirely sure why celiac disease causes these, often in the absence of typical "bowel" symptoms, we do know how[1]. Studies of the upper gut in celiac disease patients frequently show abnormal motility and peristalsis: the conveyor belt isn't working properly (The constipation that is often paradoxically a symptom of celiac disease probably has the same basis).

So many celiac patients are going to be referred not for small bowel investigation but for upper GI endoscopy, and the gastroenterologist is expecting not celiac disease, but reflux esophagitis, hiatus hernia, gastritis or peptic ulcer disease. Wouldn't it be nice—and wouldn't it make life a lot simpler for the so far undiagnosed celiac patient—if the gastroenterologist could spot villous atrophy like these other conditions?

The good news is that you can see villous atrophy down an endoscope. Well, some of the time (but more of that later). One of the most exciting developments in my career as a celiac diagnostician was when our museum piece fiber optic endoscopes were replaced by full color video scopes. Endoscopy was no longer an uncomfortable (for the endoscopist!) and hurried foray into the upper gut, hunched over with one eye peering down a clouded eyepiece, frantically trying to see everything and get the heck out before the disinfectant fumes wafting up the scope dissolved the glue holding my spectacles together.

Instead, it became a civilized stroll, which ended in a duodenum filling a ten inch TV picture in glorious color. And it became clear to me, and many other celiac specialists, that the duodenums of celiac patients didn't look quite right when they were up close and magnified in this way.

Abnormalities seen in our patients with villous atrophy[2] include mosaic mucosa (53%), scalloped folds (50%), fold loss (15%) and nodular mucosa (6%) and erosions (small ulcers) in the second part of duodenum in 7%. Occasionally the mucosa is so thin that blood vessels can be seen through it. Although uncommon in celiac disease, the finding of erosions in the second part of duodenum is of particular interest as clinicians may simply flag it up as peptic ulcer disease, even though peptic ulcers usually only affect the first part of duodenum. I've seen a few patients who had previously been wrongly diagnosed "peptic" because of this endoscopic feature.

So how have these endoscopic markers changed my practice? Around half of my new celiac patients present with dyspepsia and are recognized at endoscopy[3]. One in 60 patients (twice the background prevalence of celiac disease) referred for endoscopy from primary care with dyspepsia are diagnosed celiac because of these markers[4]. Often the story is of dyspeptic symptoms that have not responded to ulcer healing drugs, but which magically disappear on a gluten-free diet.

There are two caveats regarding endoscopic markers. While villous atrophy in adults is pretty much synonymous with celiac disease in Western Europe, elsewhere it may sometimes indicate other disease, as reported by the New York Group[5]. Secondly, the bad news is that villous atrophy can't always be spotted. We found that only 74% of villous atrophy cases had endoscopic markers[2], and as many patients had endoscopy for biopsy because we were expecting to find celiac disease, that figure may be an overestimate of routine practice. The Mayo Clinic found markers in only 59% of celiac patients from a group of anemic patients having endoscopy[6]. While 82% of our patients with subtotal or total villous atrophy had one or more endoscopic markers, the yield fell to 58% for partial villous atrophy[7]. And as you might expect, I have never seen endoscopic markers in gluten-sensitive patients with milder (Marsh I, Marsh II) histologic abnormalities that have not yet progressed to villous atrophy.

So lack of markers does not mean that there is no need to biopsy, particularly in high risk groups like patients with anemia and insulin dependent diabetes. In an ideal world, duodenal biopsy would be a routine part of every upper GI endoscopy, as already proposed by Peter Green and Joe Murray[8]. In practice, particularly in the good ol' under-funded UK National Health Service that I work for, this would have very significant resource implications. I suspect such a policy—duodenal biopsies taken at every endoscopy—implemented without a major funding initiative on my side of the Atlantic might find our already overworked and undervalued histopathologists under the cars of gastroenterologists furiously cutting through their brake lines.

In the meantime, and until the New Jerusalem of routine duodenal biopsy during endoscopy is constructed, recognition of the endoscopic markers of celiac disease, while not foolproof, represents a pragmatic way of diagnosing celiac patients who present with dyspepsia.

Sorbitol H2-Breath Test: A Simple, Non Invasive, Cheap and Effective Method to Assess Small Bowel Damage in Celiac Disease

By Antonio Tursi, M.D.

The diagnostic algorithm for celiac disease demands a screening approach based on anti-endomysium (EmA) and anti-tissue transglutaminase (anti-tTG) and, in case of antibodies-positivity, patients should undergo intestinal biopsy to confirm the presence of small bowel lesions according to celiac disease.

Unfortunately, this approach is rarely effective in clinical practice, especially in patients with mild to moderate histological lesions. In fact several recent studies have shown that 5-10% of patients affected by mild to moderate lesions of the small bowel typically seen in celiac disease actually lack EmA and anti-tTG antibodies[2-5]. In light of these scientific results, should all patients who are suspected to have, or who are at risk for celiac disease—including first degree relatives of celiacs, those with Down's syndrome or autoimmune thyroid disease, patients whose stories indicate celiac disease, etc.— undergo intestinal biopsy? This does not seem like a very reliable approach—perhaps other more non-invasive tests should be done in conjunction with serological testing to help determine which patients should undergo a biopsy. The sorbitol H_2-breath test (H_2-BT) could be exactly what is needed.

Sorbitol is a hexahydroxy alcohol that is present in many fruits such as peaches[6]. It is used as a sugar substitute in dietetic foods and as a drug vehicle. At low doses (5 grams/day) sorbitol is completely absorbed by the small bowel, and low dose ingestion does not typically produce any symptoms. However, we know that celiac disease patients often experience sugar malabsorption (as lactose malabsorption)[7] which prompted us to hypothesize that the same may be true for sorbitol.

In general terms, sugar malabsorption could be primary—congenital enzymatic/carrier deficiency, or acquired—developing after intestinal damage caused by acute gastroenteritis, medications, Crohn's disease, celiac disease, etc.[8] In the normal individual, gut bacteria are primarily located in the colon and in the distal small intestine. When sugar malabsorption is present, unabsorbed sugars in excess are available in the distal small bowel and colon for bacterial fermentation, with air excretion of H_2 and CH_4[9]. This mechanism occurs for all sugars—lactose, fructose, glucose, sorbitol—and H_2 lactose, fructose and sorbitol breath tests are commonly used to detect specific sugar malabsorption issues.

Sorbitol H_2-BT Methods

This is a simple, non-invasive, repeatable, and cheap test. To minimize basal hydrogen excretion, subjects are asked to have a carbohydrate-restricted dinner on the day before the test (for example, a meal of rice and meat) and are studied after an overnight fasting for at least 12 hours. On the testing days, patients do a mouthwash with 20 ml of chlorhexidine 0.05%; smoking and physical exercise are not allowed for 30 minutes before and during the test. End expiratory samples are collected before the patients drink the test solution—5g of sorbitol in 150/200 ml of tap water—and every 30 minutes for 4 hours using a two-bag system. The two-bag system is a device consisting of a mouthpiece, a T-valve and two collapsible bags, for collection of dead space and alveolar air. From this system, the breath sample is aspirated into a 20 ml plastic syringe. Samples are generally evaluated for H_2 using a model DP Quintron Gas Cromatograph

(Quintron Instrument Company, Milwaukee, WI). It is also possible to measure the hydrogen concentration in each collected sample by a portable breath-hydrogen analyzer (for example, EC60 Gastrolyzer Breath Hydrogen Monitor, Bedfont Scientific Ltd, Upchurch – Kent, England [U.K.]). An increase in H_2 concentration of at least 20 ppm over fasting baseline is considered positive for sorbitol malabsorption. The cut-off for calculating the validity of the test is shifted every 30 minutes, and a Response Operating Characteristics (ROC) curve is plotted on the basis of the obtained results. Results are expressed as parts per million (ppm).

Sorbitol H_2-BT and Celiac Disease

Corazza, et al., in 1988, performed the first study assessing the effectiveness of sorbitol in detecting intestinal damage in celiac disease. They showed for the first time that low dose concentrations of sorbitol (5 grams at 2%) are malabsorbed by almost all celiac disease patients[10], and these results were confirmed in a more recent study[11]. These provocative results led to the idea that it could be used as a screening tool in celiac disease, in addition to serological tests. However, these results have not been completely considered by investigators, and using sorbitol H_2-BT to screen for celiac disease was not investigated further for another four years.

In the 2001 we published a paper about the low-prevalence of anti-gliadin and anti-endomysium antibodies in a sub-clinical/silent form of celiac disease. We found that 5-20% of celiac disease patients affected by this form of the disease lack these antibodies according to histological damage[4], and we found the same results using anti-tTG[12]. Based on this research it was apparent that there was a risk of not properly diagnosing a very high percentage of celiac disease patients if their screening is based solely on serological tests. At this point we tried to use the sorbitol H_2-BT as screening tool to obtain more information on patients' intestinal absorption, and to help select patients who should undergo intestinal biopsy.

Sorbitol H_2-BT in Detecting the Sub-clinical/Silent Form of Celiac Disease

Sub-clinical celiac disease is defined by the presence of a gluten sensitive enteropathy with extra-intestinal symptoms (iron-deficiency anemia, alopecia, recurrent abortion, etc.) but without gastrointestinal symptoms, whereas silent celiac disease is defined by the presence of a gluten-sensitive enteropathy not accompanied by any symptoms, but identified during the course of screening of high-risk groups such as first-degree relatives of celiac patients, patients with insulin-dependent diabetes, Down's syndrome, IgA deficiency and thyroid disorders.

In detecting silent celiac disease sorbitol H_2-BT seems to be better than serological tests. We found that EmA were positive in 77/96 (80.80%) and sorbitol H_2-BT was positive in 94/96 (97.91%) of patients with sub-clinical celiac disease, whereas EmA were positive in 17/27 (62.96%) and sorbitol H_2-BT was positive in 26/27 (96.29%) of patients with silent celiac disease ($p < 0.001$ in both forms of celiac disease). The best cut-off value in ppm and minutes in both forms of celiac disease are higher and shorter in the severe form rather than in the mild form of intestinal damage (respectively $p < 0.001$ in both forms)[13]. Therefore sorbitol excretion seems to be closely correlated with the severity of histological lesions.

Sorbitol H_2-BT as Screening Test in Relatives of Celiac Disease Patients

The prevalence of celiac disease among first-degree relatives has been reported to be about 10-20%, and approximately 50% of the newly diagnosed cases are asymptomatic[14,15]. It is known that lymphoma and cancer deaths[16,17] occur more frequently in first-degree relatives of celiac disease patients, and it is also known that gluten withdrawal has a protective role in the complications associated with the disease[18].

However, up to 50% of celiac disease relatives show mild histological damage without evident mucosal atrophy[19-21]. Since several recent studies showed that serological tests are ineffective in detecting celiac disease in patients with mild histological damage, there is a concrete risk that a significant proportion of celiacs among relatives may be missed. Since a routine intestinal biopsy in all family members is, however, unfeasible— asymptomatic individuals would rarely accept such an approach—it is very important to identify an optimal non-invasive method of screening first-degree relatives. In this regard sorbitol H_2-BT screening seems to be better than serological tests.

In my experience, sorbitol H_2-BT is extremely effective at detecting histological damage in relatives of those with celiac disease. We found that AGA, EmA and anti-tTG showed strong positivity only when there was severe intestinal damage (Marsh IIIb-c lesions—but overall positivity was 36.73%, 38.78%, and 44.89% for AGA, EmA and anti-tTG respectively), whereas sorbitol H_2-BT showed a strong positivity in patients with only mild histological damage (Marsh I-IIIa—overall positivity was 83.67%). *A significant proportion of celiac disease patients will be missed if relatives of those with celiac disease are screened only via serology*[22].

Sorbitol H_2-BT in Assessing Histological Recovery after a Gluten-free Diet

Currently the only effective therapeutic approach to celiac disease is the gluten-free diet, and the result of a proper gluten-free diet is clinical and histological improvement.

In particular, the gluten-free diet plays a key role in preventing nutritional deficiency, especially of micronutrients, and in reducing the risk of the development of intestinal malignancies. There is great demand for highly sensitive, non-invasive tests that can be done to determine histological recovery in patients after the start of a gluten-free diet—with the ultimate goal of reducing or eliminating the need of follow-up endoscopies and biopsies.

If we consider EMA an indicator of small bowel damage, it would be expected to persist until histological recovery occurs. However, several recent studies failed to show a positive relationship between EMA and histological improvement after a gluten-free diet[23-26]. Our study confirmed these experiences, since microscopic damage persists at histological examination during the follow-up despite EMA negativity. It is difficult to explain the poor predictor value of EMA in assessing histological recovery. EMA positivity seems to be related not only to the length of intestinal involvement but also to the grade of histologic damage. Thus, when histological damage improves we can note a false EMA negativity, since histological lesions improve more slowly than EMA seroconversion. Moreover, EMA are a marker of the immunological activity related to the gluten sensitivity, it is therefore hypothesized that after a period of gluten restriction the immunological process can be quite inactive and thus EMA will subside.

Similarly, anti-tTG antibodies do not seem effective to assess histological recovery in the follow-up of celiac patients after they have started a gluten-free diet due to its poor correlation with histological damage. Anti-tTG is generated in genetically predisposed individuals by complexes formed between anti-tTG and gluten[27]. So, it is hypothesize that anti-tTG should disappear soon after gluten withdrawal, and these findings have been frequently recognized in our clinical practice, for example we sometimes see a quick subsiding of anti-tTG values soon after patients begin a gluten-free diet—in some cases within few weeks.

In my experience, sorbitol H2-BT seems to be very effective even in assessing histological recovery after gluten-free diet. We found a strict correlation between cut-off values (in ppm and minutes) of H_2 excretion and the patients' histological lesions. In particular, maximal cut-off values (in ppm and in minutes) correlate statistically with a more severe degree of intestinal damage—patients with more severe histological lesions had higher cut-off value H_2 levels and earlier peaks (in minutes). Likewise, we found that progressive histological recovery correlated significantly with decrease of maximal cut-off values (in ppm) and with the later appearance of the peak (in minutes). This is a very important finding, since it permits us to observe and to monitor the progressive improvement of the histological damage of small bowel after a gluten-free diet—*with-out any small bowel biopsy*[28,29].

Sorbitol H_2-BT in Borderline Entheropathy

A clinical problem arises when patients present with symptoms suggestive of gluten sensitivity (diarrhea, weight loss, unresponsive iron-deficiency anemia, etc.) but small intestinal biopsies reveal only minor abnormalities, particularly lymphocytosis with or without crypt hyperplasia (Marsh I-II lesions). It is hypothesized that some of these patients have borderline celiac disease. A gluten challenge may be a good choice in these patients, as it may provoke a significant worsening of the mucosal lesions, which could lead to a correct diagnosis. This approach, however, may not be necessary if we have a sensitive non-invasive method to detect such mild intestinal lesions. Serological tests are insufficient in this area. We recently found that AGA, EmA and anti-tTG were positive in 0-20% of patients showing Marsh I-II lesions, whereas sorbitol H_2-BT was positive in 18-41% of such cases[30]. Clearly this data shows that it makes sense to use Sorbitol H_2-BT to detect cases of borderline entheropathy.

Factors Affecting Sorbitol H_2-BT in Clinical Practice

Unfortunately, several factors may affect the results of sorbitol H_2-BT. First of all, sorbitol H_2-BT shows high sensitivity but low specificity. Several small bowel disorders, including Crohn's disease, are associated with excessive rates of H_2 breath excretion and then with sorbitol H_2-BT positivity[31]. Moreover, the breath tests will be positive in the setting of not only small bowel mucosal injury, but also in cases of rapid intestinal transit and small bowel bacterial overgrowth[32]. Finally, despite its low cost, the breath test is quite cumbersome, since it requires an overnight fast followed by at least 4 hours of the patient's time for testing.

Conclusion

Sorbitol H_2-BT is a simple, feasible, repeatable, cheap, non-invasive test that can accurately assess intestinal absorption. Unfortunately low specificity may affect the results and may make it difficult for us to distinguish the different causes of malabsorption using only the sorbitol H_2-BT results. On the other hand, sorbitol H_2-BT may be very helpful and seems to be very promising in the following areas:

- Identifying patients suspected of having celiac disease with mild intestinal damage, who are serologically negative for celiac disease;
- Screening relatives of patients with celiac disease;
- Monitoring dietary compliance to the gluten-free diet.

Although intestinal biopsies will remain the "gold standard" for assessing the state of small bowel, sorbitol H_2-BT is a very interesting and non-invasive test that has the potential to reveal just how large the current "black hole" in celiac disease diagnosis is. At the very least it can help diagnose patients whose complaints cause us to suspect celiac disease but who have negative blood tests - and it is an excellent method to monitor the recovery of patients who are on a gluten-free diet. It is a key part of my medical practice in the treatment of celiac disease.

How is Your Heartburn?

By Dr. Ron Hoggan, Ed. D.

Gastro-esophageal reflux disease, or GERD, is the focus of considerable medical attention at the moment. This very old problem has gotten some new attention as it has recently been recognized as a significant factor in some pulmonary diseases[1] and esophageal malignancies[2]. While some sufferers have few or no symptoms of reflux disease, most of us feel at least some degree of discomfort when a mixture of food particles and stomach acids is pushed back up the esophagus where there is less protection from harsh stomach acid. The protection diminishes the further up the esophagus the acid rises, as there is some mucous produced in the lower reaches of the esophagus nearer the stomach. The unprotected tissues further up the esophagus are burned, often causing pain, and sometimes, permanent damage[2].

We need only turn on our television sets to see the frequent and expensive advertising campaigns for the various products available to treat this widespread problem of indigestion and heartburn. If you regularly experience heartburn or indigestion, you may take one of the many drugs that are often prescribed to reduce production of stomach acid. Or you may just take one or more of the over-the-counter remedies such as Tums, Gaviscon, Rolaids, Mylanta, etc. But all of these products, whether prescribed or not, simply mask the symptoms of GERD without addressing the underlying cause.

Many of us who have gluten-induced disease have experienced some degree of relief from GERD symptoms after beginning a gluten-free diet. Prior to my diagnosis of celiac disease, I not only took prescription medications in a vain attempt to control the acidity in my stomach and throat, I also ate a huge quantity of Tums and/or Rolaids every day, all day long. The lucky ones among us experience complete, long-lasting relief from indigestion and heartburn. For those of us who aren't so lucky, the problem may result from one or more of several factors such as smoking, excessive alcohol consumption, or allergic reactions to food.

If you struggle with excess acid production and/or esophageal reflux, it may be the result of your immune system reacting to the contents of your stomach. When such immune reactions are mounted, histamine is released into the stomach, which triggers excessive secretion of gastric acid. If there isn't enough food in the stomach to absorb the acid produced, we begin to feel uncomfortable. We may eat more food to get temporary relief or we may take one or more of the remedies listed above. Weight gain and obesity are predictable results of eating more and more to control stomach acid production. Prescription and non-prescription anti-acid strategies pose a host of other health problems—from inducing vitamin/mineral deficiencies—to compromising the immune protection provided by stomach acids, to putting a lot more sugar into our diets. Whatever we choose, GERD is likely to continue until we address the underlying problem by eliminating allergenic foods from our diet.

The first step in this elimination process is to identify the foods that are triggering an immune response. There are simple, convenient IgG antibody blood tests available to help identify the specific foods that are causing your discomfort. If you are following a gluten-free diet and you continue to experience GERD, you may benefit from this testing. However, if you have been free of gluten for more than a few months, you should not expect these tests to identify any of the gluten grains (Also, such negative results should not be taken to imply that it is safe to return to eating gluten, IgG is only one of the five of this class of antibodies we produce.)

Once the allergenic foods have been identified, they should be strictly removed from your diet for at least six months. You can try re-introducing the offending foods after that time, but some immune reactions may last many years. Even six years after my own IgG food allergy testing, I must still avoid eggs, dairy proteins, and several other foods that were identified back then. The lab where my blood was tested (Immuno Labs, Ft. Lauderdale) provided information on the strength of the immune reaction to each allergenic food. From weak to strong, the reactions were numbered +1 to + 4. This has been very helpful because I was able to re-introduce most foods marked +1 and +2 after about six months.

Whether you follow a gluten-free diet or not, if you are experiencing heartburn and/or indigestion, food allergy testing may be just what you need. It has proven very helpful to my family and me.

To HAIT and Back: The Musings of a Thyroid Patient on the Vagaries of Medical Diagnosis and Treatment in America

By Edward R. Arnold

If it really is true that nobody really wants to see a grown man cry, then certainly nobody would have wanted to hang around me near the onset of a long illness whose mystery would take 14 years to solve.

It began subtly and mildly in 1989, my 43rd year. I had just finished a long and exhausting malpractice suit on behalf of my daughter, an attractive, genetically-normal child who had contracted quadriplegic cerebral palsy in a completely avoidable incident of post-natal asphyxia which had radically changed the nature of life for my spouse and me. By the time 1989 rolled around, I was thoroughly exhausted and carrying a toxic load of anger directed at an incompetent member of the medical profession who had never learned the importance of state-of-the-art skills in a profession that literally has the power of life, death, and disability.

From late 1989 on through 1990, I experienced strange episodes of profound sadness, usually of one to two hours' duration, which became increasingly disruptive to my ability to handle a job and child-care duties. Initially, these episodes seemed to come from nowhere. Later on, I found that playing certain pieces of music of which I was fond, would send me into such intense sobbing that I would be forced to pull over if this occurred while driving.

By the time 1991 rolled around, something was to be added to these periodic bouts of intense sadness. Early in that year, my daughter became very ill, keeping both my spouse and I awake at night for weeks on end. By the time the problem was diagnosed to be a dental infection and dental surgery was done, I had begun to have a sensation of "hollowness", as though I really weren't part of this world, most of the time. In late summer of that year, a series of events in which my subconscious had informed me that a friend had a serious illness, sent me into a final "dive": I simply stopped sleeping more than about two hours per night. When I first stopped sleeping, I soon noticed that even low-level use of alcoholic beverages would further interrupt sleep and throw me into a state in which I couldn't think of anything but how terrible I felt. This state of pronounced alcohol intolerance would continue for 14 years.

The final blow came in November 1991, when I went into a completely disabling panic/anxiety attack that sent me to bed, cowering. I had no alternative but to seek treatment from the psychiatric profession. Unfortunately, the first two psychiatrists prescribed drugs, which either had no effects, or had effects that seemed worse than the problem they were supposed to solve. The third psychiatrist, whom I stuck with for about six months, came up with a treatment plan that was partially effective (but certainly not restorative). I stayed with this psychiatrist until it became clear that his treatment was equivalent to Jefferson Airplane singing "one pill makes you larger, and one pill makes you small". I was being jacked up every morning by a toxic, activating SSRI anti-depressant so I could semi-function, and then dropped by benzodiazepenes every night into a non-restorative twilight sleep state.

In retrospect, the most amazing thing about these first three psychiatrists was that *not one of them ordered any tests of my endocrine function*. Treatment consisted solely of a series of benzodiazepenes, anti-depressants, mood stabilizers, and anti-psychotics, administered in a trial-and-error fashion that yanked my psyche and body chemistry around like a manic pit bull on a two-foot leash.

Throughout the latter part of 1992, I transitioned to care with my primary-care physician, mostly because I trusted him more than any of the psychiatrists I had seen up to that time. He was able to stabilize me with one of the old tri-cyclic anti-depressants, doxepin, along with low doses of Valium. Although doxepin packs a big morning hangover for many who use it, and has very strong anti-cholinergic effects, its ability to put me out at night helped me function satisfactorily for much of the 1990s, even at doses as low as 10mg, once daily in the evening.

In 1993 I consulted a highly recommended psychiatrist, who was the first psychiatrist who actually looked at my thyroid function. When my TSH was measured at 3.5, without also checking my FT3 and FT4, that doctor concluded that thyroid was not my problem. Of course, standards of thyroid diagnosis and treatment have changed radically in the 12 years since. Under the new AACE guidelines, a TSH of 3.5 would now be suspect, because studies of patients with TSH over 3.0 have shown that most progress to hypothyroidism (i.e., TSH greater than 5.5). The new AACE guidelines would mean that further testing and evaluation should be done.

Until the fall of 1997, I continued treatment with doxepin and intermittent Valium, adding the practice of meditation to help calm myself. At that time, I came back to my primary-care physician with the symptom of profound exhaustion on top of the symptoms of insomnia, anxiety, and depression I had suffered for years. Fortunately, my GP was suspicious of thyroid function, and found that my TSH was floating above 8. Since this was well above the old/traditional limit of 5.5, he was ready to start treatment, with (as would be expected of most GPs) T4-only replacement.

I began taking thyroxine (T4) shortly thereafter with high hopes. Initially, the treatment was successful: getting the added thyroxine into my system caused an immediate improvement in quality of sleep.

However, the use of T4 did not turn out to be an unqualified success. After use of T4 for about a month, it was apparent that use of thyroxine alone did not produce a full recovery—I still suffered from anxiety, which the medication seemed to be increasing.

In the meantime, hair loss became an issue. Several years earlier, I had noticed that running my fingers through my hair would produce an unpleasant sensation, almost as though the hair roots were tender. By the time of my 50th birthday, in 1996, I had noticed that my pillow was virtually coated with hair by the time I would remove it for washing. Unfortunately, nobody, including my GP, reminded me that hair loss is a prime symptom of hypothyroidism; and, like most males, I was ready to assume it was plain old male pattern baldness. By the time I was treated correctly and the hair loss stopped, I had pronounced thinning on the crown, which was too advanced to be reversed in response to the treatment of the thyroid problem.

In about 1998, I began experimentation with amino acids, which was to last for almost seven years. I found that use of tryptopan, 5-HTP, and GABA could reduce (but not correct) the worst of my symptoms. In retrospect, though, use of amino acids is a poor substitute for a well-functioning thyroid, as well as being expensive and inconvenient.

By the summer of 1999, I had reached a paradoxical situation. Experimentation had shown that my body needed on the order of 100 micrograms of thyroxine (T4) to keep my TSH down to a reasonable level. Yet taking that much T4 caused intense anxiety, requiring me to use strong sleeping medications. By late summer 1999, I had noticed another distressing symptom—my acute sense of hearing was being increasingly impacted by tinnitus. Evidently, the root cause that drove me into hypothyroidism, could also impact hearing.

It was soon after a household move in the spring of 2000, that I had a partially disabling attack of severe epicondylitis (more commonly known as tennis elbow). It was obvious that my body was no longer able to handle the short-term stresses of the hard physical work required by a move. This obvious physical symptom, accompanied by increasing periodontal and continuing mental issues, prompted me to seek other treatment.

In September 2000, I began seeing a prominent "metabolic" doctor (M.D.) who is well known for his treatment of the metabolic disorders of diabetics. This doctor has written a number of books related to dietary changes and supplements needed to stave off metabolic degeneration as one ages. I was switched to Armour thyroid, and began treatment with other hormones (primarily hydrocortisone in low doses to supplement adrenal function, and pregnenolone). I took an enormous range of nutritional supplements recommended by this doctor, and also made radical changes in diet, which I maintained for nearly two years. Unfortunately, nothing seemed to really work—I did not obtain substantial relief of my symptoms. A thyroid test in Sep 2001 still showed unsatisfactory results—my TSH was 4.7, and my FT3 was below the bottom of the normal range.

By the spring of 2002, I had decided I would have to take my care elsewhere if there were to be progress. After doing a brief telephone consult with a naturopath outside my home state, I began seeing a naturopath in my home town for whom I had obtained very positive recommendations via a web search. By March 2002, the naturopath had informed me that testing showed my hypothyroidism was due to anti-thyroid antibodies, i.e., my body was attacking its own thyroid gland. This condition is officially known as Hashimoto's Autoimmune Thyroiditis (HAIT—as I now know, HAIT is the leading cause of hypothyroidism). I found this discovery quite amazing; how come the three endocrinologists I had seen between 1998 and 2002, had not given me this information? The naturopath started me on Thyrolar (synthetic combination T3/T4) because she said that my body's ability to make T3 might have been compromised by HAIT.

Soon after beginning to see the naturopath, I learned that Dr. Stephen Langer of Berkeley, CA might have additional information on the problem I had been having with thyroid hormone causing anxiety in a hypothyroid patient. I had searched for information about this syndrome in a number of places but found nothing; for instance, the well-known book "Thyroid Solution", by Ridha Arem M.D., contains no information on the condition. So, I consulted with Dr. Langer and learned that a small percentage of people with Hashimoto's are exquisitely sensitive to even low doses of Thyrolar. In fact, the condition is rare enough that virtually no GPs, and only a few endocrinologists, know of its existence. Apparently, it does not have an official name attached to it. I decided to refer to it as "HAIT anxiety syndrome", although there are a few doctors who prefer to refer to any neurological symptoms accompanying HAIT as "Hashimoto's Encephalopathy".

I began to feel a little better between March 2002 and June 2003. I'm not sure why the message about gluten grains had not penetrated before, but by June 2003, the naturopath reminded me again that she had seen a positive result to a test for antibodies to gliadin (one of the two major proteins in gluten grains) in 2002, and that I really should consider removing gluten grains from my diet. This recommendation was based on three factors:

- I had antibodies to the protein gliadin found in wheat and other gluten grains such as rye and barley;
- I had anti-thyroid antibodies which were over the threshold that defines HAIT;
- Medicine really is an experimental science, and this experiment, in spite of its inconvenience, appeared to be worth a try.

In a numbers sense, the response of my anti-thyroid antibodies to the removal of gluten grains from my diet was slow, but gratifying. My thyroperox test started off at 25, dropped to 19 within 6 months, 7 within 10 months, and became zero in less than 2 years. I eventually concluded that the removal of gluten grains from my diet was not all that difficult, partly because I wasn't a celiac who had to worry about that last 1%. I also concluded that removal of gluten would have a positive health effect in terms of the reduced glycemic index of the foods I consumed.

My symptomatic improvement thereafter was not immediate. It soon became obvious that T3/T4 treatment is not an exact science, and the proportion of T3 to T4 needs to be closer to the human body's need, not the pig's need (Both Armour and Thyrolar have the T3/T4 ratio of one part T3 for every four parts T4, typical of the pig's biochemistry). For instance, in late 2003, my TSH had dropped very low, i.e. I had become clinically hyperthyroid due to excess T3 as revealed by a free T3 test. I have since gone through a couple more of these "yo-yo" episodes while being treated, which is a not uncommon event—thyroid treatment is as much art as science.

Cost of treatment also became a problem. By June 2004, I began seeing a highly recommended Physician's Assistant (P.A.), who was known locally to be very good at thyroid treatment, and whose clinic would accept my health insurance. I continued to see the naturopath, although at less frequent intervals, since my insurance (like most) would pay nothing for naturopathy. The P.A. and the naturopath did not completely agree on treatment methods, particularly the use of adrenal supplements (hydrocortisone and DHEA in low/biologic doses) along with thyroid supplements; but they were both in agreement that I should continue to pursue combination T3/T4 therapy. So, I blended recommendations from the two for awhile, transitioning to T3 and T4 in separate tablets of Cytomel and Synthroid, so the percentage of T3 could be altered.

I gradually transitioned off adrenal supplements during 2005, and very gradually increased my T3/T4 supplementation over the course of the year. Finally, by September 2005, I began to realize that I truly had recovered my health—I had episodes of feeling really good again! Still, my sleep was not perfect. I had discovered what Ridha Arem M.D. documented in the book *Thyroid Solution* - a return to the euthyroid state may not immediately eliminate all symptoms. After going to a small dose of the atypical anti-depressant mirtazapine, I finally could feel, every day, like I had in my 30s. Unfortunately, it had taken an agonizing 14 years to get there.

Today, I religiously take my 10 micrograms T3, and 75 micrograms T4, split into two doses each day. I also religiously avoid all traces of gluten grains in my diet because I now understand that the gluey, hard-to-digest proteins in them are a substance which can cause major metabolic disruption. Like the co-author of the book "Dangerous Grains" Ron Hoggan, with whom I have corresponded, I have come to realize that our society's over-use of a potentially toxic substance isn't just dangerous to the 1 in 133 people who have full-blown celiac disease—it can cause a very poor quality of life for the approximately 1 in 5 who have gluten intolerance. I have also come to the realization that, to those few who are unlucky enough to encounter the HAIT Anxiety Syndrome, you may require combination T3/T4 therapy to feel better; and, you may never feel as well as you did when you were young, unless you find a way to stop your immune system from waging war on your thyroid.

Most of all, 14 years after it started, I feel as though a significant part of my life has been taken from me. I was unable get joy or pleasure from life, I was unable to work effectively, and I was unable to be the kind of parent I could have been between my 45th and 59th years of life.

I never imagine that I would be looking forward to the relatively advanced age of 60. However, given that I now feel better than I did at anytime between the ages of 43 and 59, 60 looks like a good place to be.

Summary

In retrospect, the most important things I ended up learning from 14 years of very unpleasant experience are:

If you have psychiatric symptoms, e.g., depression, anxiety, panic disorder, etc., make sure your endocrine system is evaluated, with thyroid testing as the cornerstone. Beware of doctors who offer an antidepressant first thing, without endocrine evaluation.

The emotional/psychiatric effects of hypothyroidism are just as important, and just as damaging, as the physical ones. Unfortunately, many doctors focus on the physical.

If you want to get well, you have to apply all your skills and intelligence to investigating your problem, which most MD's may not understand. You may also have to turn to "alternative" practitioners.

If your TSH is above 3.0, or maybe even 2.5, and your doctor will not do more comprehensive testing (e.g. FT3/FT4), and/or try a test run of thyroid supplementation, find another doctor.

If your doctor diagnoses you as hypothyroid, demand that a test for anti-thyroid antibodies be done. If you have any antibodies, even if they are under the threshold where HAIT is considered to start, get testing for allergy to foods, and testing for allergy to common environmental toxins if food testing reveals nothing. You may find, as I did, that you won't feel as well as possible until you free your body from antibodies.

Endoscopy in Celiac Disease

By Antonio Tursi, M.D.

It has long been known that celiac disease can produce changes in the appearance of small intestine on barium contrast radiographs, one such change being so-called "loss" of duodenal folds. However, over the last two decades it has been recognized that a number of changes in the duodenum clearly associated with celiac disease can be identified endoscopically. Because it is now understood that the manifestations of celiac disease are wide and variable, and that the disease is more common than recognized in the past, the clinical significance of these endoscopic observations has been greatly amplified. Awareness of these endoscopic features may alert the endoscopist to the presence of celiac disease and the need for duodenal biopsies in patients undergoing endoscopy for symptoms unrelated to the disease as well as those with vague, non-specific manifestations.

The well established endoscopic features in the duodenum that are markers for celiac disease include: loss of folds; scalloping of folds; mucosal mosaic pattern; whilst less commonly described findings include a visible vascular pattern and micronodularity in the duodenal bulb.

1. Loss of folds

   "Loss" of folds is defined as an obvious reduction in height or number of folds in the second portion when viewed with maximal air inflation. The sensitivity and specificity of this marker range from 73 to 88% and from 83 to 97% respectively[4,5].

2. Scalloping of duodenal folds

   Scalloping occurs when multiple grooves run over the apex of a duodenal fold. Grooves in the mucosa between folds have also associated with celiac disease and likely a manifestation of the same process that leads to scalloping. The sensitivity and specificity of this marker are 88% and 87% respectively[6,7].

3. Mucosal mosaic pattern

   Mucosal mosaic pattern may be recognized both in the duodenal bulb and in the second portion of the duodenum, and its assessment may be easily performed by chromoendoscopy. Unfortunately, the sensitivity of this marker is quite low (57%)[8].

4. Micronodularity in duodenal bulb

   This marker is quite frequent in childhood and adolescent patients, but it can be also recognized in young adults[9-11].

5. Visible vascular pattern

   This marker describes a prominence of underlying duodenal blood vessels in patients with celiac disease. Unfortunately, this is the least sensitive endoscopic marker in all studies in which it was specifically evaluated[6,12,13].

All these markers are helpful in recognizing celiac disease. Moreover, in some cases specific endoscopic features can be associated with specific histological damage and may be associated with the clinical form of the disease. We found in fact that endoscopic appearance of the duodenum may be predictive of histological damage grading. Moreover, we showed that in a young patient with subclinical/silent celiac disease there is a greater probability of finding slight/mild endoscopic abnormal/mild histological damage[11].

Unfortunately, an endoscopic marker suspected for celiac disease itself is not specific for celiac disease. For example, looking at scalloping, Shah, et al., described 13 cases in which scalloping of duodenal folds was not caused by celiac disease but due to other causes (HIV-related infection, tropical sprue, giardiasis, eosinophilic gastroenteritis)[14].

On the other hand, the presence of one or more endoscopic markers increases the sensitivity and specificity ranging from 87.5 to 94% and from 99 to 100% respectively [12,15].

There is non-existing classification of endoscopic lesions in celiac disease. However, I think that it may be graded according to some simple considerations. Celiac disease is considered a crianial-caudal disease, which affects primarily the proximal segments (first the duodenal bulb and then the second and third duodenal portions) and then the distal segments of the small bowel (first jejunum and then the ileum). Therefore, we may hypothesize that endoscopic damage occurs first in the duodenal bulb and then in the distal tracts of the duodenum. For this reason, and according to other endoscopists in Italy, I proposed the following classification in 2002[11]:

- Slight/mild endoscopic damage: micronodular bulb, granular mucosa of the second duodenal portion, scalloping of duodenal folds, reduction of duodenal folds;
- Severe damage: "mosaic" pattern of the duodenal mucosa, visible vascular pattern, loss of duodenal folds.

The effectiveness of this grading system was confirmed in the same study. In fact we found that the so-called "slight-mild endoscopic damages" seen at endoscopy was associated with a mild-moderate histological damage ($p < 0.005$), while the so-called "severe endoscopic damages" was related to severe histological damage ($p < 0.0005$). Unfortunately, no Consensus Conference on celiac disease has discussed this problem yet.

New endoscopic methods

Several new endoscopic techniques have been recently developed to increase the sensitivity and specificity of endoscopy in diagnosing celiac disease.

"Immersion" technique.

The "immersion" technique consists in observing duodenal mucosa using a high-resolution, high-magnifying (x2) video endoscope that observes the villous architecture with a water film. This approach seems to be effective in allowing the visualization of duodenal villi and the detection of total villous atrophy[16]. A recent study found that this approach is highly accurate in detecting total villous atrophy in suspected celiac cases, and it seems both accurate and cost-sparing to diagnose celiac disease in subjects with marked duodenal villous atrophy, having a sensitivity, specificity, and positive and negative predicting values of 100%[17]. Moreover, this approach also seems to be effective in detecting patchy villous atrophy in celiac patients with patchy lesions[18].

Zoom endoscopy

This technique provides a very impressive magnification capability of x115. This approach may allow the macroscopic detection of unrecognized villous atrophy in patients with unsuspected celiac disease. Badreldin, et al., found recently that zoom endoscopy may be valuable in assessing degree of villous atrophy, having a positive predicting value of 83% and a negative predicting value of 77% in detecting villous atrophy[19].

Double-balloon endoscopy (DBE)

This technique will become probably the best endoscopy technique in investigating small bowel. It allows high-resolution visualization, biopsies and therapeutic interventions in all segments of the GI tract. DBE is a safe and feasible diagnostic and therapeutic tool for suspected or documented small-bowel diseases. However, it requires a long time for small bowel exploration (about 70 minutes from the oral route, and about 90 minutes by the anal route) and requires expertise personnel to obtain better results[20]. At present, the best candidates for the procedure appear to be those with obscure GI bleeding.

Wireless capsule endoscopy

Celiac disease is an inflammatory disease that involves the entire small intestine. Even in the 1960s it was documented, by using peroral biopsies, that the inflammatory atrophic process can extend a variable distance down the small intestine, not uncommonly involving the ileum[21]. These data have recently been confirmed by endoscopic studies that found ileal inflammatory changes predicting villous atrophy in duodenal biopsy specimens [22].

Wireless capsule endoscopy is a new effective and easy method to investigate small bowel. The M2A video capsule endoscope (Given Imaging Ltd; Yokneam, Israel) is a wireless capsule (11 mmx27 mm) comprised a light source, lens, CMOS imager, battery and a wireless transmitter. The slippery outside coating of the capsule allows easy ingestion and prevents adhesion of intestinal contents, while the capsule moves via peristalsis from mouth to anus. The battery provides seven to eight hours of work in which the capsule photographs two images per second (between 50,000-60,000 images all together), which are transmitted to a recorder which is worn on the belt. The recorder is downloaded into a computer and seen as a continuous video film. Since its development, additional support systems have been added, a localization system, a blood detector and a double picture viewer. All of this is intended to assist the interpreter of the film and to shorten the reviewing period.

The full range of indications for CE became apparent with time. The initial device was invented as a better diagnostic tool for small bowel pathologies (such as obscure gastrointestinal bleeding or Crohn's disease[23]). In light of this high specificity for the diagnosis of small bowel diseases, it is considered that capsule endoscopy may be of value in the diagnosis of celiac disease for patients with a positive endomysial or tissue transglutaminase antibody and who are unable to or unwilling to undergo EGDscopy[24]. The very important limit of this new technique in celiac disease is represented by the absence of histological-proven damage. It is recognized that the endoscopic signs of villous atrophy are not sensitive for the lesser degrees of villous atrophy, so partial villous atrophy may be missed by this approach[13].

On the other hand, I think that the patients who appear to be ideal candidates for capsule endoscopy are those patients who fail to respond to a gluten-free diet, or who develop alarm symptoms while on a gluten-free diet. These patients often undergo extensive radiologic, and sometimes, surgical evaluation, because of concern for the development of complications (such as lymphoma[25,26] or ulcerative jejunitis[27]. It is clear that lesions detected by capsule endoscopy in this high-risk group will require further evaluation of these abnormalities through biopsy. Capsule endoscopy may thus be used to select patients to undergo enteroscopy[28] or, more probably in the near future, double-balloon endoscopy[29].

The role of endoscopy in the follow-up of celiac disease

Data on small-intestinal recovery in patients with celiac disease are scarce and contradictory. This is especially the case for adult patients, who often show incomplete histological recovery after starting GFD. On the other hand, there are very few data about the endoscopic recovery on GFD. We recently conducted a two-year prospective study on 42 consecutive adults with newly diagnosed celiac disease. All the patients underwent endoscopy and small-bowel biopsy. A normal endoscopic appearance (absence or mucosal irregular findings, normal duodenal folds) was found in 76.2% after two-year on a GFD. Subdividing the patients according to age, patients aged from 15 to 60 years showed significant improvement within 12 months but faster in patients in patients <45 years, whereas the improvement in endoscopic findings in patients older than 60 years was not statistically significant even 24 months after starting GFD. On the contrary, histological recovery was much slower since only younger patients (5-30 years) showed significant improvement of histology within 24 months[30]. These data showed for the first time that endoscopic recovery is faster than histological recovery after starting GFD.

Conclusion

A number of studies have demonstrated a strong correlation between the endoscopic duodenal findings and celiac disease. Furthermore, absence of specific features suspected from celiac disease does not exclude celiac disease and specimens should always be obtained when there is a suspicion that the disease may be present. For this reason, capsule endoscopy should be not recommended as first endoscopic step in searching celiac disease, but it may be best used to recognize endoscopic recovery and to exclude complication in celiac patients on GFD.

The last question is: How long should we continue with endoscopic and histological follow-up? Looking at the results recently obtained from our group, my advice on follow-up could be summarized as follows: patients aged under 30 years should undergo endoscopic/histological assessment after one year; patients aged 30-45 years should be reassessed after two years; and patients aged 50 years and over should be reassessed after two years, including an immunohistological assessment to exclude refractory celiac disease.

Lung Disease, Celiac Disease, Gluten Sensitivity, and Smoking Tobacco

By Dr. Ron Hoggan, Ed. D.

The association between celiac disease and a range of respiratory diseases has long been recognized[1]. An exploration of the literature on this point brought me several new insights. For instance, I learned that elevated gluten antibodies are also an important risk factor for certain lung disorders. Although celiac disease was only slightly more frequent (one of 29 subjects had celiac disease) a whopping 40% (12 of 29) of patients with sarcoidosis showed gluten sensitivity[2]. I also learned that some researchers are even pointing to celiac disease as an underlying cause of some cases of lymphocytic bronchoalveolitis[3], which is an inflammation that narrows the airways in the lungs. Perhaps the most startling new insight I gained was that despite compliance with a gluten-free diet, patients with celiac disease continue to show signs of a mucosal defect in the lungs[4].

From a personal standpoint, although I experienced asthma and many breathing problems as a child, I have blamed my twenty-five years of smoking cigarettes for the bulk of my lung problems. While I remain confident that this is a large factor in the lung disease I have today, I am also realizing that my celiac disease is a contributing factor. I have made some important strides in improving my lung function as a result of my studies, and it is these that I would like to share with you here.

Although my memory is vague on this point, I'm sure I experienced improvement in my breathing from the celiac diagnosis and subsequent gluten-free diet. I'm also sure that food allergy testing, and subsequent avoidance of additional allergenic foods helped stabilize my breathing to the point where I have rarely experienced breathing crises in the last six years. Nonetheless, I have been limited by a very small capacity for exercise and the predictable losses in conditioning. In the process of researching ketogenic and low carbohydrate dieting for a video I am working on, I chanced upon a reference[5] to a study of healthy women that claimed a 5% increase in peak flow and a 10% improvement in pulmonary function after one week on a low carbohydrate diet[6].

I have now been following a low carbohydrate diet for more than a month. My average peak flow has increased by about 15%. Far more importantly, my tolerance for exercise has increased quite dramatically. Although I still become breathless after vigorous exercise, I can engage in mild to moderate exercise for considerable periods without any breathing difficulty. This constitutes a considerable improvement in my breathing and provides an important increase in the quality of my life.

I realize that smoking is a foolish habit to start. Despite many warnings I continued this habit for many years, until six months prior to my celiac diagnosis. I know I am fortunate in not having contracted any of the deadly diseases caused by smoking. Thus, I take solace in the research that shows that tobacco smoking is a way of self-treating the symptoms of celiac disease[7,8,9]. These publications have helped me deal with the self-recrimination that accompanies the knowledge that I created my own breathing problems. It has also led me to a deeper understanding of the powerful addiction I experienced, the illness I felt after I did finally quit, and the recognition that celiac disease has shaped a great deal of my life.

Gluten's Inflammatory Role in Celiac and Other Chronic Diseases

By Jefferson Adams

Recently, a team of doctors in the Czech Republic conducted a study of the inflammatory action of wheat gluten, and its relation to chronic diseases. Even with all of the research that has been conducted, many of the causes and mechanisms behind inflammatory and autoimmune diseases remain shrouded in mystery. Doctors just don't know what causes most autoimmune diseases or how they actually work. It is assumed that some sort of breakdown occurs in the innate and adaptive immune system that regulates the body's mucous.

On one level this makes a great deal of sense. Epithelial cells make up our skin and the linings of our respiratory, digestive and uro-genital tracts. From the moment we're born, our epithelial cells are in contact with the outside world. Germs, bacteria, and other foreign substances regularly bombard our skin.

Just the simple act of breathing brings dirt, germs, bacteria and other foreign substances in contact with the epithelial cells that line our lungs. Eating and drinking puts dirt, germs and bacteria in contact with the epithelial cells that line the digestive and uro-genital tracts.

It is the job of our mucous membranes, and the mucous they generate, to protect the epithelial cells that line our respiratory, digestive and uro-genital tracts. When the mucous layer fails, the immune system can be stressed. When the immune system breaks down or over-reacts, autoimmune ailments can result. Unlike the multiple layers of epithelial cells that form the protective layers of our skin, just a single layer of epithelial cells protects our uro-genital, respiratory and digestive tracts.

Many people are surprised to learn that the surface area of human skin averages just two square meters in size, while of the lining of the respiratory, digestive and uro-genital tracts average about 300 square meters. Again, these surfaces are mostly covered with just a single layer of epithelial cells. Yet to fend off the millions of microorganisms that regularly bombard them these tissues must be able to tell the bad from the good microorganisms and to keep the bad ones from crossing the epithelial barrier.

Unlike other food proteins, the group of proteins in wheat, known as gliadin, has the ability to cause immune cells to produce cytokines. Cytokines are proteins and peptides that function as signaling compounds. Simply put, they tell other cells what to do.

Inflammatory Activity of Gluten in Chronic Disease

In the case of celiac disease, the presence of wheat protein activates immune cells to produce cytokines that tell the cells lining the intestine to become inflamed as a means of protecting the body against what it sees as a foreign invader.

In the skin, mucosa, and lymphoid tissues there is a highly specialized kind of white blood cell called a dendritic cell. The role of dendritic cells is to initiate a primary immune response by activating lymphocytes and secreting cytokines.

Research has shown that when these dendritic cells are exposed to wheat gliadin, they cause the body to increase the production of cytokines, which in turn triggers inflammation of the mucosal layer. This pattern of activity seems to play an important part in celiac disease.

As stated earlier, this thin epithelial layer is all that protects the body from invasion by harmful intruders. It is also a place where nutrient exchange occurs. In the respiratory tract, oxygen is exchanged. In the digestive tract, nutrients are absorbed. In fact, for nutrients to be absorbed, it is necessary for there to be a degree of permeability in these cell linings.

If they kept everything out, we'd die of malnutrition, or maybe thirst. If they let everything in, we'd likely die of one disease or another. So, the body keeps up a delicate balancing act here. In fact, the body has developed a highly sophisticated system of mechanical and chemical mechanisms whose job it is to protect this single layer of epithelial cells by identifying, degrading and removing intruders, while identifying and permitting beneficial items like nutrients to pass freely into the body for processing.

In healthy folks, this process works very smoothly. The bad stuff is broken down and cleaned out, while the good stuff is permitted to cross the barrier and to carry the proper nutrients to our bodies.

Once we leave the sterile environment of the womb, billions of different bacteria begin to colonize most of our mucosal and skin surfaces. Whether a person is healthy or not, the number of foreign bacterial cells living on and in our bodies far outnumber the cells we have when we are born.

Most of these bacteria are beneficial, with the most beneficial bacteria residing in the gut. In fact, there are so many different kinds, with such high levels of specificity, that scientists haven't yet been able to cultivate all of them. These beneficial bacteria in the gut play an important role in immunity, metabolism, and other activities.

Gluten's Connection to Various Chronic Diseases

A wide range of inflammatory and autoimmune diseases are associated with celiac disease and untreated celiac patients, including a higher risk of complications from anemia, infertility, osteoporosis, and gastrointestinal cancer. Many other disorders are associated with celiac disease, including endocrine diseases like type 1 diabetes, thyroiditis, connective tissue diseases, liver diseases, and Down syndrome, along with nervous system disorders like epilepsy, ataxia, and peripheral neuropathy. One of the strongest associations with celiac disease is autoimmune diabetes. We now know that 5-10% of diabetic patients have celiac disease, a rate more than 5 to 10 times that of the general population. Almost all of these patients improve on a gluten-free diet.

It's unclear why a gluten-free diet might produce improvement in some of these people with these conditions, but one prominent hypothesis is that a percentage of folks with those conditions have compromised gut barriers that somehow permit undigested gluten that provokes an immune response.

An interesting side-note here is that mainstream researchers have recently begun to admit that diabetes, which was previously thought to be "exclusively" endocrine in nature, and heart disease, which was thought to be "purely" circulatory in nature, are both characterized by an inflammation component. In other words, inflammation of tissue, and therefore, of cells, plays an important part in both diseases. Similarly, celiac disease, which was thought to be largely gastrointestinal in nature, is increasingly showing connections to a wide range of disorders that affect nearly every major organ in the body.

Strangely, or perhaps not so strangely in light of this recent evidence, a gluten-free diet seems to have a beneficial effect on a number of chronic diseases in people who are entirely free of celiac disease.

Some patients with psoriasis and urticaria, for example, have shown improvement with a gluten-free diet, as have some patients with cryptogenic ataxia and peripheral neuropathy.

A number of schizophrenics have shown a reduction of symptoms on a gluten-free diet. Also, a number of people with rheumatoid arthritis who observe a vegan, gluten-free diet have reported improvement in their condition.

Animal models have proven to be helpful in better understanding many different diseases and to help create new and more effective treatments. There's a whole specialized area of biology called "Gnotobiology." These people specialize in working in germ-free conditions. Gnotobiologists have developed strains of animals that are reared in germ-free environments.

Imagine if you had never been exposed to any of the harmful or beneficial bacteria that colonize the human body once it leaves the sterile environment of the womb. You would make a great guinea pig for better understanding how disease might work.

Like people, once rats are born, they undergo a profound change. Intestinal micro flora have a major effect on the mucosal immune system. One of the benefits of using gnotobiotic animal models is that researchers can separate the effects of microflora and dietary antigens.

Since scientists know that applying wheat-gliadin to the gastro-intestinal tracts of conventionally raised rats of the AVN strain beginning shortly after birth results in pronounced jejunal changes, that is, celiac-associated lesions, it's beneficial if they can have a "clean" group of rats to test and compare against the conventionally raised rat group to see if there's some kinds of microflora that might provide some protection against celiac disease.

One of the things that the research team discovered is that breastfeeding seemed to be profoundly protective against the adverse effects of wheat gluten.

The research team actually looked at rat pups in which they had induced enteropathy to compare those given breast milk to those handfed on formula. Among other things, they found that rats that were suckled never showed flat mucosa so characteristic of celiac damage when exposed to wheat-gliadin.

It's unclear exactly why this is, though breast milk has so many beneficial elements to it, that it's hard to imagine it not being responsible for a great deal of immune-related development in general. Rat breast milk in particular imparts epidermal growth factor (EGF), which seems to play an important part in of the rat's jejunal cells.

The research team also studied the effects of gliadin in a model system. In fact, the team was able to take a close look at the effects of gluten on cells within the stomach cavities of mice.

In one test, a group of rats received epidermal growth factor via breast milk, while another group received straight formula with no EGF. Both were treated with wheat-gliadin. Rats without EGF showed villous atrophy, while those receiving breast milk, and thus, EGF, were protected against pathological mucosal changes and also against celiac-associated damage.

Basically, it all boils down to several things:

First, it looks very much like the way is paved for the development of celiac disease by the innate immune system when the presence of gliadin promotes functional and phenotypic maturing in dendritic white blood cells, which then leads to the gliadin peptides being presented to certain T lymphocytes, which then trigger the associated inflammation and resulting damage.

The research team concluded that it does, indeed, seem to be the unique structure of gluten and its fragments that provokes the response from the mechanisms of innate immunity. In predisposed individuals, gluten seems to more readily activate an immune response than other proteins like soy protein and egg protein.

Next, breastfeeding seems to offer some protection against gluten intolerance and associated damage.

In many cases, a gluten-free diet brings about improvement in chronic inflammatory and autoimmune diseases.

Lastly, celiac disease is just one of many inflammatory and autoimmune diseases to be associated with the intestinal damage arising from chronic exposure to gluten in gluten-intolerant individuals. Also, many inflammatory and autoimmune diseases show improvement once gluten is excluded from the diet.

CHAPTER 6:
NUTRITION: THE DIETARY, POLITICAL,
AND ECONOMIC BATTLEGROUND

Editor's note:

The pancreas secretes insulin when blood glucose levels rise. Insulin softens cell walls to allow movement of glucose into cells. If our blood glucose is in excess of our current energy needs, the insulin will move glucose into adipose cells to be stored as fat. When our diet is dominated by carbohydrates and our energy needs rise, our cells require more glucose. Thus, eating carbohydrates can start a vicious cycle of excess consumption with some fat storage. Then hunger strikes and we want to eat again. A diet dominated by fats, on the other hand, is unlikely to create this problem. This is primarily due to the reduced production of insulin. This is why a high fat, low carbohydrate diet will cause weight loss. Most readers will already be aware of the flaws in government recommendations that we eat plenty of grains.

Misguided Government Food Guides

By Dr. Ron Hoggan, Ed.D.

The USDA healthy eating guide and the Canada food guide have failed to provide accurate information that will help North Americans to maintain good health. They tout foods that are literally poisonous to people with celiac disease and gluten sensitivity, which amounts to at least 12%[1] and perhaps as much as 42%[2] of the population. And they push dairy products when 2/3 of the world's adult population is lactose intolerant[3] and this latter statistic does not include the many others who have allergies to dairy proteins. If our government agencies can be that far wrong, how useful are the rest of their dietary recommendations? In brief, they are useless to those who wish to promote longevity and good health through diet as has been reported in the large nutritional studies by Walter Willet et al. at Harvard[4] (more on this later). These political documents are little more than reflections of the powerful maneuvering of competing

177

and complimentary industries and economic forces with enormous vested interests in maintaining the status quo in our food supply. And these forces have been exercising their influence since the very first USDA food guide was published in 1898, when the first Canada Food Guide was published in 1942, and with every subsequent revision of each of these documents.

The discerning reader will notice that these food guides look more like promotional literature than objective recommendations. Yet both government bodies that publish and support these healthy eating guides firmly insist that they are valuable, science-based instructions for their respective citizens to follow. Conversely, a massive, long-term study of diet and chronic disease among more than 67,000 female health care workers, conducted at Harvard University over a period of 12 years, has clearly discredited such claims[4]. We can also challenge these claims on a purely logical level.

From an historical perspective, current nutritional claims from the USDA and Health Canada were first published in 1898 and 1942, respectively. The minor changes since 1933 in the U.S.D.A. guide and since 1942 in Canadian guide have brought little meaningful change. Thus, this information was first published decades before much of the modern scientific evidence was available to support or refute these faulty claims. Surely, once a governmental body has issued such strident 'healthy eating guides' they have a vested interest in maintaining the general thrust of their recommendations. And that is exactly what appears to have happened. Despite the plethora of discrediting research data, revisions to recommendations from the USDA and Health Canada, over the last 65-75 years, are little more than cosmetic, except for their concessions to special interest groups and other dietary dictocrats.

Examination of relevant, up-to-date scientific research shows a preponderance of discrediting evidence for two large food groups that are not just endorsed by these food guides. They push dairy and grains on us as health-promoting dietary necessities.

There is also considerable evidence that debunks the anti-fat bias of these guides. For instance, one report of a study of almost 20,000 post-menopausal women who followed a low fat diet over a period of 12 years showed that a diet low in fats and high in fruits, vegetables and grains did not significantly reduce the risk of heart disease, stroke, or cardiovascular disease[5].

I will not waste your time citing and quoting from the many congruent studies. Neither will I claim that there are no reports that support these guides. Nonetheless, there can be little doubt that North Americans are becoming more and more obese and are dying of cardiovascular disease and cancers at alarming rates despite our finely honed (and very expensive) medical systems that increase longevity through thwarting deadly injuries and infections. The primary problem is that dietary recommendations are really just political instruments and are not based on current scientific insight.

Our diets are abysmally unhealthy. Each step we take that brings us closer to the dietary recommendations of our government agencies moves us further away from the good health we seek. In my own desperation, just prior to my celiac diagnosis, I was eating bran muffins every morning, on my doctor's recommendation, and getting sicker and sicker.

Many of us with celiac disease and gluten sensitivity have been forced to re-evaluate food guide recommendations and go in search of meaningful, valid data that will help guide us to a healthier diet. Yet such individual quests are both inefficient and fraught with hazards. We need our elected representatives to set aside political and economic concerns and bring the clout of their elected offices to bear on this question. Dietary recommendations need to be based on solid science and examination of the data from both sides of conflicting views. The one-sided myopic views of special interest groups and those with vested interests in the current dietary guides need to be set aside in favor of a genuine search for answers for those of us who count on our elected leaders to exercise prudent judgment – not self-interest.

Why is Gluten Sensitivity Trivialized?

By Dr. Ron Hoggan, Ed.D.

Many individuals with celiac disease express frustration and disappointment with the cavalier attitudes and misinformation they encounter. The objective observer may wonder what our complaint is with uninformed medical practitioners. Is it the lengthy delays to diagnosis coupled with our many years of unnecessary suffering? Is it the unnecessarily premature death of one or more of our loved ones, which may have been prevented by a greater awareness of celiac disease and its many manifestations? Is it the common refusal of appropriate testing for celiac disease due to outdated perceptions of this disease? Is it the oft-heard cynicism about our diet expressed by those who have little or no experience with it? Perhaps all of these complaints contribute to the angst so often found in our community. However, I am beginning to suspect that these complaints are merely symptoms of a more sinister problem. Perhaps the underlying problem is the trivializing of gluten sensitivity and celiac disease.

I have been told, by medical pundits, that people with celiac disease are still alive to be diagnosed after many years of suffering. They go on to say that other, more important ailments must be ruled out earlier in the diagnostic process. Our symptoms, I've been told, are simply uncomfortable—not deadly.

I have also been laughed at by some of these same individuals for suggesting that neurological, psychiatric, and many autoimmune diseases can result from undiagnosed and untreated celiac disease and gluten sensitivity.

Some physicians claim that, given our awful diet, people need a powerful motive to follow it. Hence, painful or uncomfortable symptoms are useful prior to investigating celiac disease because they increase the likelihood of dietary compliance.

There is some validity to each of these excuses. It is an inconvenient diet that some celiacs ignore. Most of us do survive for decades without a diagnosis. But a pervasive, underlying theme of minimizing and dismissing celiac disease may reflect a set of preconceived notions that are deeply imbedded in our collective consciousness. As a culture, we celebrate grains as the very foundation of civilization. We learn from our earliest question about cereals that they are "good" for us. They make us strong and healthy.

Equally, almost 200 years ago, his colleagues in obstetrics "knew" that the obstetrician, Ignaz Semmelweiss, was just being silly with his pre-occupation with "invisible atomies" which he thought were spreading infections from one patient to another. Physicians were proud of their puss-infested, blood-soaked smocks. These stains attested to their hard work and dedication. The hospital staff under Semmelweiss' supervision participated in his research. They washed their hands with carbolic soap between each patient examination—and the frequency of child-bed fever dropped to a tiny fraction of the previous rate. Nonetheless, at the end of the study, Semmelweiss' ideas were dismissed and mocked as silly notions about "invisible atomies," and hand-washing came to a stop.

Today, with the benefit of microscopes and the widespread acceptance of the germ theory, Semmelweiss' "invisible atomies" are a concept that is quite easy to accept, even for elementary school students.

In another hundred years, scientists may look back on our ideas about cereals with a similar sense of superiority. The scientific evidence that condemns the foundation of our food pyramid is solid and credible. Despite that evidence, our cultural indoctrination continues to shape the thoughts and actions of those we trust to advise us on health issues. Perhaps cereals will someday be seen as a sinister conduit of disease. In the meantime, it is a challenge for us to be patient with those who continue to genuflect at the altar of cereal grains.

Mad Cows and Celiac Patients Share a Common Plight

By Ron Hoggan, Ed. D.

Just as "bovine spongiform encephalopathy," better known as mad cow disease, is thought to result from feeding infected animal parts to cattle, gluten sensitivity, dermatitis herpetiformis, celiac disease, and a host of autoimmune diseases result from feeding grains to humans. Cattle are better equipped to eat grains and we are better equipped to eat meats. And when we step outside the evolutionary food sources that shaped us, we can expect some problems—sometimes very serious problems.

Let's start by comparing human and ruminant digestive processes. Cows, for instance, have a stomach that is divided into four chambers. When grazing, cattle eat large quantities of food. They mix it with saliva and form it into boluses that they can swallow. After these boluses have been "worked on" by the micro-organisms in the first and second chambers of their four-part stomach, cattle regurgitate and chew them further, preparing them for return to the cow's stomach where much of this feed may remain for up to 5 days of further digestion. In the final chamber of the stomach, acids are secreted to aid further digestion.

Cattle spend more than 12 hours a day chewing their food. They produce more than five gallons of saliva every day, and they even utilize fermentation as part of their digestive process. The size of their digestive tracts is disproportionately large compared to that of humans. Although many infectious agents can gain entry with feed, the cow relies on the competitive advantage enjoyed by the friendly bacteria in their intestines.

By comparison, humans process food very rapidly, typically taking less than 24 hours of transit time, from mouth to anus. We have only one chamber in the stomach and a comparatively short digestive tract. Our digestive tract is the site of a large number and variety of immune processes aimed at protecting us from invading microbes.

About 10,000 years ago, humans began a dietary experiment. They started eating grains in enough quantity to warrant cultivation. Nobody knew, back then, what caused sickness or dental cavities, or even what caused people to be shorter or taller. It was not until the twentieth century that archaeologists made the connection and we began to realize that wherever grains were cultivated, within a generation or two, people became shorter by 5 or 6 inches, they also developed considerable dental cavities and bone disease.

Because the remains are only skeletal, we can't really tell what other diseases most early farmers suffered. However, archaeologists and other scientists have reported a host of evidence from Egyptian mummies indicating that this grain-dominated culture experienced considerable cardio-vascular and autoimmune disease. We also know that hunter-gatherers who consume no grains also show no signs of such diseases.

At the October, 2003 CSA/USA conference in Buffalo, Dr. Martin Kagnoff mentioned that we humans simply do not make the digestive enzymes necessary to fully digest some of the proteins found in gluten-containing grains. Just as we have been coming to realize the fallacy of dietary recommendations that encourage humans to eat grains, we have developed some other problematic economies in our food supply. For a variety of reasons, we started feeding cattle dietary protein that was largely made from the waste products of butchering other cattle. It is difficult to imagine a more effective means of communicating disease from one animal to the next.

Recently outlawed, this practice has been altered. Now, it is perfectly acceptable to feed animal parts from poultry and other species of slaughtered animals, but we are no longer allowed to feed cattle animal proteins from other cattle because it might contain the toxic prions that are implicated in Mad Cow disease.

As a consumer of beef, I am appalled at the foolishness of these "adjustments" in feeding practices for cattle. As a celiac, I am equally appalled by the continued practice of advising humans to eat enormous quantities of grains. Look at any of the food guides published by various governments of industrialized nations. I can find no part of it that is of, by, or for the people. Just as humans are not well equipped to eat grains, cows are ill equipped to eat meats. The first priority of our food scientists, producers, and our government eating guides, should be the good health of the general population.

National Institutes of Health Consensus Conference on Celiac Disease—A Historic Event

By Shelley Case, B.Sc., RD

It is well known within the celiac community that health professionals, especially physicians and dietitians, are relatively uniformed about celiac disease, including the incidence, presentations, diagnostic testing and management. As a result, many people go undiagnosed and/or misdiagnosed. A significant number also develop complications such as osteoporosis, other autoimmune disorders or lymphoma.

To address these issues, the National Institute of Diabetes and Digestive and Kidney Diseases (NIDDK) and the Office of Medical Applications of Research (OMAR) of the National Institutes of Health (NIH) sponsored a consensus conference to examine and assess the current scientific knowledge regarding celiac disease. Dr. Stephen James, Director, Division of Digestive Disease and Nutrition, NIDDK and 25 medical, government and other experts including Dr. Alessio Fasano, Dr. C. Kelly, Dr. Joseph Murray and Elaine Monarch (Celiac Disease Foundation) were members of the planning committee for the Consensus Conference on Celiac Disease which was held June 28-30, 2004 in Bethesda, MD. The conference addressed six key areas:

1.   How is celiac disease diagnosed?
2.   How prevalent is celiac disease?
3.   What are the manifestations and long-term consequences of celiac disease?
4.   Who should be tested for celiac disease?
5.   What is the management of celiac disease?
6.   What are the recommendations for future research on celiac disease and related conditions?

Invited speakers included celiac experts (17 physicians and two dietitians) from the United States, Canada, England and Finland. Each speaker was assigned a specific topic to present for 20 minutes followed by a short question period from the audience and a 13 member independent panel. The panel consisted of practitioners and researchers in gastroenterology, pediatrics, pathology, internal medicine, endocrinology, a dietitian, a geneticist, and a consumer representative. After reviewing all the scientific evidence and speaker presentations, the panel prepared a consensus statement answering the six key questions. On the third day of the conference the draft statement was presented to the audience and speakers, who then had an opportunity to provide comments and ask questions. Further revisions were made and several hours later the final document was read during a press conference. The final document, speakers' abstracts, an extensive bibliography and the three day video presentations are all available at http://consensus. nih.gov/cons/118/118cdc_intro.htm.

A Speaker's Perspective

I was honored to be one of the speakers at this historic conference. The challenge we faced as speakers was to condense a large volume of information and present it to the panel in only 20 minutes. For those who know me and have heard me speak, you will understand I was up to that challenge! Nevertheless it was a pressure-packed experience speaking in front of a prestigious panel, a large audience watching in person and on the video web cast around the world. As our presentations could have a major impact on the panel's final recommendations, it was crucial that we convey the most current and relevant information—not only in the oral presentation—but also in a written submission that is to be included in the abstract and in an in-depth article that will be compiled in a special supplement on celiac disease in *Gastroenterology*, a major medical journal.

In addition to the formal presentations made by the speakers and many members of the celiac community, those who attended this conference also had opportunities to network and share ideas, which was extremely valuable. Discussions about effective ways to disseminate all the excellent information from this conference to health professionals, people with celiac disease, and the media, was a common topic. The management of celiac disease and organizational structure of celiac organizations in other countries and the issue of oats were also discussed.

As I reflect on this event, along with the work of the American Celiac Task Force, I'm amazed and encouraged to see what can be accomplished when government, health professionals, members of the celiac community, and others, join together to pursue common goals—greater awareness, earlier diagnosis and better management of celiac disease. The Canadian Celiac Association's motto is "Together We're Better" and I believe we must continue to work together in order to be effective and reach that goal!

Could Wheat be Making You Ill? Gluten Sensitivity: A Common Unrecognized Cause of Illness

By Dr. Scot Lewey

Do you suffer from symptoms of abdominal pain, stomach aches, excess bloating, gas, diarrhea, fatigue, bone or joint pain, skin rashes, headaches, difficulty concentrating or irritability? Gluten, the major protein in wheat, barley and rye causes these symptoms in many people but most, including their physicians, are unaware that gluten is the cause and that a gluten-free diet may relieve these symptoms. Though there are diagnostic blood tests available for identifying gluten sensitivity, these tests have limitations. Many physicians are unaware these blood tests are available, including genetic tests for the risk. Most physicians are also unaware of the broad manifestations of gluten sensitivity and fail to order tests that could diagnose the cause. Sadly, the condition often goes unrecognized and untreated when it is very common and reversible by simply following a gluten-free diet. No medications or surgery are required.

Worldwide nearly 1 in 100 people have the most severe form of gluten sensitivity or intolerance known as Celiac disease though it is estimated that more than 90% are undiagnosed. Startlingly, many more than this - possibly 10-30% of people of northern European ancestry - have lesser forms of gluten sensitivity causing symptoms that will improve on a gluten free diet. The low carbohydrate diets have become popular because many have lost weight but they also frequently experienced dramatic improvements in general feeling of well being, increased energy, relief from fibromyalgia, joint aches, improved skin, fewer headaches, and improved digestive symptoms. However, many fail to gain full benefit because they don't know they are gluten sensitive and have not completely eliminated gluten from their diet since gluten is present in so many foods that we eat.

Gluten is insulinogenic, meaning it stimulates insulin release, and thereby promotes weight gain. Abnormal blood sugar regulation also often occurs. Some people will gain weight despite malabsorbing essential nutrients. It is now known that more than 10% of insulin dependent diabetics have celiac disease. What is not yet known is whether the celiac came first or the diabetes, but that they commonly occur together. Celiac disease is also commonly associated with other autoimmune conditions such as lupus, rheumatoid arthritis and thyroid problems. Celiac disease is a reversible cause of infertility, low birth weight infants, pre-term labor, and recurrent miscarriages. Untreated it is associated with a significantly increased risk of numerous cancers including all GI cancers and lymphoma. It is a common cause of unexplained anemia especially from iron deficiency and causes premature osteoporosis. Dietary elimination of gluten allows the intestine to heal so that absorption is normalized and symptoms are relieved. After five years of a gluten-free diet the cancer risk returns to normal as long as the individual remains gluten-free for life.

Classic celiac disease is diagnosed by abnormal blood tests and an abnormal intestinal appearance on biopsy. Blood tests for celiac disease include antibody tests for gliadin (AGA), the toxic fraction of gluten; endomysial antibodies (EMA); and tissue transglutaminase antibody (tTG). High antibody levels to EMA and tTG are generally accepted as diagnostic for celiac disease though some individuals with celiac disease and most with lesser degrees of gluten sensitivity may have normal levels. AGA levels have, in the past, been considered very sensitive but not specific for celiac disease. Newer assays for AGA antibodies for gluten that has undergone a chemical change called deamidation that appears to be more specific for celiac disease (Gliadin II, Inova) may be as or more accurate than EMA and tTG antibody tests.

However, lesser forms of gluten intolerance may be missed when any of these blood tests are normal or borderline and/or small intestine biopsy is normal or indeterminate. Stool antibody testing for antigliadin and tTG has been performed in research labs and published in a few studies. The commercial lab, Enterolab, now offers these tests though the former research gastroenterologist Dr. Ken Fine, who patented the test, has yet to publish the results of his findings in a peer reviewed journal. His unpublished data and the clinical experience of some of us who have used his test have indicated the tests are, to date, 100% sensitive for celiac disease. They are highly sensitive for gluten sensitivity of lesser degrees before blood tests or biopsies become abnormal but when symptoms exist. These symptoms reverse on a gluten-free diet instituted by those with abnormal stool antibody levels.

Small intestine tissue obtained by biopsy during upper gastrointestinal endoscopy has been considered the "gold standard" for the diagnosis of celiac disease since the 1950s. However, recent studies have demonstrated that some people with gluten sensitivity, especially relatives of celiacs with few or no symptoms, may have changes from gluten injury in the intestine that can only be seen on a small intestine biopsy with special stains not routinely used, or on electron microscopy done in the research setting. Immunohistochemistry stains can detect increased numbers of specialized white blood cells called lymphocytes in the intestinal lining tips or villi as the earliest sign of gluten induced injury or irritation. Electron microscopy also reveals very early ultrastructural changes in some individuals when all other tests are normal. According to published research, when people are offered the option of gluten-free diet based on these abnormalities they have usually responded favorably, whereas those who continued to eat gluten often later developed classic celiac disease.

What these studies suggest is that a "normal small intestine biopsy" may exclude celiac disease as defined by strict criteria but it does not exclude gluten sensitivity, a fact appreciated by many individuals who ultimately started a gluten-free diet based on their symptoms, family history, suggestive blood test or stool antibody test(s). Those few physicians who appreciate the concept of the spectrum of gluten intolerance or sensitivity are outnumbered by the medical majority that continues to insist on strict criteria for the diagnosis of celiac disease before recommending a gluten-free diet.

Physicians either unfamiliar with the research on celiac or who are holding onto the strict criteria for celiac as the only indication for recommending a gluten free diet unfortunately often leave many gluten sensitive individuals confused or frustrated. Some seek answers on the Internet or from alternative practitioners. Many have their diagnosis missed, challenged, or dismissed. Others are misinformed or receive in-complete information. As a result many may fail to benefit from the health benefits of a gluten-free diet because they are advised that it is not required because they have normal blood tests and/or normal biopsies.

Another source of confusion lies in the knowledge that certain genetic patterns are present in over 90% of individuals with celiac disease. Testing for such specific blood type patterns on white blood cells known as HLA DQ2 and DQ8 is increasingly em-ployed to determine if a person carries the gene pattern predisposing to celiac disease. Some use the absence of these two patterns as a way of excluding the possibility of celiac disease and the need for testing or gluten-free diet. However, there are rare reports of classic Celiacs who are DQ2 and DQ8 negative. Moreover, recent studies indicate other DQ patterns may be associated with gluten sensitivity though very unlikely to predispose to classic celiac disease.

Testing for all the DQ patterns has been advocated by Dr. Fine based on his experience with stool antibody testing that has revealed that the other DQ types are associated with elevated levels, symptoms, and positive response to gluten-free diet. According to his unpublished data, all the DQ types except DQ4 are associated with a risk of intolerance to gluten. Testing for the DQ types allows a person to determine if they carry one of the two high risk gene types for celiac disease or the other "minor" DQ type associated with gluten sensitivity but low risk for celiac disease.

Enterolab also offers the stool testing for gliadin antibodies and tissue transglutaminase antibodies as well as several other stool tests for food intolerance or colitis. Though not widely accepted, these tests have gained favor with the lay public as an option for deter-mining sensitivity to gluten or other food proteins, either despite negative blood tests and/or biopsies, or in place of the more invasive tests. Most recommend the accepted blood tests and small bowel biopsy for confirmation of celiac. The favorable reports in the lay community have been overwhelmingly positive though they can't be subjected to peer review by the medical community prior to the publication of Dr. Fine's data.

Physicians open to the broader problem of gluten sensitivity are reporting these tests helpful in many patients suspected of gluten intolerance with negative blood tests and/ or biopsies, though some are not certain how to interpret the tests. The national celiac organizations have difficulty commenting on their application without published re-search though a recent article in the British Medical Journal did show stool tests highly specific for celiac. Dr. Fine's has publicly commented that his unpublished data demonstrates those with abnormal stool tests indicating gluten sensitivity overwhelmingly respond favorably to a gluten free diet with improvement of symptoms and general quality of life.

There is no agreed-upon definition for gluten sensitivity or intolerance, especially for those who do not meet the strict criteria for celiac disease yet may have abnormal tests and/or symptoms that respond to gluten-free diet. Those individuals become confused when they realize that because they aren't diagnosed with celiac disease, they don't know where to turn for more information. Consensus in the medical community on definitions and more research in this area are greatly needed.

Under my Doctor's Nose—But Diagnosis Missed

By Prof. Rodney Ford M.B., B.S., M.D., F.R.A.C.P.

Oh dear! This week I met three parents in my clinic who are quite annoyed. Perhaps infuriated is more accurate. All three families have a child who has been unwell for years. All three children had blood tests done over the last two years by another pediatrician—these tests showed high levels of gluten antibodies (a high IgG-gliadin level) which was ignored.

Anna is nine years old. She is now gluten-free and is better: she sleeps all night, has no tummy pains, has more energy and she is enjoying life again. She is strictly gluten-free. Even small amounts of gluten upset her tummy. She says: "I feel good!"

Previously, she had tummy pains since two years of age. However, over the last few months everything got worse with very bad tummy pains and more diarrhea. Two years ago she had a blood test which showed high gluten antibodies—IgG gliadin 72 (usually less than 20 units). But her pediatrician ignored this result .

When I saw Anna I repeated her blood tests: she had persistently high gluten antibodies (IgG gliadin 60) but no evidence of celiac disease (a normal tTG).

Her parents, with a sense of irritation said: "Obviously, her diagnosis under the nose of our previous doctor, so why did he miss it? Why didn't he suggest going on a gluten-free diet at that stage? It would have stopped Anna having another two years of suffering! How frustrating! Why don't more doctors know about this diagnosis?"

Emma

I unscrambled Emma's illness recently. She is eight years old. Emma's mum sent me this thank you card:

"Dear Dr Ford, We just want to say a BIG THANK YOU for all you have done for us! Emma has been pain free from her gluten free diet! All of us are now gluten-free and we feel more energized and happier in our tummies! Your information has also helped some of my friends! Keep going and keep informing people about this important information. Thank you so, so much.

PS: Hopefully we won't have to see you again!"

Emma had been seen by another pediatrician two years ago who did blood tests showing very high IgG-gliadin antibodies at 91 units (should be less than 20) a normal tTG, and the genes associated with celiac disease (DQ2/DQ8) were not detected.

My repeat tests showed that her gluten antibodies were still very high (IgG-gliadin 86). She showed a dramatic response to the gluten-free diet. Her tummy pains and lethargy melted away. She is now a happy, vibrant eight-year-old, and with grateful parents.

Dan

Perhaps Dan's story is the saddest. He is now 12 years old. He has had constipation and leaky poos for more than five years. He smells. He is embarrassed that he has accidents in his pants. School is difficult. His parents are exasperated that Dan seems to have no control of his bowels. Dan is depressed and anxious about his terrible situation.

Yet again he was assessed by another pediatrician a few years ago. His gluten antibodies were sky high (IgG-gliadin of 94) but ignored because he had no evidence of celiac disease. Dan had to go through a lot of "behavior modification" therapy, but with no benefit—it only made him more anxious and withdrawn.

Yes, you guessed it. His repeat blood tests confirmed a gluten problem. And yes, within a few weeks of going gluten-free he is now in control of his bowels—at long last. He can now give me a smile. He has the gluten syndrome and has suffered years of unnecessary pain and embarrassment. His parents had labeled him as lazy, naughty and manipulative. He was being lined up for some more psychotherapy. Oh Dear!

Please help these children!

I often feel moments of sadness and frustration in my clinic. I hear similar stories every day. I see parents crying with relief that the answer has, at last, been found. I also see families who are angry. A gluten-free remedy is so simple and benign, yet it has not been suggested despite elevated IgG gliadin antibodies.

This complacently and blindness causes unnecessary suffering. Many of my medical colleagues continue to ignore gluten sensitivity. They are in denial. They attribute the response to a gluten-free diet to a placebo effect. They undermine their patients through telling them to go back to eating gluten because they do not have celiac disease.

The way forward is for the gluten-free community to keep spreading the word: that gluten can cause a great deal of harm to many people and it needs to be considered as a front line diagnosis. The good news is that this year some researchers in the big Celiac Foundations and Celiac Research Institutes in the USA are starting to research gluten-sensitivity. At last Gluten Syndrome is being taken seriously. We need to help all of the Annas, Emmas and Dans of this world.

CHAPTER 7:
CONTENTIOUS ISSUES WITHIN THE
GLUTEN SENSITIVE/CELIAC COMMUNITY

Who Should Follow a Gluten-free Diet?

By Dr. Ron Hoggan, Ed.D.

As you have already seen, there are many contentious issues within and regarding the celiac and gluten sensitive community. Perhaps the most contentious issue within the GS/celiac community is the question that has also been raised by some members of the media. The question asks: "who should follow a gluten free diet?" The diet has been labeled a "fad" diet by many of these members of the media[1, 2]. Implicit support of this unfortunate notion comes from some prominent members of the celiac research community who suggest that only those with biopsy proven celiac disease should follow a gluten free diet. It is therefore not surprising to see reporters who, working in the popular media, mock and deride the gluten free diet as a silly fad that has a placebo effect on those who follow it[1]. While I view this perspective as silly, it is made more contentious by the medical specialists who support it, thus making it clear that this topic warrants thorough discussion.

Historically, Dr. Willem Karel Dicke began treating celiac patients with a gluten free diet in 1936, based on the comments of a concerned mother expressed in 1932. By 1937 he was convinced, by patient recoveries, of the value of a gluten free diet for celiac patients[3]. While European gastroenterologists and pediatricians accepted Dr. Dicke's work fairly quickly, it would take years of mockery and derision before the gluten free diet would be accepted internationally, especially in the U.S.A. It was not until the early 1960s that the international medical literature reflected acceptance of this diet[4] and acceptance among gastrointestinal practitioners took decades longer.

Today, the gluten-free diet is accepted as the treatment of choice for celiac patients. Acceptance of the same diet for treatment of dermatitis herpetiformis (also known as Duhring's disease) a skin disease commonly found among celiac patients is far from complete among dermatologists even today. Some dermatologists, despite widely reported increases in risk of deadly cancers in association with the consumption of gluten among those with dermatitis herpetiformis (DH) continue to treat this gluten-induced skin condition with prescriptions for Dapsone, a drug which, unlike a gluten free diet, does not reduce the risk of malignancy in these patients.

I have listened to a presentation by one such dermatologist wherein he pointed to various difficulties with the diet to justify his failure to even suggest a gluten free diet to his patients with dermatitis herpetiformis[5]. While these patients may feel that the complications of a gluten free diet are preferable to those of malignancy, they are never given the information that would let them make their own choice in this matter. This particular presenter focused on the "unpleasant taste" of gluten free foods as his primary justification for not recommending a gluten free diet to DH patients.

More recent work has shown that a gluten free diet can, after many months of strict compliance, abolish anti-islet cell and anti-thyroid antibodies[6]. While gluten may not be an underlying factor in all cases of these diseases, it is certainly therapeutic in at least some of these individuals.

Similarly, some non-celiac, gluten sensitive individuals have been reported to experience relief from seizures on a gluten free diet[7].

Marios Hadjivassiliou, et al., have also reported that more than half of their cases of neurological disease of unknown origin have elevated anti-gliadin antibodies, while only a fraction of these have celiac disease[8]. Thus, non-celiac gluten sensitivity is associated with a wide range of neurological disease that rivals that associated with celiac disease.

Many of the gastrointestinal complaints of those with non-celiac gluten sensitivity are also alleviated by a gluten free diet[9]. Some researchers have begun to assert that celiac disease can serve as an instructive model for other forms of autoimmunity[10].

There can be little doubt that those with celiac disease are not the only individuals who can benefit from a gluten free diet. Articles by Dr. Rodney Ford, Dr. Scot Lewey, and others in this chapter make it clear that a gluten free diet can be therapeutic where an open mind and the patients' best interests are prevalent. Further evidence comes from several other sources including the high rate of cancer and mortality among gluten sensitive non-celiac patients[11]. Still other research is showing that it is the zonulin and leaky gut (and hence, gluten sensitivity) that may be conferring the increased risk of cancer and autoimmunity on celiac patients[12].

Editor's note:

What follows is the clearest, most accessible explanation of genetic testing and fecal antibody testing that I've read.

Celiac Disease Versus Gluten Sensitivity: New Role for Genetic Testing and Fecal Antibody Testing?

By Dr. Scot Lewey

Celiac disease has a prevalence of 1 of 100, or 1% of the general population. Between 90-99% of celiacs are HLA DQ2 and/or DQ8 positive. Every individual has two DQ serotypes. Because the molecular HLA nomenclature can be confusing DQ serotyping is a method for simplifying the results. There are four major types and 5 subtypes: HLA DQ1, DQ2 from each parent.

Though 35-45% of individuals of Northern European ancestry are DQ2 and/or DQ8 positive only 1% has classic celiac disease as defined by abnormal blood tests and small intestinal biopsies. Several autoimmune conditions also occur more frequently in DQ2 and DQ8 who are positive for DQ3 and DQ4. DQ1 has two subtypes - DQ5 and DQ6, whereas DQ3 has three subtypes - DQ7, DQ8 and DQ9. Each individual has two copies of HLA DQ. One DQ type is inherited from each parent of these individuals.

There is accumulating scientific evidence that many individuals are gluten sensitive and respond to a gluten free diet though they have normal blood tests and/or normal intestinal biopsies (fail to meet strict criteria for celiac disease). This is commonly being referred to as non-Celiac gluten sensitivity (NCGS). Many individuals who have NCGS are relatives of confirmed celiacs and were previously referred to as latent celiacs. Electron microscopy and immunohistochemistry studies of individuals with normal biopsies but suspected of or at risk (1st degree relatives of celiacs) have revealed ultrastructural abnormalities of the intestine and those who chose a gluten free diet usually responded and many who did not ultimately developed abnormal biopsies on long term follow-up. Seronegative celiac has also been recognized. That is, blood tests are negative, but the biopsy reveals classic abnormalities of celiac and the individual responds to a gluten free diet.

Fecal antibody testing for gliadin (AG) and tissue transglutaminase (tTG) tests by Enterolab in Dallas has revealed elevations in 100% of celiacs tested and up to 60% of symptomatic individuals without Celiac disease (NCGS) even if not DQ2 or DQ8 positive. (Fine, K unpublished data, http://www.enterolab.com). The only DQ pattern he found not associated with gluten sensitivity is DQ4/DQ4, a pattern typically found in non-Caucasians who are known to have a low prevalence of Celiac disease.

Testing for DQ2/DQ8 has been suggested as a way to exclude celiac disease. That is, if you are negative for DQ2 and DQ8, then you are very unlikely to have celiac disease. However, well documented cases of celiac disease and Dermatitis Herpetiformis (DH) have been confirmed in DQ2 and DQ8 negative individuals. Moreover, we now have the clinical experience that other DQ patterns predispose to gluten sensitivity because these individuals frequently have elevated fecal antibodies to AG or tTG and respond to a gluten free diet.

Why some people develop celiac disease or become sensitive to gluten is not well understood. Risk factors include onset of puberty, pregnancy, stress, trauma or injury, surgery, viral or bacterial infections including those of the gut, medication-induced gut injury or toxicity (e.g. NSAIDs), immune suppression or autoimmune diseases, and antibiotic use resulting in altered gut flora (dysbiosis). The severity of the sensitivity is related to the DQ type, pre-existing intestinal injury, degree of exposure to gluten (how frequent and large a gluten load an individual consumes), and immune status. Once initiated, gluten sensitivity tends to be life-long. True celiac disease requires life-long, complete gluten avoidance to prevent serious complications, cancers, and early death.

Serotypes can be determined from blood or buccal mucosal cells obtained by oral swab from several commercial labs including Prometheus, Labcorp, Quest, The Laboratories at Bonfils, and Enterolabs. Fecal IgA anti-gliadin and IgA tissue transglutaminase antibody testing is only available commercially in the U.S. through Enterolabs. The fecal AG and tTG testing may be helpful to those with normal blood tests for celiac and/or a normal small bowel biopsy but suspected of being gluten sensitive. Though the fecal antibody results are not widely accepted by many "celiac experts" numerous testimonials of individuals testing positive only on fecal tests who have responded to a gluten free diet can be found in support groups, web postings, personal communication from Dr. Fine, and this physician's clinical experience.

Editor's note:
The shift from the previous article is an enormous one. What follows is a personal experience that is uniquely informed by medical and scientific expertise. This thoughtful and engaging set of insights reveals a compelling essential truth that is most compelling.

I would have preferred that Dr. Lewey use the term 'gluten sensitivity' in place of gluten intolerance. Specific word choice aside, his message is powerful and compelling.

Gluten Sensitivity: A Gastroenterologist's Personal Journey down the Gluten Rabbit Hole

By Dr. Scot Lewey

Gluten intolerance resulting in symptoms and illness similar to celiac disease without meeting diagnostic criteria for celiac disease is a new concept. This concept of non-celiac gluten sensitivity (NCGS) or gluten related disease (GRD) may be a new paradigm that is hard for some people to swallow, especially when I suggest that it affects as much as 10% to 30% of the population.

Gluten ingestion is an avoidable, treatable, and reversible cause of illness in many people. It is contributing to the rising epidemic of autoimmune diseases. Many resist these concepts finding them either unbelievable, unacceptable or both. I believe that their rejection is neither rational nor helpful. It may be reasonable to reject them for cultural or financial reasons though I don't believe they can legitimately be rejected based on scientific grounds or experience.

Celiac disease is not rare. Celiac disease affects 1 in 100 people in the world. Yet the diagnosis of celiac disease is still frequently missed and/or delayed.

It is a common disease that is often undiagnosed or misdiagnosed. It may even be the most common autoimmune disorder. Though the risk is largely genetic, it is preventable by simply avoiding gluten. Autoimmune diseases associated with celiac disease may also be preventable by avoiding gluten.

When I was in medical school over twenty-five years ago, I was taught that celiac disease was rare. In residency we were shown photos of short, emaciated children with skinny limbs and pot-bellies. We were told that their medical history included symptoms of profuse, watery, floating, foul-smelling diarrhea, and iron deficiency anemia. The picture and story was burned into the hard drive of our brains, not necessarily because anyone believed we would see someone with celiac disease in our practice, but because celiac disease was considered rare and odd enough that it was a favorite board examination question. That image and story remains in the minds of most physicians, preventing them from seeing celiac disease in a much broader light.

When I entered subspecialty training in gastroenterology, 13 years ago, specific blood tests for celiac disease were available but still new. We were beginning to order the blood test when classic symptoms of celiac disease were seen without an identifiable cause, or if we happened to sample the small intestine during endoscopy and classic Sprue changes were seen in the intestinal biopsy. Celiac disease was still considered somewhat rare. We did not routinely biopsy the small intestine to screen for celiac disease, and genetic tests were not yet available.

It wasn't until 2003 that Fasano's landmark article reported Celiac disease affected 1 in 133 people in the U.S. Only recently has it been accepted that family members of people with celiac disease, those with digestive symptoms, osteoporosis, anemia, and certain neurological, skin or autoimmune disorders constitute high risk groups for celiac disease. They have an even higher risk of between 2% to 5%, though most physicians are unaware of these statistics. Every week, using the strict diagnostic criteria, I confirm 2-3 new cases of celiac disease. I also see 5-10 established celiac disease patients. However, for every identified celiac disease patient there are 3-10 who have clinical histories consistent with celiac disease, but who fail to meet the diagnostic criteria. Yet they respond to a gluten-free diet. Many have suggestive blood test results, biopsies and or gene patterns but some do not.

More than 90% of people proven to have celiac disease carry one or both of two white blood cell protein patterns or human leukocyte antigen (HLA) patterns HLA DQ2 and/or DQ8. However, so do 35-45% of the general U.S. population, especially those of Northern European ancestry. Yet celiac disease is present in only 1% of the same population. DQ2 or DQ8 are considered by some experts to be necessary though not sufficient to develop celiac disease. However, celiac disease without those two genes has been reported.

Other gluten related diseases including dermatitis herpetiformis, the neurological conditions of ataxia and peripheral neuropathy, and microscopic colitis have been described in DQ2 and DQ8 negative individuals. The DQ genetic patterns found in other gluten related diseases and associated with elevated stool antibody tests indicate that many more people are genetically at risk for gluten sensitivity. Furthermore, the response of numerous symptoms to gluten-free diet is not limited to people who are DQ2 or DQ8 positive.

Most celiac experts agree upon and feel comfortable advising people who meet the strict criteria for the diagnosis of celiac disease: they need to follow a life-long gluten-free diet. Controversy and confusion arises when the strict criteria are not met, yet either patient and/or doctor believe that gluten is the cause of their symptoms and illness.

Many alternative practitioners advise wheat-free, yeast-free diets, which are frequently met with favorable response to what is really a form of gluten-free diet. Similarly, the popularity and successes of low carbohydrate diets require adherence to a diet that has been credited with improvement of headaches, fatigue, bloating, musculoskeletal aches, and an increased general sense of well-being that is self-reported by many dieters. I believe this is because of the low gluten content. Gluten avoidance is clearly associated with improvement of many intestinal and extra-intestinal symptoms such as those listed above.

Many also stumble onto this association after initiating a gluten-free diet or wheat-free diet on the advice of friends or family members; dieticians, nutritionists, alternative or complementary practitioners; or after reading an article on the Internet.

Within the medical community, there seems to be an irrational resistance to a more widespread recommendation for gluten avoidance. Physicians who maintain that those who fail to meet strict criteria for diagnosis of celiac disease should not be told they have to follow a gluten-free diet will often acknowledge that many of these patients respond favorably to a gluten-free diet. Some, however, continue to insist that a gluten-free diet trial is unnecessary, unduly burdensome, or not scientifically proven to benefit those who do not have celiac disease. This position is taken despite the absence of evidence that a gluten-free diet is unhealthy or dangerous and much evidence supporting it as a healthy diet.

Those who have observed dramatic improvements, both personally and professionally, find such resistance to recommending a gluten-free diet to a broader group of people difficult to understand. Considering the potential dangers and limited benefits of the medications that we, as doctors, prescribe to patients for various symptoms, it really seems absurd to reject dietary treatments. Yet, it does not seem to cross most doctors' minds to suggest something as safe and healthy as a gluten-free diet, let alone to, at least, test for celiac disease.

My personal journey into gluten related illness began when my physician wife was diagnosed with celiac disease. I had mentioned to her numerous times over several years that I thought she should be tested for celiac disease. After her second pregnancy she became progressively more ill experiencing, for the first time in her life, diarrhea, fatigue, and chronic neuropathy. An upper endoscopy revealed classic endoscopic findings. Celiac disease blood tests were elevated, and genetic testing confirmed she was DQ2 positive. This forever changed our lives and my practice. But the story doesn't end there.

Having diagnosed myself with irritable bowel syndrome (IBS) and lactose intolerance in medical school, I had not considered gluten as a possible cause of my symptoms until my wife turned the table on me and said I should also be tested for celiac disease. My blood tests were not elevated but I was confirmed to also be DQ2 positive.

Having observed a good response to gluten-free diet in a few of my patients who had elevated stool gliadin antibody levels, I looked critically at the research behind this testing and spoke with Dr. Ken Fine before paying to have my entire family tested through Enterolab. Both my gliadin and tTG antibodies were elevated and I responded well to a gluten-free diet. I began recommending stool antibody and DQ genetic screening to patients who did not meet the strict criteria for celiac disease but appeared to have symptoms suggestive of gluten sensitivity. Contrary to some critics' claims about the stool antibody tests, there are many people who do not have elevated levels. Almost everyone I have seen with elevated levels has noted improvement with gluten-free diet, including myself.

Not only did my "IBS" symptoms resolve and lactose tolerance dramatically improve, but my eyes were further opened to the spectrum of gluten related illness or symptoms. I was already aggressively looking for celiac disease in my patients but I began considering non-celiac gluten sensitivity (NCGS) or gluten related diseases (GRD) in all my patients. What I have found is that gluten is an extremely common but frequently missed cause of intestinal and non-intestinal symptoms. Dramatic improvements in symptoms and health can be observed in patients who try a gluten-free diet.

Since only a fraction of DQ2 or DQ8 positive individuals have or will eventually get celiac disease, does that mean gluten is safe to eat if you have those gene patterns? Even if you do not get celiac disease, does continuing to eat gluten put you at risk for other autoimmune diseases, especially ones linked to the high risk gene patterns? Why do some people with these patterns get celiac disease but most do not? Do some who do not have celiac disease experience symptoms from gluten that would improve with gluten-free diet? These questions need to be answered so that people can decide whether they want to risk that gluten is causing them to be ill, or is increasing their risk of celiac disease or other autoimmune diseases.

Added to my gluten-free diet, a daily diet of scientific articles on celiac and gluten related disease has revealed that there are many clues in the literature and research indicating the existence of non-celiac gluten sensitivity or a need to broaden our definition of celiac disease. Dr. Hadjivassiliou has called for a new paradigm. He advocates that we start thinking of gluten sensitivity not as an intestinal disease but as a spectrum of multiple organ, gluten-related diseases. Mary Schluckebier, director of CSA, asks that physicians interested in this area work on forming and agreeing on new definitions for gluten related illness while pushing for more research and cooperation between medical researchers, food and agricultural scientists, dieticians, and food manufacturers.

Only those who look for NCGS and advise a gluten-free diet to those not meeting the strict criteria for celiac disease, are going to see the larger group of people who have a favorable response to a broader application of the gluten-free diet without further research. Those of us who are personally affected by gluten sensitivity or professionally involved in treating individuals with adverse reactions to gluten (or both) should support the research into the broader problem of gluten related illness. I believe that NCGS is real and will be validated in studies. Are you open to this concept and are you willing support more research in this area?

Newly Diagnosed Celiacs Need Bone Density Testing

By Dr. Ron Hoggan, Ed.D.

It was gratifying to learn, from a recent post to the Celiac Listserv, that some celiac-savvy medical practitioners are now ordering bone density testing as soon as a patient's serology indicates celiac disease. This emerging standard of care is well rooted in the medical and scientific literature and constitutes a reasonable and appropriate strategy for the effective care and treatment of celiac disease patients. Investigators have been recommending this approach for more than a decade[1,2] and these recommendations are particularly important given the more recent data showing a dramatic fracture rate among celiac patients that is seven times that of controls[3,4].

Although the sensitivity of endomysium (EMA) and tissue transglutaminase (tTG) may be open to criticism, there can be little doubt that these tests are quite specific and usually reported as close to 100%. Simply put, almost everyone who has a positive serological test result can be shown to have or be developing celiac disease. Thus, when an EMA or tTG test is positive for celiac disease, some practitioners are diagnosing celiac disease based on serology alone. (This approach remains controversial.)

Researchers have long known that celiac disease is associated with significant bone demineralization and increased risk of fractures[5]. Relevant research also shows that therapeutic intervention in celiac patients can require a very different approach than with non-celiac patients[6-7] and there is considerable variation from one celiac patient to the next[1], which practitioners must also consider.

Suspected causes of the increased bone disease and fracture risk include: reduced intestinal absorption area and compromised active transport of calcium across the intestinal barrier[3]; hyperparathyroidism, possibly as the result of cross reaction of endomysium antibodies with parathyroid tissues[8]; autoimmune hyperthyroid disease, which is frequently found in association with celiac disease[9]; excessive mineral release from the bones and excretion[3]; vitamin D deficiency[10]; along with a host of other celiac-associated possibilities. One or more of the above factors are likely contributors to the unique needs of every newly diagnosed celiac patient.

Even when bone density testing reveals metabolic bone disease, it does not reveal the exact nature of the underlying problem[3] and celiac disease patients with bone mineral losses often can not be predicted clinically[1] so testing is the only rational option. While a strict GF diet will usually have a positive impact on bone density, that improvement falls far short of control values[11]. Bone density values and trends will provide assistance in determining individual fracture risk, which is an important clinical consideration[2].

Every person, regardless of celiac disease diagnosis, is unique. It is especially important that each one should have early testing to determine their bone mineral status at diagnosis because of the very strong association between celiac disease and bone disease. Such test results enable health care providers to monitor their celiac patients' bone health and fracture risk. Simply put, if we can not see where we started from, how can we tell how far we have come or whether we are moving in the right direction? Early bone density testing is the first step in therapeutic intervention. In many cases, coupled with follow-up testing, it will be the only intervention needed.

In other cases, however, bone density testing will be the first step in a lengthy therapeutic process that may involve several changes in treatment as the individual progresses. Some patients may require magnesium supplementation as part of a therapeutic intervention for parathyroid disease[6]. Others may need treatment for autoimmune thyroid disease which afflicts more than 12.9% of newly diagnosed celiac patients[12]. Most celiac patients have been shown to have low vitamin D status[10] which, depending on a variety of factors, may indicate a need for vitamin D supplementation. Still others may require pharmacological interventions.

Alert practitioners will, in keeping with the literature, order bone density testing. Abnormal results should identify concurrent bone disease and alert the practitioner to the need for further testing to determine the exact nature of the pathology/pathologies that may be at work. Regardless of the particular cause of bone disease or abnormality, bone density testing is the very first step in each of these interventions. Follow-up bone density testing will usually provide meaningful information to direct treatment and is especially useful when juxtaposed with initial test results.

There can be little doubt that bone density testing is appropriate for newly diagnosed celiac disease patients. This practice is strongly advocated in the medical and scientific literature and promises to mitigate the sometimes ghastly consequences of bone disease, demineralization, and degeneration that are too often found in association with celiac disease. Ultimately, such testing will not only improve quality of life for celiac patients, but in combination with appropriate supplementation, dietary, and pharmacological practices, this testing will save health care dollars through reductions in acute care.

For these reasons, I was surprised to read that the insurance company of the person who posted that message to the celiac listserv had refused to pay for the bone density testing ordered by her health care practitioner on the basis of positive celiac serology. In the early days of endomysium and tissue transglutaminase testing, some insurance companies also failed to see that serological testing would one day save substantial sums of health care dollars by reducing the number of endoscopic biopsies required for a celiac diagnosis. My own diagnosis required three endoscopic biopsies. Similarly, it appears that at least one insurance company is overlooking the savings from acute care that they will accrue from the emerging standard of care in which bone density testing is ordered for all patients with positive celiac serology tests. One can only hope that they will soon recognize the real cash value such testing offers to health insurance providers.

My History with Interstitial Cystitis

By Carol Farmholtz

About 10 years ago I thought I had a bladder infection. It came on very suddenly. One day I was fine and the next day I was having all of the symptoms of a bladder infection. I went to my family doctor who prescribed Macrobid—even though I did not test positive for an infection. The Macrobid did not help at all and I was still having the bladder urges and pain. The family doctor referred me to a urologist who did so many tests I can't even remember them all but every one came out negative. He gave me one antibiotic after another even though I continued to test negative for an infection.

After one test he determined that I had fibroids on my uterus and referred me to a gynecologist who did a laparoscopy and confirmed the fibroids. He said that some of them were apparently pressing on my bladder and suggested I have a hysterectomy.

I consulted another gynecologist for a second opinion. He confirmed the fibroids so I went ahead with the hysterectomy. When I recovered from the surgery and the bladder symptoms were still the same I went back to the urologist for more tests and he eventually confirmed the diagnosis of interstitial cystitis (IC). He put me on Elmiron which is the only medication specifically for the disease. I also had two bladder distensions. Those gave me no relief either. I basically suffered through it for a year or two until I went for acupuncture and started seeing a holistic doctor. He told me to quit eating grains which I did and found relief very quickly.

Being one who wants to know what is going on with my body, and wanting to know all I could about interstitial cystitis I was on the computer researching it constantly to see what treatments were working for other people. In all of my research I only found one reference to anyone being on a gluten free diet and getting relief from it so believe me it did not surprise me whatsoever that one would not be able to find any reference connecting interstitial cystitis to gluten intolerance.

I haven't been to an urologist in a few years. My original urologist moved away and when I mentioned to the next one that the only relief I found came from a gluten free diet, he didn't really seem that interested. Other doctors I have seen didn't even know what gluten was and also seemed disinterested.

Initially, after being diagnosed with interstitial cystitis, I attended several conferences on IC and went to some support group meetings but they all seemed to revolve around drugs and most specifically Elmiron. The main website for IC research is www.ichelp. com and is sponsored by Elmiron so it is no wonder the only research they are interested in promotes using Elmiron. I have shared the story of my success using a gluten free diet for IC with other people who have interstitial cystitis and are suffering terribly. None of them have taken me seriously. I am confident this is because their doctor never mentioned it to them. Not being a doctor, who am I to be able to know how to treat this condition, even though I speak from experience? I am also sure that they think it is just too difficult to follow such a restrictive diet and would rather be treated with medications.

The holistic doctor I went to was Michael Leveque here in Central Florida. He has moved away from my area and is currently in the Ft. Myers, Florida area. When I was seeing Dr. Leveque I participated in some workshops he did and he used my case history in his presentation and also had my testimonial on his website.

The acupuncture physician I saw is Sue Leveque, DOM and the wife of Michael Leveque, who now practices in Fort Myers, Florida also. She offered other holistic services including lab testing for gluten intolerance and a variety of other nutrition related conditions. My test results, processed at BioHealth Diagnostics in California www.biohealthinfo.com revealed that I had three parasitic infections, heliocobator pylori (a bacterial infection that causes ulcers and acid reflux) and heavy metal toxicity. I was successfully treated for the parasitic and bacterial infections with antibiotics and also used a pro-biotic treatment afterwards to counteract the effects of antibiotic therapy. In addition, I had my amalgam fillings removed and went through chelation treatments to rid my body of heavy metals.

As a result of all that I have done, I am healthier now than I have been in years. And I know that the primary reason my health has improved to the point it is today is because my diet is gluten-free.

New Data on Used Oats

By Dr. Ron Hoggan, Ed.D., and Ginny Nehring

To the newly diagnosed celiac patient, beginning a gluten free diet is often overwhelming, confusing, and sometimes, depressing. Initially it may be a relief to finally have a diagnosis. All seems easy and uncomplicated when sitting in the comfort of the doctor's office. A visit to the store and the purchase of a few things that *may* be safe to eat is the time when most of us come face-to-face with the fact that life as we knew it is over.

If you are lucky and do some homework, you find that gluten is hidden in almost everything. Gluten is the protein in wheat, rye, barley and oats. Or is it? Conflicting information regarding gluten abounds. Some authorities believe oats are safe for the celiac patient, and gluten is frequently being listed as including only wheat, rye, and barley.

Too many people—especially the newly diagnosed—receive conflicting information. They aren't even sure what gluten is, and then they have to contend with the added misinformation about oats. It is a difficult situation—that sometimes gets even worse.

For instance, we are continually amazed by the number of people who think that just a "little" gluten is okay. Unfortunately, too many doctors and dieticians tell their patients that as long as their symptoms are gone they can safely have gluten occasionally. This is just plain wrong. It goes far beyond the oats debate in the literature, and it is of concern to those of us who have maintained a gluten free diet with zero symptoms and clean blood tests for many years.

But what about eating oats? According to Hogberg, et al., oats "can be accepted and tolerated by the majority of children with celiac disease."[1] This conclusion is based upon their finding that those subjects who consumed oats showed intestinal and serological recovery after one year on the diet. The indicators used to measure this recovery were blood tests and biopsies. The same group also reports that while 20% of the test subjects dropped out of the study, all subjects who stayed with the study showed no adverse effects from including oats in their diets. But what about the 20% who dropped out? How carefully were the symptoms of any of the subjects in this study monitored? Because these subjects were newly diagnosed, there was no basis for comparison with their previous experience and/or symptoms on a gluten-free diet.

In counterpoint to the Hogberg group's findings, a very different story is told by the research conducted by Peraaho et al. They looked at the impact of oats on the quality of life along with gastrointestinal signs and symptoms. They compared these findings to similar examinations of a control group of celiac patients who were eating a gluten-free diet that did not include oats[2]. While the quality of life did not differ between these groups, *those eating oats experienced significantly more frequent diarrhea*. They also experienced more severe constipation, and *a small but significant increase in intraepithelial lymphocytes was revealed in their biopsies*. The Peraaho group did report, in congruence with the Hogberg et al. findings, that the villous architecture did not differ between groups, and antibody levels did not increase among those eating oats.

Both studies are very revealing. They show us that symptoms can sometimes be more revealing than test results, and that the serological and endoscopic evidence, without counting intraepithelial lymphocytes (IELs) can only provide a crude measurement of disease. While the Marsh system for evaluating biopsies for celiac disease requires counting IELs, and is widely accepted, too many pathologists and gastroenterologists continue to rely on the villous morphology alone when they rule out celiac disease.

Peraaho et al. identified two important weaknesses in research that suggests oats are safe for celiac patients. First, the intestinal biopsy will miss a number of cases of celiac disease if IELs are not counted, so oats advocates should include IEL counts. Second, many celiacs are exquisitely sensitive to gluten, and their reactions are far more accurate than many supposedly objective tests (please bear in mind that some/many of us can be symptom-free while the disease progresses and gluten causes internal injuries). Thus, our well-being is in our own hands and a function of the extent to which we comply with the gluten-free diet.

Further, many of us are simply not able to tolerate oats. We suggest the following approach: First, ensure that your diet is absolutely gluten free, including hidden gluten and cross-contamination. Then, if the idea of adding a grain to your diet is important to you, try oats that have not been contaminated through growing, harvesting, or processing. If you remain symptom free when eating oats, enjoy. Be aware, however, that a significant portion of celiac patients clearly react to oats, and the elevation of IELs, along with the increased bowel symptoms should suggest erring on the side of caution and avoiding oats if any signs or symptoms appear.

More on the Problems with Oats in the Gluten Sensitive Diet

By Ron Hoggan, Ed. D.

Experts have decreed that pure oats are safe for people with celiac disease[1,2,3]. The definition of this disease is based on a very specific type of injury to the intestinal wall that heals following the removal of gluten from the diet. This intestinal damage, called villous atrophy, is caused by the interaction between the immune system and certain proteins found in wheat, rye, and barley. Identical proteins are not found in oats (although there is also some variation between the protein groups found in wheat, rye, and barley). Further, many newly diagnosed celiac patients have been shown to recover from their celiac symptoms while eating significant quantities of oats and their intestinal biopsies do not show signs of villous atrophy[1]. (Admittedly, the quantity of oats consumed by these study subjects does not rival the grain protein consumption in a regular, gluten-laden diet, but the quantity is significant). Therefore, this food is considered safe for celiac consumption.

Given these facts, it is not surprising that many gastroenterologists are now recommending that their patients eat oats. Some claim that patients are more likely to follow a gluten-free diet if that diet allows oats. Others point to the definition of celiac disease, which clearly requires gluten-induced villous atrophy. Still others insist that since we now know which proteins cause the villous atrophy, oats must be safe for celiac patients to consume.

There are several problems with these perspectives, beginning with the assumption that patients will be more compliant with the diet if it includes oats. I have explored the medical literature and have been unable to find a single study that investigates dietary compliance as a function of including oats in the gluten-free diet. I'd be happy to hear about such a study. But until the question is investigated, the assumption is just one more opinion afloat in a sea of unfounded beliefs about grains and diet.

Many celiac patients experience an addictive element in gluten. I have long suspected that is the result of morphine-like, opioid peptides found in the digests of gluten[4-8]. Are some peptides from oats capable of producing these opioids? Has anyone investigated that issue? Again, I can find no evidence that this issue has been studied.

Reliance on the biopsy to reveal problems with oat consumption is another relevant problem. As many of us can attest, and the medical literature reports, gluten challenges that intentionally involve ingestion of relatively large quantities of gluten often fail to reveal villous atrophy for weeks, months, and sometimes, years[9]. Many celiac patients will also agree that despite our best efforts at compliance, gluten sometimes manages to sneak into our diets, particularly in the early months of following the diet. Yet a second biopsy usually shows dramatic healing of the intestinal wall, despite these dietary errors. Clearly, the intestinal biopsy is a fairly crude tool for measuring intestinal health. Its use in exonerating oats thus becomes suspect. An even more troubling element of this issue is that there are gastroenterologists who are recommending that their patients consume breakfast cereals that contain malt flavoring, because patients consuming such small quantities of malt do not show villous atrophy[10].

Also troubling is the fact that many of the studies that support the safety of oats have not employed the Marsh system for identifying intestinal injury, a refinement that significantly increases the sensitivity of the intestinal biopsy.

The greatest weakness of the pro-oats position is the underlying assumption that we fully understand celiac disease and gluten sensitivity. This is simply not the case. The research shows that some celiacs do develop symptoms when consuming oats. While most newly diagnosed celiacs experience reduced symptoms and improved health, this may simply be the result of consuming less grain-derived protein. Researchers have long known that even partial compliance with the gluten-free diet produces health improvements in celiac patients[11].

The definition of celiac disease that requires villous atrophy followed the discovery of the beneficial impact of the gluten-free diet by more than 20 years—those in doubt about this point, please refer to the English translation of Dr. Dicke's Ph.D. thesis at http://members.shaw.ca/dicke//. Our current understanding of the disease began with the observed benefits of the gluten-free diet. Intestinal biopsies were a much later development.

A similar debate arose regarding the inclusion of wheat starch. It was long held to be a safe nutrient in the gluten-free diet in many European countries. In fact, the studies that showed a reduced risk of cancer and a variety of celiac-associated conditions were often conducted among patient groups living where wheat starch was deemed acceptable[12,13]. Yet, when wheat starch consumption was studied in Canada, against a back-drop of zero tolerance, *most* of the subjects developed signs and symptoms of celiac disease[14].

Many celiacs and gluten-sensitive individuals know that their symptoms do not fit with the conventional view of celiac disease. Some of us believe that there is a continuum of severity. Others believe that there are many sub-types of celiac disease. Still others believe, me included, that it really doesn't matter whether a person has intestinal damage. The important, defining characteristic should be whether a person is mounting an immune response against the proteins in the most common substance in our food supply.

Whatever our beliefs we turn to the experts when faced with health concerns and crises. However, those answers often rely on the medical definition of celiac disease, where villous atrophy heals in response to a gluten-free diet. In cases where the biopsy was improperly taken, or too few samples were taken, or patchy intestinal lesions were missed, or other forms of gluten-induced ailments are causing symptoms, we may not get answers that aid our health. Many individuals who are gluten sensitive will be, under such circumstances, dismissed with a diagnosis of IBS.

Given the facts, we have several hurdles to overcome before we can, in my opinion, render an informed judgment about the safety of oats. We need a much better understanding of gluten-induced disease in all of its manifestations. We also need a definition of celiac disease that is more useful to the patient who is experiencing symptoms of gluten sensitivity/celiac disease. As part of this, we also need a test that is more accurate, and can identify celiac disease after beginning the diet—a challenge that many of us face. Until we have overcome these hurdles, any pronouncement regarding the safety of oats is premature.

Further research is, in my opinion, the greatest need of the celiac community. We need to know more, not just about celiac disease, but about the whole range of nutritional and pathological impacts of eating grains. In my own quest, I have learned from the experiences of other celiac patients. Each new facet of my own experience has been illuminated by someone else's story. I have come to understand ADHD as a frequent companion of celiac disease. Learning disabilities are also common among celiacs. Behavioral disturbances are the norm, and speech problems are common. My understanding continues to grow as I hear from others who struggle with gluten sensitivity.

Despite its usefulness, this patient-to-patient network of information sharing is not enough. We need well designed, well executed research. We need a better understanding of our disease and how to protect future generations from the current, inaccurate assumptions about grains. The oats question is only one facet of a much larger need for more information and better testing methods.

Gluten isn't *really* gluten

By Dr. Ron Hoggan, Ed. D.

Technically speaking, gluten is a group of sub-groups of storage proteins found in the endosperm of many plant seeds. Arguably, gluten is found in corn, rice, wheat, rye, barley, and other grass-related seeds. However, the meaning of the term 'gluten' is quickly shifting in our language to include only the storage protein groups found in wheat, rye, barley, and various hybrids of these grains. This narrowing of the meaning of this term is perhaps due to the recent explosion of public and scientific awareness of gluten sensitive enteropathy, or celiac disease. Sub-groups of gluten have been found to induce excessive zonulin production which causes increased intestinal permeability and may well be at the root of most autoimmune diseases.

CHAPTER 8:
ESTABLISHING AND MAINTAINING A HEALTHY GF LIFESTYLE

Consider Camps for Your Gluten-Free Little One (Being gluten-free shouldn't change your summer plans)

By Danna Korn

For a kid, absolutely nothing compares to the excitement of counting down those last few days before school is out for summer, and life goes from routine and imprisoning to lazy and carefree. That's right – sing it now – *school's out for summer!*

We parents, admittedly, have some mixed emotions about summer break. We eagerly await the mornings free of chaos and last-minute-I-have-nothing-to-wear tantrums, evenings without battles over homework, and afternoons when kids will have more time to play, and maybe even to help around the house and yard (a mom can dream, can't she?).

But summer break is a catalyst for new battles, such as trying to explain to our kids that yes, it is your summer vacation, and yes, it is supposed to be relaxing, but 16 hours of television is still too much. The first few days are what I call freebies. We all enjoy the lack of structure, allowing our little ones to sleep as long as they'd like (but why is it that on school days they whine that they could have slept until noon, and during summer break they're up at the crack of dawn?), and even buying into the oh-so-well-presented argument that this is just the first (second, third) day of vacation, and it's the only day they'll watch TV all summer—promise! Energized by the contagious enthusiasm of summer break, we pack weeks worth of fun into the first few days, and revel in every minute of family freedom.

And then…by about day four…you hear those dreaded two words that can, in and of themselves, induce critically high blood-pressure levels faster than anchovies on crackers: *I'm bored!*

Most parents go into the summer with good intentions and the best-laid plans for staving off the boredom blues. Fun-but-educational math and science workbooks, fun family fitness programs, and a well-stocked arts and crafts cabinet can sound like a good idea, but kids (and adults!) just want to have fun. The difference is that adults have responsibilities and obligations, and can't usually put our lives on hold for three months. They, however, can – and should.

But my kids are gluten-free….

Oh, good point. That just means you may have to be a smidge more creative, but basically, if your child can't eat gluten, your options for battling boredom are just the same as everyone else's. Yep. Just the same. You may have to be a little more creative, and you'll undoubtedly need to spend time educating those around you. But it's well worth the time and energy to provide your child with some of life's greatest summer experiences and memories.

You may want to consider summer camps. Both day and away camps offer tremendous opportunities and experiences. There are some wonderful specialty camps for celiac kids, but don't feel that your options are limited to those. Do you think it's too hard because of your child's diet? Think again!

Day Camps/Away Camps—Gluten-Freedom!

Sending your child away to camp is difficult. Oh—don't misunderstand me—it's not difficult because of the diet. It's saying good-bye that's the hard part!

Whether you choose day camps or away camps is up to you. From a dietary standpoint, the concept is the same. You may want to take all the worry out of it and send your child to a camp specially designed for celiac kids. Three are listed at the end of this article. But don't think you're limited to specialty camps. You can send them to any camp if you keep a few important things in mind:

Educate counselors/cooks in advance.

If possible, meet with the head counselor in person to discuss your child's dietary requirements. Ideally, you should meet with the nutritional director or chef, too. You'll probably be surprised at how receptive they are. Most camps are accustomed to accommodating conditions such as diabetes or severe allergies, and are glad to learn the intricacies of the gluten-free diet.

Make sure you give them plenty of time to make arrangements for your child's dietary needs. Meet several weeks in advance so they can plan, prepare, understand, and adapt menus. Remember to discuss preparation techniques, so they understand how to avoid cross-contamination during preparation and serving.

Send reference information.

Make sure the counselors and cooks have printed copies of safe and forbidden food lists. They can be found at www.Celiac.com, or send them with a copy of *Kids with Celiac Disease*. These resources will be important if there are questions about ingredients or special treats, and if they take the time to read more about celiac disease, you will have educated someone on the subject, and that is also important.

Make sure your child understands his diet.

If you've read *Kids with Celiac Disease* or heard me speak, you know that I'm a downright nag when it comes to giving your child control of his diet. It's crucial! But in this case, it's also key to ensuring a safe and enjoyable camp experience. Remember, if you don't give your child control of his diet, his diet may control him.

Send food.

Don't rely upon the camp to provide specialty gluten-free foods like bread and pasta. They're expensive and difficult to get, but more importantly, it's not up to others to accommodate your child's diet (another "nagging point" of mine). Be sure to send mixes for cookies, brownies, and other treats, if they have the facilities to prepare them. These days, the specialty mixes you can buy are so good that your child's treats are likely to be the hit of the camp.

More than simply a great way to beat the summertime boredom blues, sending your child to camp can be a huge growing-up experience. Oh—and the kids will do some growing up, too!

Focus on Flax

By Shelley Case, B.Sc., RD

Flax is widely grown across the Canadian prairies and northern USA, with Canada being the world's top producer. It is harvested for a variety of purposes. The stems are used in the production of linen cloth and fine quality papers. Flaxseeds are sold whole or ground and incorporated into a number of food products or packaged for individual consumer use. Flax oil is an edible oil produced by cleaning, cracking and pressing flaxseeds under controlled temperatures and sold as a "cold-pressed oil" that is bottled in dark colored bottles and refrigerated. The seeds are also used for industrial purposes to make linseed oil, which is produced by using solvents to extract the oil from the seed during the crushing process. Sold in raw or boiled form, linseed oil is a main ingredient in paints, stains, coatings and linoleum floorings.

Flax has been consumed throughout history for its nutritional and health benefits. It is loaded with dietary fiber, vitamins, minerals, protein and other healthy substances.

"F" is for fiber

Flax contains two types of dietary fiber- soluble and insoluble. Soluble fiber can lower blood lipid levels and helps regulate blood sugar levels. Insoluble fiber acts as a bulking agent and promotes regularity and may also reduce the risk of colon cancer. Three tablespoons of ground flax contains 6 grams of total dietary fiber.

"L" is for lignans

Lignans are naturally occurring compounds found in a variety of plant foods. Flax is the richest source of lignans, containing 75 times more than any other plant food. Lignans are referred to as phytoestrogens and have weak estrogen-like properties. Recent research has revealed that lignans may protect against hormone-sensitive cancers such as breast cancer.

"A" is for Alpha-Linolenic Acid (ALA)

Flaxseed is rich in ALA, an omega-3 fatty acid. Omega-3 fatty acids play a role in reducing the risk of heart disease by lowering blood fat levels and making blood platelets less sticky, thereby reducing the risk of blood clots. They also have been cited as beneficial for people with immune system aliments.

"X" is for excellent

Flax is high in vitamins and minerals such as Vitamin B6, folic acid, potassium, iron, calcium, magnesium, phosphorus, and zinc. Flax is also a rich source of plant protein.

DIETARY FLAX

Whole Flaxseed

- The whole seed provides dietary fiber, which pass undigested through the body, and act as a laxative.
- They can be stored at room temperature for up to one year.
- Add them to a variety of recipes for a pleasant change in texture and flavor.

Ground Flax

- Flaxseeds can be ground in a coffee grinder or food processor. You can also purchase "milled/ground" flax available in vacuum-sealed packages from health food stores or grocery stores. When the seeds are ground you receive the maximum nutritional benefits from flax including dietary fiber, alpha-linolenic acid (ALA), lignans, protein and other nutrients.
- Use ground flax immediately or store in an opaque container in the fridge or freezer for up to 90 days. For optimum freshness it is best to grind flax as you need it.
- Ground flax has a light, nutty flavor and can be added to hot or cold cereals, muffins, cookies, breads, pancakes, waffles, meat loaf, burgers, casseroles, soups, salads, yogurt, frozen yogurt, ice cream, pudding or a fruit smoothie blender drink. Remember that baked goods with flax will brown more readily.
- As with any new high fiber food, start slowly, 1-2 teaspoons, and make sure you consume enough fluids. To get the health benefits from ground flax, use 1-4 tablespoons/day.
- One tablespoon of ground flax contains 25 calories, 2.5 grams of fat, 2 grams of dietary fiber and 2 grams of ALA.

Flax Oil

- The oil is rich in alpha-linolenic acid. However it does not contain all the other nutritional components such as dietary fiber, protein, and lignans.
- Flax oil needs to be refrigerated at all times and once opened must be used within six to eight weeks, as it goes rancid after that time.

Omega-3 Enriched Eggs

- Hens fed a specially formulated flaxseed diet produce an omega-3 rich egg. These eggs contain 8-10 times more alpha-linolenic acid (ALA) than a regular egg.

Flax in Gluten-Free Products

- Several companies are adding flax to their products. Some examples are bars and bagels from Enjoy Life Foods, fortified rice pasta from Pastariso, fortified potato and rice pasta from Pastato, Omega Smart nutritional snack bars, sunflower flax rice bread and Kinni-Kwik sunflower flax bread and bun mix from Kinnikinnick Foods.

People with gluten intolerance need to keep nutrition a top priority, and flax can be a healthy addition to the gluten-free diet!

Unique Gluten-Free Grains

By Danna Korn

Variety, it's been said, is the spice of life. So what's a person to do when they're told to eliminate wheat and/or gluten from their diet? Most turn to rice, corn, and potatoes—an adequate set of starches, but ones that are sorely lacking in nutrients, flavor, and imagination.

The superheroes of gluten-free grains are often referred to as "ancient" or alternative grains, which are loaded with nutrients and unique, interesting flavors. The following is a condensed excerpt from my newly published book, _Wheat-Free, Worry-Free: The Art of Happy, Healthy, Gluten-Free Living_.

"Alternative" Grains: The Superheroes of Gluten-Free Grains

If you're an adventuresome eater, you're in for a treat. In searching for alternatives to wheat, rye, or barley, you'll discover a variety of wheat-free/gluten-free grains that you may never have heard of before, many of them loaded with nutrients and robust flavors not found in typical grains like wheat and rice. If you're not the adventurous type and you just long for the ease of a few tried-and-true favorites, you'll find them here as well.

Perhaps you fall into still another category—you've been eating a wheat or gluten-free diet for a while and you think you already know everything there is to know. Okay, what's quinoa, and how the heck is it pronounced? Is teff wheat-free? Do Job's Tears have religious significance? If you don't know the answers to these questions, or if you think 'ragi is a spaghetti sauce and 'sorghum' is what you get when you have your teeth cleaned, it's time to move on to lesson one.

Alternative Grains and Non-Grains

Even if you can't eat wheat, rye, barley, or oats, there are several other grains, fruits, and legumes that are not only acceptable alternatives to them, but they also happen to be loaded with flavor and nutrients. Here are some of the many choices available to those on a wheat and gluten-free diet:

- Amaranth
- Buckwheat/groats/kasha
- Cassava (arrowroot)
- Chickpea (garbanzo)
- Job's Tears
- Millet
- Montina
- Oats (oats can be contaminated with other grains)
- Quinoa
- Ragi
- Rice (only brown rice is whole grain)
- Sorghum
- Soy
- Tapioca
- Taro root
- Teff

Many of the proteins found in these alternatives are a great source of complex carbohydrates. The fuel from these carbohydrates, found in plant kingdom starches, produces what nutritionists call a protein-sparing effect, which means the body can meet its energy requirements without dipping into its protein reserves.

Several of these alternative grains and non-grains are high in lysine, an amino acid that controls protein absorption in the body. Because this amino acid is absent from most grains, the protein fraction of those grains is utilized only if eaten in conjunction with other foods that do contain lysine. All high protein grains are better utilized by the body when they are eaten with high-lysine foods such as peas, beans, amaranth, or buckwheat.

Amaranth (WF/GF): Loaded with fiber and more protein than any traditional grain, amaranth is nutritious and delicious, with a pleasant peppery flavor. The name means "not withering," or more literally, "immortal." While it may not make you immortal, it is extremely healthful, especially with its high lysine and iron content.

Buckwheat (groat; kasha) (WF/GF): It sounds as though it would be closely related to wheat, but buckwheat is not related to wheat at all. In fact, it's not even a grain; it's a fruit of the *Fagopyrum* genus, a distant cousin of garden-variety rhubarb, and its seed is the plant's strong point. The buckwheat seed has a three-cornered shell that contains a pale kernel known as a "groat." In one form or another, people have used groats as food since the 10th century B.C.

Nutritionally, buckwheat is a powerhouse. It contains a high proportion of all eight essential amino acids, which the body doesn't make itself but are still essential for keeping the body functioning. In that way, buckwheat is closer to being a complete protein than any other plant source.

Whole white buckwheat is naturally dried and has a delicate flavor that makes it a good stand-in for rice or pasta. *Kasha* is the name given to roasted hulled buckwheat kernels. Kasha is toasted in an oven and tossed by hand until the kernels develop a deep tan color, nutlike flavor, and a slightly scorched smell.

Be aware, however, that buckwheat is sometimes combined with wheat. Read labels carefully before purchasing buckwheat products.

Millet: Millet is said by some to be more ancient than any grain that grows. Where it was first cultivated is disputed, but native legends tell of a wild strain known as Job's Tears that grows in the Philippines and sprouted "at the dawn of time."

Millet is still well respected in Africa, India, and China, where it is considered a staple. Here in the United States, it is raised almost exclusively for hay, fodder, and birdseed. One might consider that to be a waste, especially when considering its high vitamin and mineral content. Rich in phosphorus, iron, calcium, riboflavin, and niacin, a cup of cooked millet has nearly as much protein as wheat. It is also high in lysine—higher than rice, corn, or oats.

Millet is officially a member of the Gramineae (grass) family and as such is related to montina.

Montina (Indian Rice Grass): Indian rice grass was a dietary staple of Native American cultures in the Southwest and north through Montana and into Canada more than 7,000 years ago, even before maize (corn) was cultivated. Similar to maize, montina was a good substitute during years when maize crops failed or game was in short supply. It has a hearty flavor, and is loaded with fiber and protein.

Quinoa ("KEEN-wah"): The National Academy of Science described quinoa as "the most nearly perfect source of protein from the vegetable kingdom." Although new to North Americans, it has been cultivated in the South American Andes since at least 3000 B.C. Ancient Incas called this annual plant "the mother grain," because it was self-perpetuating and ever-bearing. They honored it as a sacred food product, since a steady diet appeared to ensure a full, long life; and the Inca ruler himself planted the first row of quinoa each season with a gold spade.

Like amaranth, quinoa is packed with lysine and other amino acids that make a protein complete. Quinoa is also high in phosphorus, calcium, iron, vitamin E, and assorted B vitamins. Technically a fruit of the *Chenopodium* herb family, quinoa is usually pale yellow in color, but also comes in pink, orange, red, purple, and black.

Quinoa's only fault is a bitter coating of saponins on its seeds. The coating comes off with thorough rinsing prior to cooking, and some companies have developed ways to remove the coating prior to delivering quinoa to stores.

Sorghum (milo): Sorghum is another of the oldest known grains, and has been a major source of nutrition in Africa and India for years. Now grown in the United States, sorghum is generating excitement as a gluten-free insoluble fiber.

Because sorghum's protein and starch are more slowly digested than that of other cereals, it may be beneficial to diabetics and healthy for anyone. Sorghum fans boast of its bland flavor and light color, which don't alter the taste or look of foods when used in place of wheat flour. Many cooks suggest combining sorghum with soybean flour.

Soy and Soybeans: Like the ancient foods mentioned at the beginning of this section, soy has been around for centuries. In China, soybeans have been grown since the 11th century B.C., and are still one of the country's most important crops. Soybeans weren't cultivated in the United States until the early 1800s, yet today are one of this country's highest yielding producers.

Soybeans are a legume, belonging to the pea family. Comprised of nearly 50 percent protein, 25 percent oil, and 25 percent carbohydrate, they have earned a reputation as being extremely nutritious. They are also an excellent source of essential fatty acids, which are not produced by the body, but are essential to its functioning nonetheless.

Teff (WF/GF): Considered a basic part of the Ethiopian diet, teff is relatively new to Americans. Five times richer in calcium, iron, and potassium than any other grain, teff also contains substantial amounts of protein and soluble and insoluble fiber. Considered a nutritional powerhouse, it has a sweet, nutty flavor. Teff grows in many different varieties and colors, but in the United States only the ivory, brown, and reddish-tan varieties can be found. The reddish teff is reserved for purveyors of Ethiopian restaurants, who are delighted to have an American source for their beloved grain.

A Word About Sprouted Grains

Some people believe that "sprouted grains," even ones that contain gluten such as wheat, are gluten-free—not true! The sprouting process sparks a chemical reaction that begins to break down gluten, so some people who are slightly sensitive to gluten may find that they can tolerate sprouted grains better, but too many of the peptides that are reactive for celiacs are still present, so sprouted grains are not safe for people with celiac disease or gluten intolerance.

Learning to Decipher Customer Service-Speak

By Danna Korn

You've found a food you'd really like to eat. You've read the label, and it looks as though the product might be gluten-free. You're drooling! You can dig in, right? Wrong. It's a good idea to call the manufacturer to confirm that there aren't hidden sources of gluten.

Years ago, when we would call manufacturers and ask them if their products were gluten-free, they would either suspect us of making a crank call and hang up, leave us on "hell-hold" for 35 minutes while they "checked" (a euphemism for when they put you on hold and hope you hang up), or respond with a confident, "Oh no, honey, there's no sugar whatsoever!"

Before you bother calling the manufacturer, read the label. If there is an obviously unsafe ingredient, don't waste your time or theirs. Tune in to the person on the other end of the phone. Do they sound like they understand what you're talking about? Are they giving you conflicting information? Can you trust what they say?

Fortunately, most product labels have a toll-free phone number listed on the packaging. I highly recommend carrying your cell phone in the grocery store with you, so that you can call quickly while you're still there—before you buy a product.

These days, most customer service representatives actually know what we're talking about most of the time, and can offer a knowledgeable answer that instills confidence that the answer is accurate, albeit sometimes not all that helpful. When you call a company to find out if its product is wheat or gluten-free, you'll get one of four responses:

No, our product is not gluten-free:

Do not interpret this as meaning, "No, our product is not gluten-free." I realize that's what they said, but it may not be what they mean. Probe deeper by asking, for example, "Can you tell me what in your product has gluten in it? I read the label and didn't see anything questionable." One time when I asked this, the woman told me it was "whey" that contained gluten. Penalty flag! Whey doesn't contain gluten! This is when you need to realize that you're talking to someone who doesn't understand the concept, and you should ask to be transferred to a quality control supervisor.

Sometimes this response is accurate, and either an ingredient wasn't clearly called out on the label (unfortunately, this still occurs from time to time), or you were calling about a questionable ingredient only to find out it's a good thing you called. Following are the standard replies and their possible meanings:

We can't verify its status:

Translation: "It's wheat-free/gluten-free, but we're covering our rear ends because we don't want someone to sue us." Sadly, in our litigious society, it may actually be a founded fear that they have.

Of course, this response—"we can't verify its status"—could actually mean what it says—that they can't verify the status. Usually they'll tell you this is because they get their additives from other sources, and even though they claim to be gluten-free, Company A doesn't want to be responsible in case Company B used gluten. The risk factor in either case is probably low.

Every now and then, this response is given because they have an "If we tell you what's in our product, we'd have to shoot you" mentality. Assure them that you're not trying to steal their oh-so-treasured secret-sauce recipe, but that you have a serious medical condition that requires you to know if there are certain ingredients in the food you eat. Sometimes you just can't get an answer, in which case you fall back to the golden rule: When in doubt, leave it out!

Yes, it is gluten-free:

This doesn't necessarily mean, "Yes, it is gluten-free." You have to judge for yourself whether or not they truly understand the concept. Sometimes they'll follow it up with, "There are no sources of wheat, rye, or barley, and there are no questionable additives.

Therefore it's safe for someone with celiac disease, gluten intolerance, or wheat allergies." Ah, you just want to kiss these people.

Other times, when pressed, they get squirmy. If you say, for instance, "Oh, okay, then I can assume the modified food starch is derived from a non-gluten source?" and they give you an audible "blank stare," you might want to dig a little deeper before trusting their answer.

Huh?

Thankfully, this isn't a common response anymore, but it does happen. Politely try to explain what types of ingredients might be in the product you're calling about, and if it doesn't "click," ask to speak to a quality control supervisor or nutritional expert.

Of course it's helpful and sometimes necessary to be specific in some cases, saying, "I'm calling to see if this product is gluten-free, which means it doesn't contain wheat, rye, or barley." Not only is this clarification helpful for them, but you may have educated one more person about gluten.

Many times, one of the added benefits of calling, even if the product you were calling about turns out not to be okay, is they'll offer to send you a list of their wheat-free/gluten-free products (sometimes they even toss in a few coupons). Always take them up on it, and save the lists for future reference.

It's important to learn from your answers. If there was an ingredient on the label that you had never heard of, and you talked with a knowledgeable customer service representative who told you that product was gluten-free, take note. That means the ingredient is gluten-free, too. Add it to your own copy of the safe and forbidden list, and remember for future label-reading experiences.

Excuse me for a moment while I put on my Miss Manners hat, but it's important to be polite, professional, and appreciative when you call manufacturers. Not only will you get much better service, but we need them! We need them to comprehend the gravity of our questions and to understand how important it is to be 100 percent sure that the answers they give us are accurate. We need them to realize that they can't guess at their answers, and that we very much appreciate that they understand what we're asking.

Calling manufacturers can be a pain, for sure, but it's an important part of living and loving the gluten-free lifestyle. Not only is it a good habit for you since ingredients change frequently, but it sends companies the message that if their labeling was clarified, we wouldn't bother them so often! It also tells them that millions of people avoid wheat or gluten, and maybe they'll think twice before using an ingredient that has a wheat source when they have the option to use one that is wheat and gluten-free.

Should the Entire Family be Gluten-Free?

By Danna Korn

In the 13 years I've been involved in the wonderful world of "gluten freedom," one of the questions I've been asked most frequently is whether or not the entire family should be gluten-free. For parents who have kids on the gluten-free diet, this seems to be a natural instinct—*if Johnny can't eat gluten, none of us will*. But I'm not sure that having the entire family go gluten-free is the best thing—unless, of course, it's for health reasons (I, for example, *choose* a gluten-free diet because I believe it's healthier). This is one of those questions that has no correct or incorrect answer, so I'll share with you, for what it's worth, my personal perspective on the issue.

Pros:

It's easier when the whole family is gluten-free, because you're making only one version of every meal, as opposed to two or three. There is less risk of contaminating safe foods because there aren't any "unsafe" foods in the house. Preparation is easier, and there's no need for the gob drop or any other tricky food-preparation maneuvers. Finally, from a psychological standpoint, you avoid having some people feel ostracized when their food is made separately and they're eating different foods from the rest of the family.

Cons:

It's more expensive and sometimes more labor-intensive for everyone to eat specialty foods (Try not to be a "saver." Sometimes, after spending $3 each for sugar ice cream cones, I'll find myself guarding them like a hawk. I've accumulated several boxes of untouched stale cones now). Feeding the whole family home-made gluten-free bread at nearly five dollars per loaf, when three out of four family members *could* be eating a commercial brand, has an impact on the family's time and finances.

More important, especially if children are involved, forcing the entire family to be gluten-free because of one person's dietary restrictions can put a strain on relationships. Sometimes this works in both directions. In my family, for instance, my daughter would resent being forced to be on a 100 percent gluten-free diet (we're pretty close to that anyway) just because that's how her brother Tyler eats. Interestingly, though, it works the other way too. Tyler doesn't *want* his sister to be deprived of a bagel, nor does he resent her for being able to eat one (especially because the gluten-free bagels we buy over the Internet are so good these days!). Resentment is almost inevitable at some level if family members are forced to give up their favorite foods for one member of the family—at least when kids are involved.

The last reason against a gluten-free family is probably the most compelling one, and is the primary reason I haven't forced my whole family to be gluten-free: it's not reality. Again, this is more important when a child in the family has the restricted diet, because the reality is that this world is filled with gluten, and most people on this planet eat it—lots of it. These children need to learn how to handle the fact that, for the rest of their lives, they'll be surrounded by people eating gluten. If that makes them feel bad, sad, or mad, that's okay. What better place to learn to deal with those unpleasant emotions than in the loving environment of their own home? They may be more tempted to cheat because the food is in their home and others are eating it; again, there may be no better place to deal with temptation and learn to resist it than in the loving environment of their own home.

The compromise:

In no way am I advocating someone waving a Krispy Kreme donut in your face singing, "Nah-nee-nah-nee-nah-nee…you can't eat this" in an effort to build character. With the excellent gluten-free products available today, it's easier than ever to compromise by eating *relatively* gluten-free. Try to buy salad dressings, condiments, spices, and other foods and ingredients that are gluten-free when you can. For foods like pasta, bread, and pizza, you can make two varieties, one of which of course is gluten-free and prepared carefully to avoid contamination.

Cost aside, I don't see any reason to bake "regular" cookies and baked goods anymore. The gluten-free mixes are so incredible that my kids and their friends prefer them to "the real deal." They're easy enough that the kids can make them themselves, and it's a psychological upper for my gluten-free son when his sister and friends can't get enough of "his kind" of cookies.

You'll probably find that because it's easier to make one meal than two, you'll gravitate toward gluten-free menus. With good menu planning, and a kitchen well-stocked with gluten-free condiments and ingredients, it's likely that your entire family will inadvertently become mostly gluten-free without realizing it, and without the resentment that might have developed if the issue had been forced.

If your family does end up mostly gluten-free, or if you eliminate gluten completely, remember that anyone who is going to be tested for celiac disease (and all family members should be) must be eating gluten for at least several weeks prior to doing any tests for celiac disease.

To Eat or Not to Eat

By Shelley Case, B.Sc., RD

Starch—the single word "starch" on a US or Canadian food label is considered the common or usual name for cornstarch. Starches from other sources must be labeled accordingly such as "potato starch", "tapioca starch" or "wheat starch". It is very difficult to completely remove all traces of protein during the manufacture of food-grade starch. Wheat starch contains varying amounts of gluten. Some European products labeled "gluten-free" are made from Codex Alimentarius quality wheat starch. North American celiac organizations do not recommend that celiacs consume wheat starch-based products.

Modified Food Starch

There are specific regulations for how food starches can be modified. However, there is no requirement for the identification of the name of the plant sources of the modified food starch on US or Canadian food labels. Corn, tapioca, potato, wheat or other starches can be used by the food industry. Corn is the most common source of North American modified food starch, with potato, tapioca or rice used occasionally. To be 100% certain, it is best to contact the company to determine the source of the modified food starch.

Dextrin

Dextrin is partially hydrolyzed starch by heat alone or by heating in the presence of food-grade acids and buffers. A variety of starches such as corn, milo, potato, arrowroot, rice, tapioca or wheat can be used. In North America, dextrin is almost always derived from corn or tapioca; however, contact the company to confirm the source of dextrin.

Maltodextrin

Corn, waxy maize, potato, rice or wheat can be used in the production of maltodextrin. North American maltodextrin is usually derived from corn or potato; however, wheat is often used in European products, and occasionally in some North American products. The US Code of Federal Regulations for maltodextrin (Sec. 184.1444) state it is derived from corn, potato or rice starch. The FDA also permits the use of other starches including wheat. If wheat is used, it must be labeled "wheat maltodextrin".

Caramel Color

Caramel color is manufactured by heating carbohydrates, either alone, or in the presence of food-grade acids, alkalis and/or salts, and is produced from fructose, dextrose (glucose), invert sugar, sucrose and/or starch hydrolysates and fractions thereof. Although gluten-containing ingredients [malt syrup (barley) and starch hydrolysates] can be used in the production of caramel color, they are not used according to food processors in North America. Corn is used most often, as it produces a longer shelf life and a much better product.

Venturing Out of the House: Restaurant Realities

By Danna Korn

Even the most seasoned wheat-free/gluten-free eater (forgive the pun—"seasoned eater") may feel a little uncomfortable venturing out of the home. It's true that your risk of getting unsafe foods *does* increase when you leave home, but most people agree that the life experiences of eating at restaurants while traveling, or even just the social aspects or convenience of eating at a restaurant on any given day or night, are well worth it.

In reality, when you eat at restaurants, some chefs will "get it" and work to ensure a safe meal for you, and others won't. Going to restaurants isn't really about eating as much as it is the ambience, the company, and, well, okay—the convenience. Focus on those primary reasons for going to a restaurant, and make the food secondary, even if there's very little you can eat. If you've heard me speak or read my books, then you've followed my advice and stuffed yourself before you left the house, so you're not hungry anyway.

Defensive Dining

It's been said that the best offense is a good defense, which probably applies to restaurant excursions as well as it does to the football field. I'm not encouraging you to be offensive; in fact, quite the opposite. It's not, after all, the waiter's or chef's responsibility to accommodate your diet. If they do, be prepared to leave a big tip, because their job descriptions definitely do not include understanding the intricacies of this diet. Nor should you fill them in on all the minutiae surrounding the diet.

A brief education is all they should need, because you should already have narrowed down the choices on the menu that look as though they might be safe, or at least may be prepared in a way that would make them safe. It's okay to ask that your food be prepared in a special manner—people do that all the time even when they are not on a special diet.

Most important, you need to be aware of specific foods and ingredients to avoid when eating out. Some things are more likely to be okay than others, and you should make it easier on yourself by choosing items that are more likely to be wheat-free/gluten-free.

Plan Ahead

Your days of eating at Italian restaurants with ease are probably behind you (although many Italian dishes are made with polenta, which is gluten-free). Pizza joints: also not likely. Chinese: possibly. Don't set yourself up for disappointment by selecting restaurants that will fill you with frustration by the very nature of their menu selection. Instead, choose restaurants with a large selection, or choose a restaurant based on its ethnicity or culture because it's likely to offer more wheat-free/gluten-free foods. Thai foods, for instance, are often gluten-free, since they use fish sauce instead of soy sauce for a lot of their marinades and seasonings (although some fish sauces can also contain wheat). Study your ethnic foods so you know the ingredients they contain and can make good choices when it comes to restaurant selections.

Knowing what to order is just as important as knowing where to go. Consider, for instance, an American-style restaurant like Denny's or Sizzler. For breakfast, you're better off contemplating the eggs (beware: many restaurant eggs are from a mix that contains gluten), hash browns (be sure to check), and bacon (check again) than you are the Waffle-Mania, even if it *is* only $3.95. For lunch or dinner, you can almost always find a restaurant that will offer you a burger (no bun), fries, and a salad (no croutons).

Be aware of things that are likely to be problematic. For instance, most sushi is okay, but some of the products, such as imitation crabmeat, usually contain wheat, while other sushi items can contain soy sauce, which usually also has wheat. Cajun cooking often uses beer to cook shrimp and other shellfish, and of course beer is off-limits on a gluten-free diet.

Make it easier on yourself by choosing foods that are more likely to be safe for you. What you end up with may not be your first choice, and you may find yourself longing for the days when you could order from a menu with your eyes closed. Don't whine about what you can't have, and focus on the things you can. Remember, eating out isn't about the food. It's about the atmosphere, the company, and the fact that *you're* not cleaning up.

Talk to the Waiter and Ask the Right Questions

Sometimes talking to the waiter is an exercise in futility. If you realize this is the case, either order what you deem to be safest, order nothing at all, or leave.

A cooperative waiter or waitress, on the other hand, is your first line of defense in keeping bad food away. Make friends. Be kind. Tip well. After you've picked what you think could be a safe menu selection or could be made into one, ask questions. Don't be shy; it's not rude or uncommon for people to ask questions, even when they're not accommodating a restrictive diet. Ask if the hamburger patty is 100 per-cent beef or if it has fillers; ask if the eggs are all-egg, or if they have fillers; check to make sure the fries aren't coated with breading, seasonings, or anything else that would make them off-limits. Check sauces and marinades; even if you mention that you can't eat wheat or gluten, people rarely realize, for instance, that soy sauce usually contains wheat.

Once you've made your menu selection, the waiter isn't dismissed. At this point it gets a little awkward because you've probably already asked a lot of questions, but there are a few more to ask, because how the food is prepared is also important. You need to make sure that the hamburgers aren't grilled on the same rack as the buns, and that the croutons aren't just plucked out of your salad, but rather that they were never put in. You even need to ask about the oil the fries are cooked in, because if they're cooked with breaded foods, you really shouldn't eat them.

At this point, even the most patient of waiters is likely to be giving you a stiff smile with that "Is there anything *else* you'd like to know?" expression. Offer to talk to the chef, if it would make things easier. Chefs, although not often edu-cated in the fine art of accommodating restricted diets, are usually interested in them nonetheless, and are usually quite fascinated when you talk to them about the wheat-free/gluten-free diet. Each time you talk to a chef, you're educating him or her and making it easier for the next wheat-free/gluten-free patron who comes along.

Do Your Homework

Many national chain restaurants have lists of their wheat-free/gluten-free products available by phone or on their Websites. Collect lists from your favorite restaurants and fast-food chains, and keep them in a folder for future reference. You may even want to consider putting them in a three-ring binder that you keep in the car.

Once you've done all the work to find restaurants that work for you, by all means don't worry about getting in a rut. There's nothing wrong with "tried and true" when your only other option is "guessed and now I'm sick." Don't get too complacent, though, because just like products at the grocery store, menu items at restaurants sometimes change ingredients. Check frequently, and remember that even if you think it's safe, if something makes you sick, don't eat it!

BYOF (Bring Your Own Food)

It probably wouldn't be too cool for a group of eight to walk into a lovely Italian restaurant, with everyone carrying their entire meal in a brown paper bag, simply to enjoy the ambience. But if you go to a restaurant and bring a small amount of food with you—even if it's the main course—it's certainly not rude. Some (but not many) restaurants have regulations about preparing food, and are allowed to serve only foods that they've prepared. Most, however, have no problem if you bring in your own pizza and ask them to heat it for you.

If you do bring your own food, make sure you it's wrapped in aluminum foil to avoid contamination during the heating process. Pizza ovens, for instance, sometimes have convection fans that can blow the flour from other pizzas around the oven, contaminating yours. If you bring bread and ask them to toast it for you, they're likely to put it in the slot of a toaster, contaminating it with "regular" crumbs and ruining your pristine bread. In that case, you might want to explain that it can't be put in a toaster, but if they have a toaster oven or broiler (that isn't blowing flour around), that would be wonderful. If you're asking them to microwave something, of course, they'll just remove the aluminum foil. The most important thing to remember if you're bringing your own food is to leave a big tip.

Sprechen Sie Gluten?

When eating at restaurants of different cultures and ethnicities, it's a good idea to know the language, especially if the restaurant is staffed by people who speak a language other than your own. Learn the important words to best communicate your special needs. For instance, in Spanish the word for flour is *harina*, but that can refer to corn flour or wheat flour, so you need to know that the word for wheat is *trigo,* and corn is *maize.* Some restaurant cards come in a variety of languages. Additionally, some Websites offer translation capabilities (see http://babelfish.altavista.com/tr).

Tipping

I'm aware of the redundancy in my continuous references to tipping and the importance of being extra generous at tip-time, but I believe it bears repeating. When it comes to asking people to accommodate the gluten-free diet, it seems imperative that we express our gratitude to those who generously oblige our requests. As awareness of this diet increases over the next few years, it will be more common for restaurateurs to understand these restrictions and accommodate them. Anything we can do as a community to enhance their understanding and acceptance will benefit us all in the long run.

Have fun!

Now that you're armed with some basic restaurant realities, remember rule #1: Have fun! Don't live your life in a bubble just because you have a dietary restriction. Bon *Appétit*!

Putting the Pieces Back Together

By Roy S. Jamron

You have just been diagnosed with celiac disease. Wonderful! Now all your gastro problems, aches and pains and fatigue and food allergies will go away. All you need to do is maintain a gluten-free diet—NOT!

Many, if not most, who are gluten intolerant have quickly found our various health problems, sadly, do not go away simply by eliminating gluten from our lives. In fact, our health problems may increase over time. Many futilely and desperately search in vain for "hidden" gluten which they are sure must be present in something they missed causing them problems.

If you are among the lucky ones whose health fully recovers after starting a gluten-free diet, great! The fact is, your gastrointestinal tract and immune system may have been under attack for years. Malabsorption is likely to have caused years of vitamin, mineral, and amino acid deficiencies resulting in damage to your body systems. You may have acquired various other autoimmune conditions along the way. If you are diagnosed over age 40, your body systems may be slowing down and not able to fully recover. The mix of beneficial bacteria and microorganisms which inhabit your gut may have become altered, depleted, or in complete disarray. Your stomach may no longer be producing a sufficient quantity of stomach acid, affecting your ability to digest food and absorb essential vitamins and minerals. Intestinal permeability and perhaps a thymus gland impaired by mineral and vitamin deficiencies may have resulted in the acquisition of multiple food allergies and intolerances. Vitamin B12 deficiency could have caused permanent neurological damage. Bones may have weakened. There may be weak, brittle and malformed finger and toe nails, skin rashes, bruising, and inflammation. Fatigue and muscle pains may be present. The list goes on. So what can one do?

Low Stomach Acid

After a diagnosis of celiac disease or gluten intolerance, you should first immediately assess if you have a low stomach acid condition. Low stomach acid or hypochlorhydria will continue to cause malabsorption problems and vitamin, mineral and amino acid deficiencies. Hypochlorhydria can lead to multiple food allergies. Low stomach acid also allows potentially harmful bacteria and microorganisms to colonize the stomach where they should not be at all. The stomach cells which produce stomach acid also produce a substance called "intrinsic factor" which is necessary to allow the intestine to absorb vitamin B12. If you have low stomach acid, intrinsic factor may be low and you may not be able to absorb vitamin B12 sufficiently. In this case, sublingual or "under-the-tongue" vitamin B12 tablets can be taken to improve absorption. In some cases, vitamin B12 injections are necessary to prevent pernicious anemia.

During digestion, stomach acid levels normally increase. The higher acid level results in a secretion of hormones which, in turn, signal the pancreas to release digestive enzymes and acid-neutralizing bicarbonate ions into the small intestine to complete the digestion of contents leaving the stomach. Maintaining a normal stomach acid level is, thus, crucial for digestion in both the stomach and intestine. Low stomach acid is also present in the vast majority of heartburn sufferers, and improper digestion due to low acid is the cause of most heartburn. Taking acid suppressors for heartburn is exactly the wrong thing to do if you have low stomach acid. Taking an acid supplement to normalize digestion can actually prevent heartburn in most cases. An excellent reference on stomach acid is the paperback book _Why Stomach Acid Is Good for You_ by Jonathan V. Wright, M.D. and Lane Lenard, Ph.D.

Low stomach acid can be treated by taking digestive enzymes and an acid supplement, such as betaine HCl, with every meal, likely for the rest of one's life. There are many digestive enzyme formulations available, and the choice depends on your individual metabolism. I prefer the pricey but high-quality fungal derived enzymes from Enzymedica, and take one Carbo capsule with every meal. The Carbo formulation has a modest level of protease enzymes. High levels of protease can cause a burning sensation in the bowels in some people, including myself, which normally goes away after a few weeks of use. Since I am mostly vegetarian, my need for protease to digest meat and proteins is reduced. Betaine HCl is available in tablet form, or as 10-grain capsules containing powdered betaine HCl, which works faster. You need to adjust the number of betaine HCl capsules to suit your low acid condition, and this usually means taking more than just one or two capsules with each meal. The number is adjusted by increasing it until you experience a warm sensation in your stomach, and then backing off by one capsule. I take three 10-grain capsules with breakfast and lunch, and six with dinner. I buy quantities of 250 capsule bottles of Solaray High Potency HCl from a discount health food company over the internet at a very reasonable price. Enzymedica products can also be purchased at discount over the internet.

Treating hypochlorhydria greatly reduced or eliminated my allergic responses to numerous foods.

A quick and simple test for low stomach acid makes use of fresh baking soda. You should not be taking antacids or acid suppressors to perform this test. Stomach acid and baking soda react to form carbon dioxide gas. First thing in the morning, before eating or drinking, add one quarter teaspoon of baking soda to an eight ounce glass of water. Mix, drink, and start timing for up to five minutes. You should normally belch within two to three minutes if your stomach acid level is adequate. Rapid and repeated belching may mean excessive stomach acid is present. Late or no belching indicates low stomach acid. Acid levels can be confirmed by measuring stomach pH using a small radio capsule (Heidelberg capsule) that is swallowed, a test which some gastroenterologists or naturopathic doctors can perform.

Probiotics

Probiotics provide beneficial microbes to help replace and restore order to the bacteria and micro flora which reside in the gastrointestinal tract. Celiac disease, hypochlorhydria, immune system disorders, and accompanying gastrointestinal distress can wreak havoc on the balance and mixture of the beneficial and necessary micro flora of the gut. Low stomach acid permits entry of undesirable and pathogenic bacteria. Malabsorption results in an excess of undigested nutrients in the gut, feeding and promoting an overabundance of undesirable bacteria species. Taking a probiotic supplement helps to re-colonize the gastrointestinal tract with beneficial bacteria which, in turn, displace the undesired bacteria.

Probiotics come in the form of foods, such as yogurt and kefir containing live cultures of beneficial bacteria, or in capsule, tablet, liquid or powdered form. Choosing a probiotic may not be easy. Research on probiotics is a very young field, and which species of bacteria provide the greatest benefit remains uncertain. You may need to try a number of different probiotic products to find one that best suits your needs.

A probiotic containing a mixture of a number of different bacteria species might be more likely to provide the bacteria combination that works for you. Ideally, a dose of probiotic should provide billions, 10, 20, or even 30 billion or more bacteria, to effectively colonize the bowel. Probiotic capsules which provide such a high dosage are expensive. A good yogurt or kefir is a much more cost effective probiotic providing many billions of bacteria per serving.

Yogurt and kefir are both fermented milk products, but kefir contains yeast in addition to bacteria. Sensitivity to yeast is a common problem among celiacs, and, hence, kefir may not be suitable for everyone. Soy yogurt and kefir are also available if you are sensitive to dairy products. Some health food stores can provide yogurt and kefir made with sheep or goat's milk if cow's milk is a particular problem. Labels on some probiotic products warn that flu-like symptoms may result during the first few weeks of use and recommend a lower dose until the symptoms disappear.

Personally, I consume a plain yogurt, without gelatin or corn syrup, preferring Nancy's Yogurt. I had a six month bout of diarrhea after a prolonged summer cold. I had been taking a probiotic capsule, and decided to switch to yogurt to provide a larger and cheaper dose of bacteria. The website for Nancy's Yogurt, which contains six live bacteria cultures, was the only one which provided a bacteria count from an independent laboratory. Nancy's Yogurt seemed to be instrumental in finally clearing up the diarrhea problem for me. I consume a heaping tablespoon of yogurt on each of two rice cakes every morning and two heaping tablespoons on my salad at dinner. Depending on the age of the yogurt, this provides up to over 30 billion bacteria per two tablespoon serving. I have also tried Stonyfield Farms Yogurt, which also contains six bacteria cultures, but the product is "runny" compared to Nancy's firm texture. I have not yet tried Mountain High Yogurt, containing five bacteria cultures, which may be another good alternative. I suggest you contact yogurt makers about their bacteria content if you try other brands. However, such information is not always reliable.

Nails

Your nails are a barometer to your health and provide a good visual aide in recognizing vitamin and mineral deficiencies and other problems. White spots and poor nail growth can indicate a zinc deficiency. Thin, brittle, spoon or concave shaped nails, and ridges running lengthwise indicate possible iron deficiency. A deficiency in vitamin A can cause slow growing brittle nails lacking pink a glow underneath. Vitamin C, folic acid, or protein deficiency can cause hangnails. A deficiency of B vitamins causes fragility, with horizontal or vertical ridges. A deficiency of vitamin B12 leads to excessive dryness, very rounded and curved nail ends, and darkened nails. Splitting, thin, chipping, or peeling nails may mean low stomach acid or low sulfur amino acid. White bands across the nails can indicate a protein deficiency. Probiotics can help fend off nail fungal infections by displacing yeasts and fungi in the gut. A host of medical problems such as thyroid, kidney, and diabetes conditions can be indicated by various malformations and discolorations of the nails. For more on these medical conditions try reading _Nail Abnormalities: Clues to Systemic Disease_ by Robert S. Fawcett, M.D., M.S., Sean Linford, M.D., Daniel L. Stulberg, M.D.

I developed a problem with nails deteriorating on the edges of the large toe nails and on one edge of the thumb and index finger of the right hand. In addition, for years I had a chronic periodic swelling and inflammation of the toes around the toe nails. When I began taking betaine HCl for hypochlorhydria, the nail deterioration seemed to stop, but there was little or no nail growth to repair the damage. Searching the internet for solutions, I came across websites which suggested that supplementing with MSM (methylsulfonylmethane) frequently resulted in increased nail growth as well as improved hair condition. MSM is a sulfur compound, and numerous health benefits have been claimed for it for which I cannot vouch. Sulfur is a component of keratin, and keratin is a protein important for the maintenance and growth of nails, hair and skin. MSM has a bitter taste, but it does not leave an aftertaste. The powder can be mixed with fruit juice, if desired. I began taking one half teaspoon of powdered MSM in a glass of water once daily, and soon noticed an apparent increase in nail growth after a few weeks. Encouraged, I began to take one half teaspoon MSM twice daily, in the morning and evening. I also began taking 500 mg L-methionine, an essential sulfur amino acid, twice daily. This increased nail growth even more, and, quite unexpectedly, within two weeks the chronic periodic swelling and inflammation of the toes completely ceased and has never returned to this day (I also noticed my hair seemed softer and had more luster, but, hey, us males aren't supposed to care about such things). I started taking MSM in January 2003.

I've had a few relapses resulting in some temporary nail deterioration, especially during the six month bout of diarrhea. Consuming yogurt seemed to help clear up the nail problem as well as the diarrhea. I also now have further increased my take of MSM powder to a heaping teaspoon in water twice daily with no side effects noticed. After nearly two years my nails are almost completely normal and healthy. Only the slow growing large toe nails still show any obvious signs of the prior condition, and they are nearly fully grown back and healthy. I buy MSM powder in 35 oz (1000 g) containers at discount over the internet.

Vitamins, Minerals and Amino Acids

Our intestines have been damaged. We may have low stomach acid. We may be vegetarian. Our metabolisms differ. Our lifestyles differ. All of these factors affect how nutrients are absorbed and how much of each nutrient we require. Does that multivitamin/multi-mineral supplement supplying the recommended daily allowance (RDA) of vitamins and minerals really meet your needs? Remember, these are the amounts needed to maintain a healthy normal individual. You need to look at your own condition to determine the amount of vitamins and minerals you need. This is no easy task. I am still trying to deal with it myself. Wouldn't it be nice if there were some little meter we could poke ourselves with, much like the glucose meter used by diabetics, that could tell us which vitamins and minerals and amino acids were low and what and how much we needed to take?

After first being diagnosed with celiac disease, you are probably deficient in numerous nutrients. Once on a gluten-free diet, many of these deficiencies will return to normal levels. Some may not. In addition, some nutrients, such as vitamin B12, may not be sufficiently absorbed via the intestine, and must be take sublingually or by injection. Paradoxically, some of the very nutrients needed to repair the intestine so that it can absorb them are not being absorbed because of the damage to the intestine.

Deficiencies may require higher than RDA amounts, at first, which must be reduced, later, to avoid overdosing. Without some form of testing and monitoring to determine our need for and levels of nutrients, there is no good way to manage our nutrient needs. I have already suggested that your nails can provide a clue to some deficiencies. Are there tests which can help us decide what we need?

Yes, there are tests which can provide you with serum levels of many nutrients. But these tests can add up and become very costly if tests are done for many nutrients and if follow up tests are performed. Some clinical labs offer package deals which might not be a bad idea for an initial assessment of your health condition. For example, one online service, http://blood-check.com/tests.htm offers an Initial Profile test for $199 which they state is: "Best suited for first-time clients who wish to understand all aspects of their health, and for established clients who wish to document their total wellness. Includes: Total Cholesterol, HDL, LDL and Ratios, Triglycerides, Glucose (Diabetes), Kidney, Liver, & Heart functions, Potassium, Calcium, Uric Acid, Electrolytes, Iron, TIBC with Ferritin reflex (anemia) PLUS a CBC (Complete Blood Count), and a Thyroid (TSH) level." Since iron anemia, diabetes, and thyroid conditions often accompany celiac disease, this initial profile seems like a good idea.

This company offers numerous other tests (over 5,600), some cheap, some expensive, for example: B12- $117.50, B12 with Folate- $236.25, Total Iron- $7.50. I do not think your insurance company is going to be willing to pay for a multitude of tests and follow up tests. A few well-chosen tests may fit within your budget. If you have the means, having the test information is better than not having it. Also, if you can find and afford a good doctor or clinical nutritionist or naturopath to work with you, so much the better. If doctors and tests are not within your means, self-education and trial and error is an alternative approach.

Besides books and libraries, the internet has a wealth of helpful websites on nutrition and nutrients. One of the best websites is the Linus Pauling Institute's Micronutrient Information Center at http://lpi.oregonstate.edu/infocenter/ which provides an excellent source of information on vitamins, minerals and some other nutrients. These websites also offer good information on vitamins and minerals:

http://www.drlera.com/vitamins/vitamins.htm
http://www.drlera.com/minerals/minerals.htm
http://www.springboard4health.com/notebook/

Amino acids, the building blocks of protein, are also important. 22 amino acids are used in human metabolism. Some amino acids can be synthesized by the body, but there are 8 essential amino acids which can only be obtained from diet. The following website provides a good overview of the amino acids:

http://www.springboard4health.com/notebook/cat_proteins.html

Additionally, you need to know how much of these nutrients your diet may be providing. The USDA National Nutrient Database for Standard Reference provides a comprehensive list of nutrients from a huge database of foods and food products:

http://www.nal.usda.gov/fnic/foodcomp/Data/SR17/sr17.html

Just remember that the amount of a nutrient given for a food does not represent how much of that nutrient your body will actually absorb. In some cases, the food may have a very high nutrient content, but only a very small percentage will actually be absorbed because the nutrient is not in a readily absorbable form.

By noting your symptoms and health condition and comparing them to symptoms caused by nutrient deficiencies, you may be able to determine or guess which nutrients you may be lacking. As similar symptoms can be caused by deficiencies of any number of other nutrients, the task is not easy. You may be able to correct the deficiency by including in your diet foods rich in the particular nutrient. You may need to take the nutrient as a supplement to insure sufficient absorption. You also must determine the dose of supplementation you require. In order to be able to assess whether the supplementation is improving your symptoms and health, you must add only one supplement at a time and make no major changes to your diet, and it may take days or weeks or months to note if the symptoms improve. This process can easily become tedious, time-consuming, expensive, and frustrating. If you have narrowed down possible nutrient deficiencies, you may opt to get tested for those particular nutrients.

Vegetarians also have special needs, as there are some nutrients better provided by animal products in the diet. The American Dietetic Association has a comprehensive paper on Vegetarian Diets which discusses these nutritional needs:

http://www.eatright.org/Public/GovernmentAffairs/92_17084.cfm

Vegetarians must make sure their diets are sufficient in protein (essential amino acids), iron, zinc, calcium, vitamin D, riboflavin, vitamin B12, vitamin A, n-3 fatty acids, and iodine. Higher RDA levels and supplementation of some of these nutrients may be necessary to maintain proper levels. Malabsorption caused by celiac disease compounds the likelihood of deficiencies.

Here is an example of tracking down a deficiency problem. A symptom I have been dealing with is fatigue. I take a multivitamin/mineral supplement, sublingual vitamin B12, plenty of vitamin C, plus additional supplements. At first, I suspected adrenal fatigue and achieved some limited relief from fatigue by drinking salted water several times daily to replace lost sodium caused by an insufficient level of the hormone, aldosterone, produced by the adrenals which regulate sodium retention in the kidneys. But lately, salted water is not having much affect, possibly because my aldosterone level is improving. In addition to fatigue and lack of energy, I was experiencing episodes of daytime drowsiness while driving to work. In a self-experiment supplementing with tin in the form of stannous chloride, I actually seemed to have completely cured myself of daytime drowsiness. However, fatigue still remains a problem. See:

"Can Tin Prevent Falling Asleep at the Wheel?"

Evaluating my supplements and considering which nutrient deficiencies are likely to cause fatigue, I noted that my multivitamin/mineral supplement provides only 10 mg iron. The RDA of iron for adult males is 8 mg and for pre-menopausal adult females is 18 mg. However, vegetarians face a lower bioavailability of iron from their diets. In meat, iron is available in a "heme" form that is more readily absorbed than the inorganic form of iron found in plants. Red meat and spinach both have a high iron content. 20% of the heme iron available in a lean steak is absorbed, but only 2% of the iron in cooked spinach is actually absorbed. The iron RDA for vegetarians is 14 mg for men and 33 mg for pre-menopausal women. Physical activity can also deplete iron stores. Sports activities, exercise, and heavy labor can raise the daily requirement for iron. Any bleeding causes iron depletion. A loss of one ml of blood results in a loss of 0.5 mg iron. Low stomach acid results in poor iron absorption and intestinal damage from celiac disease often causes iron deficiency. Other dietary factors also affect how much iron is absorbed. Vitamin C consumed in the same meal as non-heme iron improves the absorption of the non-heme iron by up to 50%. Heme iron also increases the absorption of non-heme iron. Tea, coffee and certain types of fiber (e.g. phytates) can inhibit the absorption of iron.

Taking a look at myself, I am mostly vegetarian. I have low stomach acid. My intestines may still be impaired from celiac disease, and reactions to food intolerances or allergies could also impair absorption. I sometimes experience loss of blood from rectal bleeding through an anal fissure as a result of bowel distress. I do a long series of stretching exercises every morning, and my work involves moderate physical activity. Suddenly, a supplement providing only 10 mg of iron daily seems totally inadequate for my needs. Iron deficiency could definitely explain my fatigue. Recently, I have begun daily supplementation of iron in the form of 28 mg iron from ferrous gluconate in addition to the 10 mg of iron I already take. It is too soon to tell if iron supplementation is improving my fatigue, but I do seem to be a little less fatigued. Hopefully, I will see continued improvement.

Food Allergies and Intolerances

Multiple food allergies often accompany celiac disease. In addition, temporary intolerances to dairy products and sugars may result from celiac disease. Enzymes which digest lactose and various other forms of sugar are produced in the lining of the small intestine. Production of these enzymes is impaired by damage to the intestine from celiac disease. Sugars and lactose are thus not properly absorbed. Low stomach acid, if present, also results in incomplete digestion of proteins, fats and carbohydrates. Damage to the intestine results in the intestine being less capable of absorbing nutrients. An accumulation of undigested sugars, and other nutrients, promotes an over-abundance of intestinal bacteria and other micro flora which feed on the ready supply of unabsorbed nutrients. The secretions and toxins generated by these micro flora can cause gas, discomfort, and other symptoms of intolerance and bowel distress. Intestinal damage also increases intestinal permeability or "leaky gut". Undigested and normally harmless food proteins can "leak" into the blood stream and into other body systems where they may be identified as intruders, initiating allergic and immune responses.

I have come to believe that the thymus gland may also be involved in the acquisition of food allergies. The thymus is located behind the breastbone and is responsible for the generation of T cells, critical to the function of the immune system. Until quite recently, it was thought the thymus stopped producing T cells after puberty when the thymus begins to shrink. However, it is now known the thymus continues to produce T cells in adults and throughout life. Certain regulatory T cells help the immune system decide whether foreign proteins should be tolerated or attacked. If these regulatory T cells are not in sufficient supply, allergic reactions to harmless proteins may result. The thymus is particularly sensitive to malnutrition. Hence, malabsorption from celiac disease or low stomach acid may adversely affect the thymus and its ability to produce regulatory T cells, thus leading to or contributing to multiple food allergies.

Maintaining a gluten-free diet allows the gut to heal. In most cases, the intestine will again produce the enzymes to digest lactose and other sugars, and these intolerances may go away. Intestinal permeability will decrease, and food allergies and sensitivities may lessen. The thymus may also recover from malnutrition, if not too severely damaged. If you have low stomach acid, food allergies will continue to be a problem unless you take acid supplementation (e.g. betaine HCl) and digestive enzymes with every meal. Some food allergies or sensitivities may not completely go away.

To help speed healing, it is probably best to avoid foods which are causing problems. If you have a reaction shortly after consuming the food, typically less than 30 minutes, it may be easy to determine the offending food. Some foods may cause a delayed reaction. It may be hours or even days or weeks before antibody production reaches a level high enough to cause a noticeable reaction. This makes identification of the offending food difficult. Elimination diets can be used to identify which foods are safe and which are not. Stick with eating a few basic foods that you know you can tolerate well, and then add suspected foods to your diet one at a time, allowing sufficient time—days or longer if necessary—to observe a possible reaction. Elimination diets are tedious. Some tests are available which can help to identify possible food sensitivities. These tests include the skin prick test, the RAST (Radioallergosorbent test), the ELISA (Enzyme-Linked Immunosorbent Assay) test, and the newest test, the ImmunoCAP® Specific IgE test (a fluoroenzyme-immunoassay (FEIA)). See:

http://www.future-drugs.com/admin/articlefile/ERMD040303.pdf

The skin prick test is performed in a doctor's office, a prick for each allergen being tested, and can be expensive. RAST testing uses a blood sample to test for the amount of specific IgE antibodies present. ELISA testing also uses a blood sample, but tests for specific IgG antibodies instead of IgE antibodies (associated with true allergies.) IgG reactions can typically occur hours or days after encountering a food or antigen. The ELISA test can be useful in identifying foods which cause delayed reactions. ELISA tests which can test for 190 or so food sensitivities in one blood draw are available for a relatively modest cost. However, the reliability of ELISA tests depends on the laboratory performing the test, and results between different laboratories vary greatly. RAST test results also vary from lab to lab. RAST tests are being replaced by ImmunoCAP® tests. The ImmunoCAP® Specific IgE test is much more accurate and reliable than the RAST test, and test results are consistent from lab to lab. Costs for ImmunoCAP® or RAST tests can add up as the cost increases for each different allergen being tested for.

When I first put myself on a gluten-free diet after years of chronic diarrhea and learning about celiac disease, within a few days I had the first solid bowel movement I could remember in years. But the elation was short-lived. For months afterward, my bowel movement kept changing form from solid to liquid, and the chronic diarrhea kept reappearing. Then, finally, my first breakthrough came. The growing season for melons ended. When melons were no longer a part of my diet, the chronic diarrhea finally disappeared. I had made my first discovery that other foods besides gluten were causing me problems. I began to pay close attention to any reaction or bowel distress that occurred after eating any foods. Soon I was finding foods I had been freely consuming daily and all my life were creating reactions. Fruits were especially troublesome. In response to apples, pears, bananas, oranges, tangerines, hot chocolate, popcorn and more, I was sniffling, experiencing throat irritation, a general malaise, fatigue, and bowel distress within 20 minutes after ingestion. I started to eliminate these foods from my diet. Since childhood, I have had a chronic throat-clearing problem, and, now, decades later, I finally learned the throat-clearing was due to a sensitivity to corn. I eliminated all corn and products containing corn from my diet, and the throat-clearing finally stopped. Every time I eliminated one food, however, I soon found myself sensitive to a new food. Finally it got to the point where I was reacting to almost everything I ate, even to potatoes and rice cakes. You can imagine the desperation I felt standing in the supermarket produce aisle, one day, hopelessly searching for something I could safely eat.

Meanwhile, on the internet I noted that some people were reporting that taking digestive enzymes had allowed them to consume foods they had not been able to eat for years without getting ill. Enzymes were theorized to break down proteins into pieces too small to cause reactions. That sounded reasonable to me. So I went to a health food store and bought some digestive enzymes, Enzymedica Digest, to be specific. Taking one capsule with each meal, the effect was immediate. I quickly found myself able to consume at least some foods again without reaction. All seemed to be going well for about a month, until I again started reacting to an increasing number of foods. Now what was I supposed to do?

Back to the internet! This time I learned about hypochlorhydria, low stomach acid. Back at the health food store, I bought betaine HCl. Taking betaine HCl and digestive enzymes with every meal once again caused the food sensitivities to go away—and this time *stay* away. I still keep melons, citrus fruit, and corn, as well as gluten, out of my diet. I rotate other fruits so I do not consume them on consecutive days. I find that new foods I have never eaten before can cause me problems. Montina (Indian rice grass flour) and sorghum flour cause me to have a sore throat reaction. I tried to add avocados to my diet, which I have never eaten before. After eating a couple of avocados a week for a few weeks, I broke out in hives for the first time in my life, an experience I do not want to repeat. I guess the tolerance mechanism of my immune system is now so screwed up that my immune system will no longer tolerate the introduction of any new foods into my diet. As long as I stick with old dependable foods, betaine HCl, and digestive enzymes, I seem to be on the road to recovery.

Health Basics

While all or some of the above mentioned suggestions may help you fully recover from celiac disease, it is still important to remember the basics of keeping healthy—and that is to eat a healthy diet, keep the weight off, keep active, and exercise regularly. Celiac disease has been associated with diabetes, so it is even all the more important to keep those sugary junk foods and simple carbohydrates under control and out of your diet. In addition to improving mobility and muscle tone, exercise can just plain make you feel better and help keep your bowel movement regular. For years I have been doing daily morning yoga-like stretching exercises, becoming ever-more flexible and able to obtain extreme positions as well as great balance control. I began the stretching exercises when I developed pains and cramping in my legs and it became uncomfortable just to bend my legs at the knee. My ankles would also easily buckle while walking up stairs. That was many years ago, and the leg pains and other aches are long gone. I am much more flexible now than I was as a teenager in high school. I find that the exercise almost always helps to induce a bowel movement.

Conclusion

It took me years to diagnose myself as being gluten intolerant and five more years to discover the steps toward recovery I have presented here. I am still not completely well, but, little by little I am improving. If I had not taken these steps, I would hate to think of the condition I would be in now. If I had had this knowledge years ago and acted on it—think of all the suffering and discomfort I could have avoided. It is my hope that you will use and find this information helpful to speed your recovery so your suffering will not be prolonged needlessly. Feeling ill is no way to live a life.

Planes, Trains, and Automobiles: Gluten-free Travel Tips

By Danna Korn

There's no point in enjoying the improved health and vitality you'll experience on a gluten-free diet if you're just sitting at home pining away for excitement because you're afraid to venture too far away. You have to live life to its fullest—you should be livin' la vida loca! There's no reason whatsoever to limit or, worse yet, give up travel because of this diet. Traveling wheat-free/gluten-free might be a little intimidating at first, but really, it just takes a little more planning, and sometimes an extra suitcase or two.

Pre-Travel Checklist

Before you leave, research your destination: Check with a support group in the area you're visiting to see if they have a list of celiac-friendly restaurants or grocery stores. Also search the St. John's Celiac Listserv archives for frequent posts about gluten-free-friendly restaurants. You might want to go to the Internet and look up your destination city to see if they have one or more health food stores. If they do, call the store(s) and ask what gluten-free products they carry—if you have a favorite product, ask them to order it for you before your trip so they will have it in stock when you arrive.

Be aware of legal considerations when crossing borders: Some countries have laws about what foods can be imported. Make sure you know what the laws are, and don't try to bring foods with you that might be confiscated. My family and I had an — umm — interesting experience at the Mexican border when we brought gluten-free pancake mix in an unmarked, vacuum-sealed plastic bag.

Know the language (at least key words): Learn at least a few key words of the language spoken in the country you'll be visiting. Make sure you can say wheat, flour, and other key words. Bring restaurant cards written in the language(s) of the country you're visiting (see www.celiactravel.com), or use translation software (i.e., http://babelfish.altavista.com/tr) to create your own.

Ask for rooms with a kitchenette, or stay in a condo: Even a small kitchenette with a microwave, refrigerator, and sink will make your life a little easier.

Ship food to yourself: If you're traveling a long distance or are going to be gone for a long period of time, consider shipping some of your favorite products to your ultimate destination so they're waiting for you when you arrive.

Carry a "kitchen in a suitcase": If you're accustomed to making your breads, cookies, and other baked goods from the mixes that you order online or find in specialty stores, bring them with you, as it may be difficult to find them at your ultimate destination. Bring your specialty tools or appliances, too, like your bread slicer, if you plan on cooking while you're away.

Grab your gadgets: Manufacturers offer some ultra-convenient travel gadgets these days, even for the traveling eater. Most sporting goods stores carry a small refrigerator (there are several brands) that plugs into the cigarette lighter of your car, making it easier to bring yogurt and other perishables on long drives. And we all know how toasters can present a problem since "regular" toast seems to spray its crumbs everywhere, contaminating them for gluten-free eaters. A travel toaster available on the Internet:

(www.fsmarketplace.company.uk/traveltoasters) eliminates the worry—just take your own and you're set.

BYOF: Even gluten-free bread travels well if you slice it and pack it in a hard plastic storage container. Hard-to-find cereals, pretzels, and favorite treats—even pre-baked frozen cookies—make great snacks en route or when you arrive. Don't forget to pack food for the trip itself, as well as food for your stay at the destination.

There are grocery stores everywhere you go: When you arrive at your ultimate destination, stop in at the local grocery store and stock up on some of the basics. Don't forget to buy aluminum foil and re-sealable bags, which work well to store leftovers from restaurants, or any foods that you may have brought with you.

Remember your restaurant rules: Use the tips mentioned in my books or in past issues of Scott-Free for eating out at restaurants, since you'll probably be eating out more than you do when you're at home. If you're traveling to certain places in Europe, you might be pleasantly surprised to find that in some countries like Sweden McDonald's offers two types of hamburger buns: gluten-free and "regular."

Getting There

When planning how and what you're going to eat on your trip, you have to first decide where you're going and how you're going to get there. How much and what you bring depends on whether you're taking planes, trains, or automobiles.

Driving: Driving allows you the most flexibility, and is easiest when you're trying to accommodate a restricted diet. If you're driving in the United States, there will most certainly be national fast-food chains all along the way. Even if you don't want to rely on greasy burgers and fries as a staple for your entire drive, you know that you have a backup—just in case. National restaurant chains (even those that are not of the fast-food, greasy-burger variety) have branches in all major cities—find out which restaurants are along your driving route (you can check www.mapquest.com or a similar Website), and check the restaurants' Web sites or contact them for their lists of wheat-free/gluten-free products (this is where your three-ring binder with restaurant lists that you leave in the car comes in handy). There are also commercial gluten-free restaurant guides available, such as the one at www.celiac.com.

Most importantly, BYOF. You will probably bring snack foods to munch on while you drive, so just make sure you're loaded with snacks that are easy to eat in the car, travel well, and of course, meet your dietary restrictions (and don't forget the paper towels or wet wipes!).

Flying, cruising, and riding the rails: There's less flexibility in how and where you can eat when you're at the mercy of a commercial airliner, ship, or train—but you still have a number of options. Many commercial airlines offer a selection of specialty meals, including gluten-free ones. Be careful, though, and read the labels if the food has them, because sometimes our gluten-free meals have come with fluffy, doughy bagels (that obviously aren't gluten-free). If mistakes are made, don't be mad. They tried, and at least they considered having a gluten-free meal as an option. Be glad they made the attempt, and consider writing a polite, gratuitous letter to the food supplier offering information on what's gluten-free and what isn't.

These days, airlines restrict the number of carry-on bags, so you'll have to be more efficient in packing snacks and meals for the flight. Snack items that you might include in a sack lunch usually make good take-along foods for the airplane.

Cruise ships always have executive chefs. They're accustomed to accommodating restricted diets, some of which can have dangerous consequences if mistakes are made, so they take the subject very seriously. By contacting the administrative offices of the cruise line several weeks in advance, you can arrange for the chef to provide you gluten-free meals throughout your cruise.

Trains are tougher, since most of the foods found in café cars are usually along the lines of packaged sandwiches, croissants, pastries, and other oh-so-not-nutritious goodies. I highly recommend bringing food on the train, and not just because of your restricted diet, if you know what I mean.

Hidden Sources of Gluten: My "Nearly Normal" Gluten-Free Life

By Jules E.D. Shepard

When I walked out of the doctor's office in West Virginia in 1999 with my diagnosis in hand, I felt a confusing mixture of relief at finally knowing what in the world was wrong with me and dismay at learning there was nothing left that I could eat! Celiac disease. I had never heard of it, yet all the tests showed that I definitely had this autoimmune disorder which prevented me from ever again eating wheat, barley or rye.

I had spent nearly 10 years suffering through untold and embarrassing doctors' tests and misdiagnoses as well as riding a roller coaster of nasty gastrointestinal symptoms. Bouncing between specialists at major hospitals got me nowhere for those many years, as they had no idea what was the cause of my ailments. Finally, through luck or fate, I happened upon a doctor in Huntington, West Virginia who pieced together my symptoms correctly. The good news was that I at last knew something could be done about my symptoms; the bad news was actually trying to do it! Having to transition immediately from my steady diet of pizza, pasta, and bagels to rice, beans and bananas proved necessary but incredibly difficult, especially since there were virtually no palatable gluten-free recipes, ready-made foods or mixes. As with most things, what seemed at the time like an ending was actually a beginning —it was just a little hard to see at the time.

Even as a little girl, I had loved baking! My EasyBake Oven was broken-in early, as my mother patiently let me experiment at a very young age. When I was 16, I went to Malaysia as a foreign exchange student and saw unspeakable things that caused me to become a life-long vegetarian. I could eat almost nothing my host family ate, so I survived primarily on bread and things I could make for myself. I was determined to persevere in this situation where I was the unwelcome minority. It became a matter of physical as well as emotional survival. It was an experience that brought unexpected rewards and helped me to know the value of determination and problem solving—traits I would certainly need later to handle living with celiac disease.

In college, the mainstays of my diet were pastas and breads; I also often baked for friends who loved being treated to homemade cookies, cakes, muffins and brownies. Baking was even an outlet for my creativity during law school and a great stress-reliever too! I ultimately baked so much that I ended up selling my excess treats to the law school café!

Creating recipes in the kitchen has always been part of who I am—to make and share things that others enjoy is one of my greatest pleasures. But then I woke up one day as an undergraduate and was sick. I was never the same again. It was like the final drop had dripped into a sink full of water and from then on, the sink would overflow with even the smallest addition. I couldn't go out on dinner dates, go out to eat with friends, enjoy Thanksgiving dinner with family, participate in a birthday party, or share any other social activity that involved food in any way (doesn't everything?!) without getting sick. It took almost ten years to find out that the culprit was the main ingredient in the things I most loved to eat and make!

I was in the midst of planning my wedding when the diagnosis came; just about the only things I could eat at the reception were fruit, some steamed vegetables and the (proverbial) icing on the cake. All my dreams of wowing my new husband with great cooking and baking were sabotaged as I began to experiment in the restrictive world of gluten-free cooking. Recipes from special cookbooks called for ingredients that were next to impossible to find and yielded results that were mostly inedible. My husband and I both worked long hours—he as an Assistant United States Attorney and I as an Assistant State Prosecutor—but there was no fast food I could eat, and even regular restaurant menus were mine fields of hidden gluten. Trying to bake for holidays was one disaster after another. My husband began to ask, "Is this gluten-free, honey?" and when the answer was yes, he would politely decline.

All I wanted was for my life to be "normal" again. Several things happened at about the same time which gave me direction and which have made all the difference in my life and, I hope, in the lives of many others! When I was diagnosed, my mother made it her mission to find recipes for things I could still enjoy eating and she created a binder of these recipes that we both began to expand. We started a collection of recipes from everyone from personal friends to people we met at the health food store. I found it a challenge to try recipes and to improve upon them by modifying them in my own ways.

About a year and a half after the diagnosis, we moved to Baltimore and I discovered I was pregnant. Now, added to my new job in a new place with new doctors was the very serious challenge of maintaining proper nutrition for pregnancy and breast feeding. This caused me to shift all my efforts into high gear. I wanted to revolutionize gluten-free cooking into something even non-celiacs would enjoy.

Several years of experimenting with various grains and flours culminated in my creation of a mixture that could successfully and safely replace all purpose wheat flour. The primitive binder of recipes we had begun blossomed into lots of delicious concoctions. As others, celiac and non-celiac alike, repeatedly asked for recipes and doggie bags, I realized how important it was to share my hard work and successes with others trying to live normally without wheat and gluten. I could create fabulous things to eat, teach others what I had learned about our disease and how to manage it, and meet lots of new people along the way!

I've been able to accomplish all these things by sharing my cookbook/guidebook called <u>Nearly Normal Cooking for Gluten-Free Eating</u> and by consulting with other celiacs and those with food allergies. I have met some amazing people along the way and helped them meet our challenge head-on and overcome it in fun and creative ways.

So, there really is a higher purpose for my diagnosis. I took a mighty circuitous route, but only because I have celiac disease am I now in a place where I can help others and do the things that I love best at the same time. It has been loads of work, but I persevere knowing that I'm cooking not only for me and my family, but for millions of others who can now live a healthy, gluten-free and truly "nearly normal" life!

CHAPTER 9:
TAKING ACTION

Advocating on Behalf of Persons with Celiac Disease – Doing It Well

By Cynthia Kupper, RD, CD

For many years Gluten Intolerance Group™ (GIG) has advocated on behalf of persons with celiac disease. Advocacy can include the increase of celiac disease awareness, the improvement of knowledge and educational materials distributed by any number of organizations, sitting on boards and committees of coalitions on behalf of persons with celiac disease or dermatitis herpetiformis, and fighting to pass legislation that will improve the quality of life for persons with gluten intolerance.

Advocacy is important work. It takes skill and the desire to work as a team. At times the work can also be slow and frustrating. According to Kay Holcombe's presentation at the 2002 GIG™ Annual Education Conference in Winston-Salem, North Carolina, anyone can learn to be an effective advocate. Ms. Holcombe is a lobbyist with Policy Directions, Inc. in Washington DC. She has years of health care and label reform experience. At the conference Ms. Holcombe offered the following advice for how to become an effective advocate:

- *Keep your agenda short and to the point* — When you advocate you should have no more than three agenda items or points to cover. Know what they are, what you want, and how you are going to get your message across. When you try to make too many points during a presentation it can lose its power and influence.
- *Be knowledgeable about the issue* — It is important to thoroughly understand an issue before you discuss it with your congressperson. If you do not understand the issue well enough you cannot answer questions about it or understand how it will impact people. The last thing you want to do is to lose your congressperson's respect because do not know what you are talking about or are confused.

- *Be honest* – The rule here is: do not try to mislead them. Their staff will do extensive research and will know if you are being less than honest.
- *Send a consistent message* – Nothing can hurt your cause more than to have several people who advocate it but do not say the same thing about it. Everyone must use the same words in the same manner. The message should be short, simple and consistent. Even slight deviations in your message could convey to representatives that you are not united. Everyone must 'Speak with One Voice.'

Ms. Holcombe also advised that success in advocacy work is often measured in small victories, and not necessarily in an all-out victory. A good example of this is the ingredient label reform bill currently being considered by congress. The original bill required that seven major allergens (including wheat) be clearly labeled on all food products. Through an extensive letter writing campaign, partnerships with other influential groups and expert testimony, additional language was added to the bill so that it also included "other grains containing gluten (rye, barley, oats and triticale)." This was a great victory for us—even if the bill does not ultimately pass. We got them to understand that gluten in food is an important issue for many people.

Other celiac organizations have also joined GIG™ to do advocacy work. Currently most of our advocacy work is national in scope, but we also work on state issues. To "speak with one voice" in order to be effective advocates is an important lesson that provides celiac organizations in the U.S. with an opportunity to show unity for a common cause. While not always an easy task, it is an important goal that will benefit all persons with gluten intolerance.

To learn more about the advocacy efforts of GIG™ contact us at info@gluten.net or www.gluten.net. We are currently working on national issues that could affect people with gluten intolerance in the following areas: quality of life, extra cost of food reimbursement, product labeling, research, professional and public awareness and education, and restaurant regulations.

Gluten-Free for 12 Years: A 14-year-old Boy's Perspective

By Danna Korn

When Tyler was diagnosed with celiac disease at the age of 18 months, I wanted desperately to talk to a kid—one who *could* talk—about what it's like to have celiac disease.

Do you feel gypped? Does it make you sad? Do you feel "different" from the other kids?!? I was heartbroken—grief-stricken—I had a long way to go before I would evolve into the cheerleader I hope I've become in helping people live—*and love*—the gluten-free lifestyle.

Oh, sure, friends and family told me "it would be okay," the way friends and family do in tough situations. But I felt they were just placating me—after all, what did they know? They hadn't even *heard* of celiac disease before I had explained the diagnosis. And to be honest, I didn't care much at that time about what adults thought of the situation—I wanted desperately to hear from a kid: "Look at me—I turned out just fine!"

That was nearly 13 years ago, and there weren't any kids who had celiac disease—none that I knew of, anyway. So we blazed our own trail, working hard to approach our unique challenges with optimism each and every step of the way.

Recently, I was reminded of the way I felt when Tyler was first diagnosed, when a woman with tears in her eyes approached me after one of my talks. "I know you talk about how we can all learn to live and love this lifestyle, and I appreciate your suggestions for raising happy, healthy, gluten-free kids—but," she seemed shy and embarrassed to continue, looking at the floor as she asked, "would you mind if I talked directly to Tyler?"

But of course! How could I have forgotten? That *need* to talk to a child who had been through it was so compelling at first—and *now* Tyler *could* talk! Sure you can, was my automatic reply, knowing that my 14 (and-a-half) year-old-I-at-least-like-to-pretend-that-everything-you-do-annoys-me son would be less than thrilled to take the call.

I would love for Tyler to write an article telling you how celiac disease is no big deal in his life. He did so a few years ago for my first book, "*Kids with Celiac Disease,*" when he wrote Chapter One: "What it's like to be a kid with celiac disease," but that was when he was only ten. That was *before* he turned into a teenager and had to start pretending not to want to do the things we ask him to do.

The truth is that this has never been a big deal for Tyler. We gave him control of his diet from day one, which I believe is crucial. We have always maintained an optimistic, yet realistic approach, with Tyler and his non-celiac but oh-so-supportive sister Kelsie, her being our guiding light in terms of inspiration and positive attitude.

One day, a few months after he had been interviewed on a local TV station, Tyler was approached by a woman who attended one of our R.O.C.K. (Raising Our Celiac Kids) parties. I watched with curiosity and felt somewhat protective and guarded as this woman I didn't know quickly approached him and took one of his hands in both of hers in what seemed to be an affectionate gesture. "Tyler, you have changed my life," she said boldly. Then 13 years old, he did what most 13-year-old boys might do, and said nothing—shooting an anxious glance my way, looking for guidance, but I was as bewildered as him. She began to get tears in her eyes as she continued. "I'm 65 years old. Three months ago, I was as sick as I could be. I had been to dozens of doctors, and had a list of symptoms a mile long. Everyone thought I was crazy—I even had to quit my job, because I was so sick. I truly wanted to die. Then I saw you on TV talking about celiac disease. I insisted on being tested, and was positive for celiac disease. I've been gluten-free ever since, and feel absolutely wonderful." With that, she gave him a bear hug, and he shot me a glance that I couldn't read.

I've learned not to embarrass my kids (well, sometimes I do it intentionally, but that's another story), so I said nothing, and Tyler went about his business. Several minutes later, Tyler approached me with a beaming smile. "Mom, *now* I know why you do this! It feels *really good* to help other people!"

He has since decided that he's blessed to have celiac disease, because it has provided him with an opportunity to reach out and help others—an act that even at his young age he realizes is as satisfying for him as it is for those he helps. Quite a perspective for a teenage boy, if I may brag about him a little!

So while I would love for Tyler to write an article about this, those of you who have teenagers understand that it would be easier to teach my dog quantum physics than to have him sit down and write an article—so you'll have to take my word for it. Thankfully, at this point, Tyler is a happy, healthy, gluten-free young man who thinks a lot more about baseball and his friends than he does about the restrictions of his diet. Other kids, teens, and young men and women I've met over the years have been equally optimistic and inspiring. So rest easy, parents—your kids will, in fact, be just fine... and I really *do* know this!

The National Gluten-Free Diet Project

By Cynthia Kupper, RD. CD.

It can be very confusing to person newly diagnosed with gluten intolerance to sort through all the information that abounds about celiac disease and the gluten-free diet.

The information is inconsistent—support groups are not saying the same things—why is there a difference? No wonder celiacs are confused.

Fundamentally, all the national support groups in the U.S. have missions that are similar—to serve and support persons with gluten intolerance. The five national groups: Celiac Disease Foundation (CDF), Gluten Intolerance Group® (GIG®), Raising Our Celiac Kids (R.O.C.K.), Celiac Sprue Association, Inc. (CSA/USA), and American Celiac Society all list this as their primary objective. So, what is the difference between them? Very little. All five have a network of support groups throughout the country—Chapters, Connections, and Partners. All provide local and national literature and support. All are 501(c)(3) nonprofit organizations. Some groups are larger than others, but size alone does not determine the quality or value of the work that each does. Unfortunately, there will always be disagreements between similar organizations, and what constitutes a gluten-free diet seems to be where U.S. national groups disagree. Three groups follow the American Dietetic Association gluten-free guidelines, while the others do not.

The controversy surrounding the gluten-free diet began about 25-30 years ago when the first gluten intolerance support groups began to form. At that time medical experts on celiac disease and the gluten-free diet were few and far between, and support groups were forced to develop their own gluten-free dietary guidelines. Some of the recommendations were based on the meager scientific information available at that time, and other recommendations were based on speculation, assumption, antidotal evidence or hearsay.

Over the years the field of nutrition has seen fad diets come and go. If a disease treatment includes a diet, the thinking has often been 'if some restriction is good, more is better.' There have been some very restrictive diets developed over the years that most people fail to maintain. One example of this is the dramatic change in recommendations for the diabetic diet. Somewhere along the way, the gluten-free diet became one of those diets where it got more and more restrictive—without sound scientific evidence and reasoning for it.

In the last ten years, medical professionals—researchers, medical practitioners, dietitians and pharmacists have become more interested in and aware of celiac disease. Research data collected during this time has changed the face of celiac disease and the gluten-free diet. Health care professionals have developed expertise in all areas related to gluten intolerance diseases. Some dietitian experts now spend their time working solely in the area of gluten intolerance. These people have the ability to make sound recommendations about the diagnosis, care and treatment of celiac patients, including recommendations about the gluten-free diet.

Several years ago dietitians with expertise in gluten intolerance and the gluten-free diet began scrutinizing the original diet recommendations, and investigating the rationale and science behind those recommendations. They soon began to question the validity of the original recommendations. Their exhaustive research has helped to reshape the gluten-free diet into what became the revised 2000 American Dietetic Association Gluten-Free Diet recommendations. These dietary revisions were the result of joint work and partnerships among many researchers in the U.S. and Canada whose work has modernized the gluten-free diet.

The gluten-free diet has changed over the years, just as nearly every aspect of what we know about celiac disease has changed. Do today's support groups still have the role of dictating what the gluten-free diet is—even when experts in the field have made new recommendations? As more and more celiac centers are created, support groups are finding that their roles are also changing. They no longer have to make decisions about what constitutes a gluten-free diet, but instead only have to disseminate information that has been prepared by experts. Change is difficult, but resistance to change can cause confusion, discontentment, lack of respect for support groups and professionals, anger and sometimes—outright hostility.

Some have questioned the American Dietetic Association's gluten-free dietary recommendations, and have suggested that their science was weak or flawed. In response to this, and in response to the outcry by support group members and the medical community for a single, standard gluten-free diet, the National Gluten-Free Diet Project (NGFDP) has been created. The NGFDP will be the work of dietitians in Dietitians in Gluten Intolerance Diseases (DIGID) and a multi-disciplinary professional team.

The final product will address areas of controversy and make recommendations based on sound science and well-documented research. Research information will be evaluated according to standards used for rating all research in the medical community. Will the NGFDP end the controversy? Not if people are not willing to accept science, but it will clearly provide a diet accepted by celiac professionals. To facilitate an agreement for the diet all national support groups will be invited to have input into the process.

DIGID dietitians are a highly energetic group of dietitians with expertise in the gluten-free diet. Soon they will have a published referral list for support group members, a speaker's bureau and other exciting products and information.

Giving Advice and Information—What is Your Risk?

By Cynthia Kupper, RD, CD

Support group leaders and members do it every day. Organization leaders do it. We all supply information and advice to fellow sufferers, 'newbies' and the public. We all understand how important it is to have someone to talk to, to get the information and our questions asked by someone 'who knows' what they are talking about. What if the information you give is wrong? What if the person you are talking to takes your advice and gets sick? Or is hospitalized and thinks it is because of what you told them? Are you at risk? Absolutely!

There is a fine line between offering information based on your knowledge and experience, and making it sound authoritative. There is a difference between suggesting someone consider being tested for celiac disease and saying they must be tested. There is a difference between being protected legally for what you say and not being protected.

Professionals carry medical malpractice insurance for a reason. People in our society tend to be lawsuit-happy. Doctors, nurses, dietitians and other health care professionals would not dream of taking the risk of providing information without protection. Yet every day, support group leaders and fellow celiac sufferers take risks without giving it a second thought. Are you at risk of being sued when you do that? Yes. It is not uncommon to see non-profit agencies and people acting as their officers or agents getting sued for misrepresentation or for giving bad information. If a group or agency is not adequately covered by insurance, the individuals of the group can be personally sued.

If you are not a health care professional, or even if you are and are not covered by medical malpractice insurance, you need to protect yourself. Here are some tips for protecting yourself, while working to help people with gluten intolerance diseases. This information is not a guarantee that a suit will not be filed against you, but offers a measure of protection, just in case.

1. **Create a statement of authority**. Then use it each time you work with someone or offer advice. This will identify up-front that you are: 1) a volunteer and 2) <u>not</u> a medical expert. It might be something as easy as: "I am a volunteer and not a medical expert, but I can share with you some of the information I find helpful (or I have read, etc)."

2. **Use Disclaimers on materials**. Many support groups do this already. Add a disclaimer to printed materials, the bottom of your emails, etc., that indicate the information is not meant to be medical advice and that a person's medical team should be consulted regarding treatment, diagnostic and medical concerns.

3. **Use medical advisors** to review statements, printed information, etc, for accuracy. Not many smaller groups have medical advisors readily available to them, so consider accessing the medical advisors of national organizations, reputable health institutions and organizations. Keep your documentation that the information was reviewed, by whom, and when. If you state that information was reviewed for medical accuracy, be ready to back it up by providing information about who reviewed it and when. Medical reviewers should be experts in the appropriate areas of medicine—dietitians for nutrition information, doctors or researchers for medical information, and pharmacists for drug information. While many people feel they have developed expertise in celiac disease, medical credentials add credence to being an expert. Be sure to date publications. Old information is bad news.

4. **Consider insurance coverage.** There are a number of ways to protect you with insurance. You do need to know what the insurance covers.

   a. Check to see if your home-owners policy has a volunteer package—sometimes called Volunteers of America. This package often covers persons as they do volunteer activities.

   b. As an organization consider Directors and Officers insurance. This insurance protects directors and officers of your group while doing business for the group. It does not necessarily cover giving bad advice. If you have this type of insurance, you should have a copy of the policy in your office and readily accessible to review. Be sure your organization is listed as being covered on the policy.

   c. Get event insurance for special activities such as walks, dinners, and fund raising events. This insurance protects you for that activity only. It must have your group name on it and the event. If it does not, your event isn't protected. It is not difficult to obtain this type of insurance if you have an existing general liability insurance policy.

All nonprofit, charity organizations, regional and local support groups are at risk for lawsuits. As we have seen in the past couple years, even the largest non-profits are not immune to lawsuits. Yet many people are lulled into believing 'it can't happen to me.' While it may never happen to you, you are at risk and you need to consider the amount of risk you are willing to accept. If your group is sued and doesn't have insurance, are you ready to lose your personal assets on behalf of the organization?

CONCLUSION:

The information offered in this book is just as objective as any other dietary, scientific, or medical document. Put another way, it is as political as documents from these other fields. Despite protests to the contrary, politics and economics play an enormous role in the selection, collection, and interpretation of any scientific data. Frankly, it is only human to pay more attention to issues that may affect our lives or livelihoods than to issues that appear to have no such impact. Thus, we are all more likely to notice or ignore specific data based on how it supports, or fails to support, our own beliefs or hypotheses. Such factors ultimately determine professional prestige and have a large impact on earnings and a variety of factors that enhance or diminish the quality of life for medical and dietary researchers. Politics and economics may not be the motivators that get these people up in the morning and draw them to work each day, but money and power play an important role in most peoples' lives, including those of scientists.

Thus, when we read or hear about new scientific achievements or findings, some individual or research team is not only in the spotlight but stands to make money or gain professional prestige. The very fact that we are hearing about their discovery or innovation suggests that the individual or team has made significant gains in their area. It is unavoidable that, in the process of working toward their new discovery, these individuals had to ignore some data they encountered. That is in the very nature of the process of discovery. As we focus on one issue or phenomenon, data or events from adjacent events and processes are ignored. It could hardly be otherwise.

The research team, whose ideas have formed this book, has functioned no differently. The essential differences lie in the recognition that the ideas presented here are, to some degree, biased, and in the choices that led to the final assembly and presentation of those ideas. We are offering an assortment of opinions, paradigms, and biases regarding a single disease-causing agent, in a single unified document.

The spirit that has driven the production of this volume has provided an equal voice to several competing and/or contradictory perspectives. Our intent has always been to provide the reader with information from many sides of a question and empower readers to make their own evaluations. Such a democratic approach does not make for easy reading, as the reader is engaged in the process of evaluation throughout.

As editors, our biases have also played a large role in the selection, ordering, and presentation of the many paradigms offered here. In the process, we have fallen far short of offering a complete menu of the varying perspectives on the gluten syndrome. Nonetheless, it is, we hope, a significant step toward democratizing a field that is notoriously narrow and undemocratic. The editing process has put us in awe of the richness and complexity of perspectives regarding the health problems caused by gluten for some, perhaps many, possibly most, human beings.

It is now more than seventy-five years since gluten grains were first shown to have a deleterious impact on the health of some individuals, although celiac disease was then considered to be quite rare. This particular gluten-driven disease is now recognized to afflict about 1% of the population although most of these individuals remain undiagnosed due to the slow response of the medical community to this relatively new information.

More recently, non-celiac gluten sensitivity has been found in between 10% and 12% of the general population through serum anti-gliadin antibody testing alone. Gliadin is a family of proteins that forms a sub-group of gluten, the storage proteins that provide food for grains as they germinate.

Dr. Rodney Ford has proposed both here, and in the medical literature, that the disease entities of celiac disease and non-celiac gluten sensitivity be referred to as the 'gluten syndrome' and we support that paradigm. Although in its infancy, recognition of the gluten syndrome is a large step toward developing a broader understanding of gluten as a factor in a wide array of deadly and/or debilitating ailments.

Simply put, the presence of AGA antibodies in about 12% of the general population clearly demonstrates that these people are leaking undigested and/or partly digested gluten proteins into their bloodstream, from whence they will be distributed throughout the body and brain. It has long been known that when many human cells placed in direct contact with gluten proteins in test tubes, our cells are damaged or destroyed. Hudson and colleagues reported this finding in *The Lancet* in 1976.

Whatever the specific mechanism by which this damage occurs there can be little doubt that at least as much as 12% of the population are not well equipped to consume these ubiquitous foods. As testing methods improve, we may find that many more of the approximately 40% of the population who are genetically predisposed to the gluten syndrome may be harmed by eating gluten.

Conclusion

As mentioned in previous chapters, more recent findings indicate that patients with gluten sensitivity may be at greater risk of early death and/or developing many types of cancer.

Many research projects are currently under way and are beginning to plumb the depths of gluten's impact on humans. For instance, an off-label use of the opioid blocker, Naltrexate, is now being advocated as a treatment for some cases of autoimmune disease. This could be blocking the action of opioid peptides from gluten that are reaching the brains and altering brain function in some gluten sensitive individuals.

A new drug called Larazotide will soon be on the market. It captures and wastes the excessive zonulin production that occurs in response to gluten ingestion among patients with celiac disease and other autoimmune diseases. This product is aimed at interrupting the process that leads to leaky gut and allows harmful gluten peptides access to the bloodstream.

Other researchers are developing agents that will pre-digest gluten, breaking the bonds between amino acids that form harmful protein fragments and are indigestible in the human gut. Still others are engaged in the cultivation of gluten that lacks these harmful peptides.

However, most of the above research (with the exception of Larazotide) is aimed at celiac disease alone. In the last two decades, we've come a long way with celiac disease, and that's great. Now we need widespread recognition of gluten sensitivity, as indicated by anti-gliadin antibodies or symptoms that are relieved by a GF diet.

The most recent findings at the University of Maryland, under Alessio Fasano, M.D. show that zonulin is a precursor of heptaglobulin 2, an inflammatory marker that has long been recognized as elevated in a number of autoimmune diseases including type 1 diabetes, multiple sclerosis, and a variety of cancers, as well as in many allergies.

Whatever the future reveals, it is our fervent hope that our efforts in putting together this body of sometimes conflicting information, the reader will be rewarded by further growth of general and medical recognition of gluten grains as disease-causing agents that threaten much of the world's population.

SOURCES:

Chapter 1

Life with Celiac Disease or Gluten Sensitivity

1. Mearin ML, Catassi C, Brousse N, Brand R, Collin P, Fabiani E, Schweizer JJ, Abuzakouk M, Szajewska H, Hallert C, Farré Masip C, Holmes GK; Biömed Study Group on Coeliac Disease and Non-Hodgkin Lymphoma. European multi-centre study on coeliac disease and non-Hodgkin lymphoma. Eur J Gastroenterol Hepatol. 2006 Feb;18(2):187-94.

2. Anderson LA, McMillan SA, Watson RGP, Monaghan P, Gavin AT, Fox C, Murray LJ. Malignancy and mortality in a population-based cohort of patients with coeliac disease or 'gluten sensitivity'. World Gastroenterol 2007; Jan 7, 13(1): 146-151

3. Cascella NG, Kryszak D, Bhatti B, Gregory P, Kelly DL, Mc Evoy JP, Fasano A, Eaton WW. Prevalence of Celiac Disease and Gluten Sensitivity in the United States Clinical Antipsychotic Trials of Intervention Effectiveness Study Population. Schizophr Bull. 2009 Jun 3.

4. Addolorato G, Leggio L, D'Angelo C, Mirijello A, Ferrulli A, Cardone S, Vonghia L, Abenavoli L, Leso V, Nesci A, Piano S, Capristo E, Gasbarrini G. Affective and psychiatric disorders in celiac disease. Dig Dis. 2008;26(2):140-8. Epub 2008 Apr 21.

5. Hä ser W, Gold J, Stein J, Caspary WF, Stallmach A.Health-related quality of life in adult coeliac disease in Germany: results of a national survey. Eur J Gastroenterol Hepatol. 2006 Jul;18(7):747-54

Chapter 2

Celiac Disease – Gluten Sensitivity What's The Difference?

1. Cooke W, Holmes G. <u>Coeliac Disease</u>. Churchill Livingstone, New York, N.Y. 1984.

2. Fasano A. Celiac disease—how to handle a clinical chameleon. N Engl J Med. 2003 Jun 19;348(25):2568-70.

3. Fasano A, Berti I, Gerarduzzi T, Not T, Colletti RB, Drago S, Elitsur Y, Green PH, Guandalini S, Hill ID, Pietzak M, Ventura A, Thorpe M, Kryszak D, Fornaroli F, Wasserman SS, Murray JA, Horvath K. Prevalence of celiac disease in at-risk and

not-at-risk groups in the United States: a large multicenter study. Arch Intern Med. 2003 Feb 10;163(3):286-92.

4. Hadjivassiliou M, Grunewald RA, Davies-Jones GA. Gluten sensitivity as a neurological illness. J Neurol Neurosurg Psychiatry. 2002 May;72(5):560-3.

5. Braly J, Hoggan R.. <u>Dangerous Grains</u>, Penguin-Putnam-Avery, New York, N.Y., 2002.

6. Anderson LA, McMillan SA, Watson RGP, Monaghan P, Gavin AT, Fox C, Murray LJ. Malignancy and mortality in a population-based cohort of patients with coeliac disease or 'gluten sensitivity'. World Gastroenterol 2007; Jan 7, 13(1): 146-151

7. Cascella NG, Kryszak D, Bhatti B, Gregory P, Kelly DL, Mc Evoy JP, Fasano A, Eaton WW. Prevalence of Celiac Disease and Gluten Sensitivity in the United States Clinical Antipsychotic Trials of Intervention Effectiveness Study Population. Schizophr Bull. 2009 Jun 3.

The Anemia and Celiac Disease Connection

1. Anemia, Vital and Health Statistics, Series 10, No. 200 , 1996. <_http://www.cdc.gov/nchs/fastats/anemia.htm> Accessed 9/10/03

2. Fasano A, Berti I, et al. Prevalence of Celiac Disease in At-Risk and Not-At-Risk Groups in the United States Arch Intern Med. 2003;163:286-292.

3. Guandalini S. Celiac disease. School Nurse News. 2003 Mar;20(2):24-7.

4. Sood A, Midha V, et al. Adult celiac disease in northern India. Indian J Gastroenterol. 2003 Jul-Aug;22(4):124-6.

5. Sachdev A, Srinivasan V, et al. Adult onset celiac disease in north India. Trop Gastroenterol. 2002 Jul-Sep;23(3):117-9.

6. Dobru D, Pascu O, et al. The prevalence of coeliac disease at endoscopy units in Romania: routine biopsies during gastroscopy are mandatory (a multicentre study). Rom J Gastroenterol. 2003 Jun;12(2):97-100.

7. Zipser RD, Patel S, et al. Presentations of adult celiac disease in a nationwide patient support group. Dig Dis Sci. 2003 Apr;48(4):761-4.

8. Cranney A, Zarkadas M, et al. The Canadian celiac health survey – the Ottawa chapter pilot. BMC Gastroenterol. 2003; 3 (1): 8.

9. Ransford RA, Hayes M, et al. A controlled, prospective screening study of celiac disease presenting as iron deficiency anemia. J Clin Gastroenterol. 2002 Sep;35(3):228-33.

10. Howard MR, Turnbull AJ, et al. A prospective study of the prevalence of undiagnosed coeliac disease in laboratory defined iron and folate deficiency. J Clin Pathol. 2002 Oct;55(10):754-7.

11. Brooklyn TN, Di Mambro AJ, et al. Patients over 45 years with i on deficiency require investigation. Eur J Gastroenterol Hepatol. 2003 May;15(5):535-8.

12. Sanders DS, Patel D, et al. A primary care cross-sectional study of undiagnosed adult coeliac disease. Eur J Gastroenterol Hepatol. 2003 Apr;15(4):407-13.

13. Dahele A, Ghosh S. Vitamin B12 deficiency in untreated celiac disease. Am J Gastroenterol. 2001 Mar;96(3):745-50.

14. Dickey W. Low serum vitamin B12 is common in coeliac disease and is not due to autoimmune gastritis. Eur J Gastroenterol Hepatol. 2002 Apr;14(4):425-7.

15. Iron-deficiency anemia in women. Harvard Women's Health Watch, Nov 2002, Vol. 10 Issue 3, p3.

16. Anemia Patient Education Sheets. Mayo Clinic website. www.mayoclinic.org. Accessed 9-5-03.

17. Annibale B, Severi C, et al. Efficacy of gluten-free diet alone on recovery from iron deficiency anemia in adult celiac patients. Am J Gastroenterol. 2001 Jan;96(1):132-7.

Unraveling Fibromyalgia

Links:

FM Monograph - Fibromyalgia: Symptoms, Diagnosis, Treatment & Research. (See "Learn about Fibromyalgia" - Overview)

http://www.fmpartnership.org

The Scientific Basis for Understanding Pain in Fibromyalgia - Robert Bennett, MD, FRCP

http://www.myalgia.com/Scientific%20basis.htm

Your Liver Functions

http://janis7hepc.com/Your%20Liver%20Functions.htm

The Liver Detoxification Pathways

http://www.liverdoctor.com/03_detoxpathways.asp

Toxicology - an introduction to occupational and environmental toxicology

http://www.agius.com/hew/resource/toxicol.htm

Xenoestrogens and Breast Cancer: Nowhere to Run

http://www.fwhc.org/health/xeno.htm

Olestra seen as antidote to toxins

http://www.cincypost.com/2005/01/04/oles010405.html

Yo-yo Diet Redistributes Hexachlorobenzene in Body Tissue

http://www.the-aps.org/press/journal/04/36.htm

Adipose tissue at entheses: the rheumatological implications of its distribution. A potential site of pain and stress dissipation?

http://ard.bmjjournals.com/cgi/content/full/63/12/1549

References:

1. Frissora CL, Koch KL. Symptom overlap and comorbidity of irritable bowel syndrome with other conditions. Curr Gastroenterol Rep. 2005 Aug;7(4):264-71.

2. Wallace DJ, Hallegua DS. Fibromyalgia: the gastrointestinal link. Curr Pain Headache Rep. 2004 Oct;8(5):364-8.

3. Zipser RD, Patel S, Yahya KZ, Baisch DW, Monarch E. Presentations of adult celiac disease in a nationwide patient support group. Dig Dis Sci. 2003 Apr;48(4):761-4.

4. FM Monograph - Fibromyalgia: symptoms, diagnosis, treatment & research. National Fibromyalgia Partnership, Inc. 2004.

5. Bennet RM. Chronic widespread pain and the fibromyalgia construct. Oregon Health Sciences University, Portland, Oregon.

6. Neumann L, Buskila D. Epidemiology of fibromyalgia. Curr Pain Headache Rep. 2003 Oct;7(5):362-8.

7. Simms RW. Fibromyalgia is not a muscle disorder. Am J Med Sci. 1998 Jun;315(6):346-50.

8. Simms RW. Is there muscle pathology in fibromyalgia syndrome? Rheum Dis Clin North Am. 1996 May;22(2):245-66.

9. Blanco LE, de Serres FJ, Fernandez-Bustillo E, Kassam DA, Arbesu D, Rodriguez C, Torre JC. Alpha1-antitrypsin and fibromyalgia: new data in favour of the inflammatory hypothesis of fibromyalgia. Med Hypotheses. 2005;64(4):759-69.

10. Blanco I, Canto H, de Serres FJ, Fernandez-Bustillo E, Rodriguez MC. Alpha1-antitrypsin replacement therapy controls fibromyalgia symptoms in 2 patients with PI ZZ alpha1-antitrypsin deficiency. J Rheumatol. 2004 Oct;31(10):2082-5.

11. Aldonyte R, Jansson L, Janciauskiene S. Concentration-dependent effects of native and polymerised alpha1-antitrypsin on primary human monocytes, in vitro. BMC Cell Biol. 2004 Mar 29;5:11.

12. Bristow CL, Patel H, Arnold RR. Self antigen prognostic for human immunodeficiency virus disease progression. Clin Diagn Lab Immunol. 2001 Sep;8(5):937-42.

13. Shapiro L, Pott GB, Ralston AH. Alpha-1-antitrypsin inhibits human immunodeficiency virus type 1. FASEB J. 2001 Jan;15(1):115-122.

14. Simms RW, Zerbini CA, Ferrante N, Anthony J, Felson DT, Craven DE. Fibromyalgia syndrome in patients infected with human immunodeficiency virus. The Boston City Hospital Clinical AIDS Team. Am J Med. 1992 Apr;92(4):368-74.

15. Buskila D, Gladman DD, Langevitz P, Urowitz S, Smythe HA. Fibromyalgia in human immunodeficiency virus infection. J Rheumatol. 1990 Sep;17(9):1202-6.

16. Wagnerova M, Wagner V, Kriz J, Wokounova D, Madlo Z, Slesingerova B. The morbidity of children with decreased serum levels of alpha 1-antitrypsin in an air pollution area. Czech Med. 1980;3(4):280-8.

17. Davison S. Coeliac disease and liver dysfunction. Arch Dis Child. 2002 Oct;87(4):293-6.

18. Duggan JM, Duggan AE. Systematic review: the liver in coeliac disease. Aliment Pharmacol Ther. 2005 Mar 1;21(5):515-8.

19. Abdo A, Meddings J, Swain M. Liver abnormalities in celiac disease. Clin Gastroenterol Hepatol. 2004 Feb;2(2):107-12.

20. Bennett RM. Adult growth hormone deficiency in patients with fibromyalgia. Curr Rheumatol Rep. 2002 Aug;4(4):306-12.

21. Van Konynenburg RA. Is Glutathione depletion an important part of the pathogenesis of Chronic Fatigue Syndrome. Paper presented at the AACFS Seventh International Conference, Madison, Wisconsin, October 8-10, 2004

22. Duyff RF, Van den Bosch J, Laman DM, van Loon BJ, Linssen WH. Neuromuscular findings in thyroid dysfunction: a prospective clinical and electrodiagnostic study. J Neurol Neurosurg Psychiatry. 2000 Jun;68(6):750-5.

23. Sategna-Guidetti C, Volta U, Ciacci C, Usai P, Carlino A, De Franceschi L, Camera A, Pelli A, Brossa C. Prevalence of thyroid disorders in untreated adult celiac disease patients and effect of gluten withdrawal: an Italian multicenter study. Am J Gastroenterol. 2001 Mar;96(3):751-7.

24. Neeck G, Riedel W. Thyroid function in patients with fibromyalgia syndrome. J Rheumatol. 1992 Jul;19(7):1120-2.

25. Lowe JC, Reichman AJ, Honeyman GS, Yellin J. Thyroid status of fibromyalgia patients. Clinical Bulletin of Myofascial Therapy, 3(1):47-53, 1998.

26. Lowe JC, Honeyman-Lowe GS. Thyroid disease and fibromyalgia syndrome. Lyon Méditerranée Médical: Médecine du Sud-Est., 36(1):15-17, 2000.

27. Malik R, Hodgson H. The relationship between the thyroid gland and the liver. QJM. 2002 Sep;95(9):559-69.

28. Kelly GS. Peripheral metabolism of thyroid hormones: a review. Altern Med Rev. 2000 Aug;5(4):306-33.

29. Wu G, Fang YZ, Yang S, Lupton JR, Turner ND. Glutathione metabolism and its implications for health. J Nutr. 2004 Mar;134(3):489-92.

30. Kidd PM. Glutathione: systemic protectant against oxidative and free radical damage. Altern Med Rev 1997;1:155-176.

31. Benjamin M, Redman S, Milz S, Buttner A, Amin A, Moriggl B, Brenner E, Emery P, McGonagle D, Bydder G. Adipose tissue at entheses: the rheumatological implications of its distribution. A potential site of pain and stress dissipation? Ann Rheum Dis. 2004 Dec;63(12):1549-55.

32. Rajala MW, Scherer PE. Minireview: The adipocyte--at the crossroads of energy homeostasis, inflammation, and atherosclerosis. Endocrinology. 2003 Sep;144(9):3765-73.

33. Trayhurn P, Wood IS. Adipokines: inflammation and the pleiotropic role of white adipose tissue. Br J Nutr. 2004 Sep;92(3):347-55.

34. Fantuzzi G. Adipose tissue, adipokines, and inflammation. J Allergy Clin Immunol. 2005 May;115(5):911-9

35. Riordan SM, McIver CJ, Thomas DH, Duncombe VM, Bolin TD, Thomas MC. Luminal bacteria and small-intestinal permeability. Scand J Gastroenterol. 1997 Jun;32(6):556-63.

36. Pedersen SB, Kristensen K, Hermann PA, Katzenellenbogen JA, Richelsen B. Estrogen controls lipolysis by up-regulating alpha2A-adrenergic receptors directly in human adipose tissue through the estrogen receptor alpha. Implications for the female fat distribution. J Clin Endocrinol Metab. 2004 Apr;89(4):1869-78.

37. Dieudonne MN, Leneveu MC, Giudicelli Y, Pecquery R. Evidence for functional estrogen receptors alpha and beta in human adipose cells: regional specificities and regulation by estrogens. Am J Physiol Cell Physiol. 2004 Mar;286(3):C655-61.

38. Cassidy A, Milligan S. How significant are environmental estrogens to women? Climacteric. 1998 Sep;1(3):229-42.

39. Starek A. Estrogens and organochlorine xenoestrogens and breast cancer risk. Int J Occup Med Environ Health. 2003;16(2):113-24.

40. Daston GP, Gooch JW, Breslin WJ, Shuey DL, Nikiforov AI, Fico TA, Gorsuch JW. Environmental estrogens and reproductive health: a discussion of the human and environmental data. Reprod Toxicol. 1997 Jul-Aug;11(4):465-81.

41. Waxman J, Zatzkis SM. Fibromyalgia and menopause. Examination of the relationship. Postgrad Med. 1986 Sep 15;80(4):165-7, 170-1.

42. Sverdrup B. Use less cosmetics--suffer less from fibromyalgia? J Womens Health (Larchmt). 2004 Mar;13(2):187-94.

43. Moser GA, McLachlan MS. A non-absorbable dietary fat substitute enhances elimination of persistent lipophilic contaminants in humans. Chemosphere. 1999 Oct;39(9):1513-21.

44. Geusau A, Tschachler E, Meixner M, Sandermann S, Papke O, Wolf C, Valic E, Stingl G, McLachlan M. Olestra increases faecal excretion of 2,3,7,8-tetrachlorodibenzo-p-dioxin. Lancet. 1999 Oct 54(9186):1266-7.

45. Geusau A, Abraham K, Geissler K, Sator MO, Stingl G, Tschachler E. Severe 2,3,7,8-tetrachlorodibenzo-p-dioxin (TCDD) intoxication: clinical and laboratory effects. Environ Health Perspect. 2001 Aug;109(8):865-9.

46. Redgrave TG, Wallace P, Jandacek RJ, Tso P. Treatment with a dietary fat substitute decreased Arochlor 1254 contamination in an obese diabetic male. J Nutr Biochem. 2005 Jun;16(6):383-4.

47. Jandacek RJ, Anderson N, Liu M, Zheng S, Yang Q, Tso P. Effects of yo-yo diet, caloric restriction, and olestra on tissue distribution of hexachlorobenzene. Am J Physiol Gastrointest Liver Physiol. 2005 Feb;288(2):G292-9.

48. McLean SA, Williams DA, Harris RE, Kop WJ, Groner KH, Ambrose K, Lyden AK, Gracely RH, Crofford LJ, Geisser ME, Sen A, Biswas P, Clauw DJ. Momentary relationship between cortisol secretion and symptoms in patients with fibromyalgia. Arthritis Rheum. 2005 Nov;52(11):3660-9.

49. Petersen AM, Pedersen BK. The anti-inflammatory effect of exercise. J Appl Physiol. 2005 Apr;98(4):1154-62.

50. Pedersen BK, Hoffman-Goetz L. Exercise and the immune system: regulation, integration, and adaptation. Physiol Rev. 2000 Jul;80(3):1055-81.

51. Steensberg A, Fischer CP, Keller C, Moller K, Pedersen BK. IL-6 enhances plasma IL-1ra, IL-10, and cortisol in humans. Am J Physiol Endocrinol Metab. 2003 Aug;285(2):E433-7.

52. Steensberg A, Toft AD, Schjerling P, Halkjaer-Kristensen J, Pedersen BK. Plasma interleukin-6 during strenuous exercise: role of epinephrine. Am J Physiol Cell Physiol. 2001 Sep;281(3):C1001-4.

53. Keller P, Keller C, Robinson LE, Pedersen BK. Epinephrine infusion increases adipose interleukin-6 gene expression and systemic levels in humans. J Appl Physiol. 2004 Oct;97(4):1309-12.

54. Johnston DE. Special considerations in interpreting liver function tests. Am Fam Physician. 1999 Apr 15;59(8):2223-30.

Food Cravings, Obesity and Gluten Consumption

1. Marsh, Michael N. Personal communication. 1999.

2. Ferrara, et al. "Celiac disease and anorexia nervosa" New York State Journal of Medicine 1966; 66(8): 1000-1005.

3. Gent & Creamer "Faecal fats, appetite, and weight loss in the celiac syndrome" Lancet 1968; 1(551): 1063-1064.

4. Wright, et al. "Organic diseases mimicking atypical eating disorders" Clinical Pediatrics 1990; 29(6): 325-328.

5. Grenet, et al. "Anorexic forms of celiac syndromes" Annales de Pediatrie 1972; 19(6): 491-497.

6. Dickey W, Bodkin S. Prospective study of body mass index in patients with coeliac disease. BMJ. 1998 Nov 7;317(7168):1290.

7. Murray, J. Canada Celiac Assoc. National Conference. 1999.

8. Howard BV, Van Horn L, Hsia J, et al. Low-fat dietary pattern and risk of cardiovascular disease: the Women's Health Initiative Randomized Controlled Dietary Modification Trial. JAMA. 2006 Feb 8;295(6):655-66.

Our Adipose Prisons

1. Taubes G, Good Calories. Bad Calories. Alfred A. Knopf. New York, 2007. 16-17
2. Williams A, One Teen's Gastric Surgery. People. Dec. 17, 2007. 107-110
3. Dickey W, Kearney N., Overweight in celiac disease: prevalence, clinical characteristics, and effect of a gluten-free diet. Am J Gastroenterol. 2006 Oct;101(10):2356-9.
4. Murray, J. American Celiac Society conference, Mt. Sinai Hospital, NYC, 1997 and Canadian Celiac Association National Conference, Calgary, 1999.
5. Celiac Disease Foundation 2001
6. Fine K, personal communication.

Chapter 3

Eating to Learn: How Grains Impact on Our Ability to Focus, Comprehend, Remember, Predict, and Survive

1. Kozlowska, Z: (1991). Results of investigation on children with coeliakia treated many years with gluten free diet Psychiatria Polska. 25(2),130-134.
2. Paul, K., Todt, J., Eysold, R. (1985) [EEG Research Findings in Children with Celiac Disease According to Dietary Variations]. Zeitschrift der Klinische Medizin. 40, 707-709.
3. Grech, P.L., Richards, J., McLaren, S., Winkelman, J.H. (2000) Psychological sequelae and quality of life in celiac disease. Journal of Pediatric Gastroenterology and Nutrition 31(3): S4
4. Reichelt, K., Sagedal, E., Landmark, J., Sangvic, B., Eggen, O., Helge, S. (1990a). The Effect of Gluten-Free Diet on Urinary peptide Excretion and Clinical State in Schizophrenia. Journal of Orthomolecular Medicine. 5(4), 169-181.
5. Reichelt, K., Ekrem, J., Scott, H. (1990b). Gluten, Milk Proteins and Autism: DIETARY INTERVENTION EFFECTS ON BEHAVIOR AND PEPTIDE SECRETION. Journal of Applied Nutrition. 42(1), 1-11.
6. Reichelt, K., Knivsberg, A., Lind, G., Nodland, M. (1991). Probable etiology and Possible Treatment of Childhood Autism. Brain Dysfunction. 4, 308-319.
7. Hoggan, R. (1997a). Absolutism's Hidden Message for Medical Scientism. Interchange. 28(2/3), 183-189.
8. Caterson ID, Gill TP. Obesity: epidemiology and possible prevention. Best Pract Res Clin Endocrinol Metab. 2002 Dec;16(4):595-610.
9. Hennessy AR, Walker JD. Silent hypoglycaemia at the diabetic clinic. Diabet Med. 2002 Mar;19(3):261.
10. Kue Young T, Chateau D, Zhang M. Factor analysis of ethnic variation in the multiple metabolic (insulin resistance) syndrome in three Canadian populations. Am J Human Biol. 2002 Sep-Oct;14(5):649-58.

11. Wahab PJ, Meijer JW, Dumitra D, Goerres MS, Mulder CJ. Coeliac disease: more than villous atrophy. Rom J Gastroenterol. 2002 Jun;11(2):121-7.

12. Catassi C, Ratsch IM, Gandolfi L, Pratesi R, Fabiani E, El Asmar R, Frijia M, Bearzi I, Vizzoni L. Why is coeliac disease endemic in the people of the Sahara? Lancet. 1999 Aug 21;354(9179):647-8.

13. Langleben DD, Acton PD, Austin G, Elman I, Krikorian G, Monterosso JR, Portnoy O, Ridlehuber HW, Strauss HW. Effects of Methylphenidate Discontinuation on Cerebral Blood Flow in Prepubescent Boys with Attention Deficit Hyperactivity Disorder. J Nucl Med. 2002 Dec;43(12):1624-1629.

14. 2: Kim BN, Lee JS, Shin MS, Cho SC, Lee DS. Regional cerebral perfusion abnormalities in attention deficit/hyperactivity disorder Statistical parametric mapping analysis. Eur Arch Psychiatry Clin Neurosci. 2002 Oct;252(5):219-25.

15. Lou, H., Henriksen, L., Bruhn, P. (1984). Focal cerebral hypoperfusion in children with dysphasia and/or attention deficit disorder. Archives of Neurology. 825-829.

16. De Santis A, Addolorato G, Romito A, Caputo S, Giordano A, Gambassi G, Taranto C, Manna R, Gasbarrini G. Schizophrenic symptoms and SPECT abnormalities in a coeliac patient: regression after a gluten-free diet. J Intern Med. 1997 Nov;242(5):421-3.

17. Knivsberg AM. Urine patterns, peptide levels and IgA/IgG antibodies to food proteins in children with dyslexia. Pediatr Rehabil. 1997 Jan-Mar;1(1):25-33.

18. Case records of the Massachusetts General Hospital. Weekly clinicopathological exercises. Case 43-1988. A 52-year-old man with persistent watery diarrhea and aphasia. N Engl J Med. 1988 Oct 27;319(17):1139-48.

19. Hadjivassiliou M, Boscolo S, Davies-Jones GA, Grunewald RA, Not T, Sanders DS, Simpson JE, Tongiorgi E, Williamson CA, Woodroofe NM. The humoral response in the pathogenesis of gluten ataxia. Neurology. 2002 Apr 23;58(8):1221-6.

20. Hadjivassiliou M, Grunewald RA, Davies-Jones GA. Gluten sensitivity as a neurological illness. J Neurol Neurosurg Psychiatry. 2002 May;72(5):560-3. Review.

21. Husby, V., Jensenius, C., Svehag, S.(1985). Passage of Undegraded Dietary Antigen into the Blood of Healthy Adults. Scandanavian Journal of Immunology. 22, 83-92.

22. Ma A, Chen X, Zheng M, Wang Y, Xu R, Li J. Iron status and dietary intake of Chinese pregnant women with anaemia in the third trimester. Asia Pac J Clin Nutr. 2002;11(3):171-5.

23. Kapil U, Bhavna A. Adverse effects of poor micronutrient status during childhood and adolescence. Nutr Rev. 2002 May;60(5 Pt 2):S84-90. Review.

24. Youdim MB, Yehuda S. The neurochemical basis of cognitive deficits induced by brain iron deficiency: involvement of dopamine-opiate system. Cell Mol Biol (Noisy-le-grand). 2000 May;46(3):491-500.

25. Otero GA, Aguirre DM, Porcayo R, Fernandez T. Psychological and electroencephalographic study in school children with iron deficiency. Int J Neurosci. 1999 Aug;99(1-4):113-21.

26. Guesry P. The role of nutrition in brain development.

27. Prev Med. 1998 Mar-Apr;27(2):189-94. Review.

28. Bruner AB, Joffe A, Duggan AK, Casella JF, Brandt J. Randomised study of cognitive effects of iron supplementation in non-anaemic iron-deficient adolescent girls. Lancet. 1996 Oct 12;348(9033):992-6.

29. Soewondo S. The effect of iron deficiency and mental stimulation on Indonesian children's cognitive performance and development. Kobe J Med Sci. 1995 Apr;41(1-2):1-17.

30. McCarthy AM, Lindgren S, Mengeling MA, Tsalikian E, Engvall JC. Effects of diabetes on learning in children. Pediatrics. 2002 Jan;109(1):E9.

31. Bertini M, Sbarbati A, Valletta E, Pinelli L, Tato L. Incomplete gastric metaplasia in children with insulin-dependent diabetes mellitus and celiac disease. An ultrastructural study. BMC Clin Pathol. 2001;1(1):2.

Chapter 4
Challenging the Gluten Challenge

1. Kuitunen P, Savilahti E, Verkasalo M. Late mucosalrelapse in a boy with coeliac disease and cow's milk allergy. Acta Paediatr Scand. 1986 Mar;75(2):340-2.

2. Bardella MT, Fredella C, Trovato C, Ermacora E, Cavalli R, Saladino V, Prampolini L. Long-term remission in patients with dermatitis herpetiformis on a normal diet. Br. J. Dermatol. 2003 Nov;149(5):968-71.

3. Shmerling DH, Franckx J. Childhood celiac disease: a long-term analysis of relapses in 91 patients. J Pediatr Gastroenterol Nutr. 1986 Jul-Aug;5(4):565-9.

4. Chartrand LJ, Seidman EG. Celiac disease is a lifelong disorder. Clin Invest Med. 1996 Oct;19(5):357-61.

5. Rostami K, Kerckhaert J, von Blomberg BM, Meijer JW, Wahab P, Mulder CJ. SAT and serology in adult coeliacs, seronegative coeliac disease seems a reality. Neth J Med. 1998 Jul;53(1):15-9.

6. Hudson DA, Cornell HJ, Purdham DR, Rolles CJ. Non-specific cytotoxicity of wheat gliadin components towards cultured human cells. Lancet. 1976 Feb 14;1(7955):339-41.

7. Anderson LA, McMillan SA, Watson RGP, Monaghan P, Gavin AT, Fox C, Murray LJ. Malignancy and mortality in a population-based cohort of patients with coeliac disease or 'gluten sensitivity'. World Gastroenterol 2007; Jan 7, 13(1): 146-151

8. Cascella NG, Kryszak D, Bhatti B, Gregory P, Kelly DL, Mc Evoy JP, Fasano A, Eaton WW. Prevalence of Celiac Disease and Gluten Sensitivity in the United States Clinical Antipsychotic Trials of Intervention Effectiveness Study Population. Schizophr Bull. 2009 Jun

9. Fasano A, Surprises from Celiac Disease. Scientific American Aug. 2009

So Why Do Celiacs Still Need a Biopsy?

1. Dickey W, McMillan SA, Hughes DF. Sensitivity of serum tissue transglutaminase antibodies for endomysial antibody positive and negative coeliac disease. Scand J Gastroenterol 2001; 36: 511-4.

2. Wahab PJ, Crusius JBA, Meijer JWR, Mulder CJJ. Gluten challenge in borderline gluten-sensitive enteropathy. Am J Gastroenterol 2001; 96: 1464-69.

3. DiTola M, Sabbatella L, Anania MC, Viscido A, Caprilli R, Pica R, Paoluzi P, Picarelli A. Anti-tissue transglutaminase antibodies in inflammatory bowel disease: new evidence. Clin Chem Lab Med. 2004;42(10):1092-7.

4. Oxentenko AS, Grisolano SW, Murray JA, Burgart LJ, Dierkhising RA, Alexander JA. The insensitivity of endoscopic markers in celiac disease. Am J Gastroenterol. 2002 Apr;97(4):933-8.

5. Dickey W, Hughes DF, McMillan SA. Disappearance of endomysial antibodies in treated celiac disease does not indicate histological recovery. Am J Gastroenterol 2000; 95: 712-4.

6. Meijer JWR, Wahab PJ, Mulder CJJ. Histologic follow-up of people with celiac disease on a gluten-free diet: slow and incomplete recovery. Am J Clin Pathol 118(3):459-63, 2002 Sep.

7. Dickey W, Hughes DF, McMillan SA. Patients with serum IgA endomysial antibodies and intact duodenal villi: clinical characteristics and management options. Scand J Gastroenterol 2005: in press

8. Barker CC, Mitton C, Jevon G, Mock T. Can tissue transglutaminase antibody titers replace small-bowel biopsy to diagnose celiac disease in select pediatric populations? Pediatrics. 2005 May;115(5):1341-6

Screening Children of Short Stature for Celiac Disease
1. Bhadada, S. Bhansali, A., Kochhar, R., Shankar, A., Menon, A., Sinha, S., Dutta, PP., and Nain, C. Does every short stature child need screening for celiac disease? Gastroenterology [OnlineEarly Articles]. doi:10.1111/j.1440-1746.2007.05261.x

Chapter 5

Magnesium Helps Rebuild Bones in Celiac Disease

1. Marsh MN. Bone disease and gluten sensitivity: time to act, to treat, and to prevent. Am J Gastroenterol. 1994 Dec;89(12):2105-7.
2. Rude RK, Olerich M. Magnesium deficiency: possible role in osteoporosis associated with gluten-sensitive enteropathy. Osteoporos Int. 1996;6(6):453-61.
3. Kumar V, Valeski JE, Wortsman J. Celiac disease and hypoparathyroidism: cross-reaction of endomysial antibodies with parathyroid tissue. Clin Diagn Lab Immunol. 1996 Mar;3(2):143-6.
4. Embry AF, Snowdon LR, Vieth R. Vitamin D and seasonal fluctuations of gadolinium-enhancing magnetic resonance imaging lesions in multiple sclerosis. Ann Neurol. 2000 Aug;48(2):271-2.

Diabetes Mellitus: More than a Complication of Celiac Disease

1. MacFarlane AJ, Burghardt KM, Kelly J, Simell T, Simell O, Altosaar I, Scott FW. A type 1 diabetes-related protein from wheat (Triticum aestivum). cDNA clone of a wheat storage globulin, Glb1, linked to islet damage. J Biol Chem. 2003 Jan 3;278(1):54-63.

Additional Food Allergies - Incomplete Recovery or Refractory Sprue?

1. Pizzuti D, Bortolami M, Mazzon E, Buda A, Guariso G, D'Odorico A, Chiarelli S, D'Inca R, De Lazzari F, Martines D. Transcriptional downregulation of tight junction protein ZO-1 in active coeliac disease is reversed after a gluten-free diet. Dig Liver Dis. 2004 May;36(5):337-41.
2. Lanzini, et al. Incomplete recovery of intestinal mucosa occurs very rarely in adult coeliac patients despite adherence to gluten-free diet. Aliment Pharmacol Ther 2009: 29, 1299-1308
3. Baker AL, et al. Refractory sprue: recovery after removal of non-gluten dietary proteins. Ann Intern Med. 1978 Oct;89(4):505-8.
4. Volta U, et al. Antibodies to dietary antigens in coeliac disease. Scand J Gastroenterol. 1986 Oct;21(8):935-40.
5. Mandal A, Mayberry J. Elemental diet in the treatment of refractory coeliac disease. Eur J Gastroenterol Hepatol. 2001 Jan;13(1):79-80.
6. Kemeny DM, Urbanek R, Amlot PL, Ciclitira PJ, Richards D, Lessof MH. Subclass of IgG in allergic disease. I. IgG sub-class antibodies in immediate and non-immediate food allergy. Clin Allergy. 1986 Nov;16(6):571-81.
7. Paranos S, et al. Lack of cross-reactivity between casein and gliadin in sera from coeliac disease patients. Int Arch Allergy Immunol. 1998 Oct;117(2):152-4.

8. Scott H, et al. Immune response patterns in coeliac disease. Serum antibodies to dietary antigens measured by an enzyme linked immunosorbent assay (ELISA). Clin Exp Immunol. 1984 Jul;57(1):25-32.

Immunoglobulin Deficiency and Celiac Disease

1. Guandalini S, Gupta P. Celiac disease - a diagnostic challenge. Clin Appl Immun Rev 2002; 2:293-305.
2. Guandalini S, Gupta P. Celiac disease - a diagnostic challenge. Clin Appl Immun Rev 2002; 2:293-305; Fasano A, et al. Prevalence of celiac disease in at risk and not-at-risk groups in the United States 2223; 163:286-292.
3. Wolber R, et al. Lymphocytic gastritis in patients with celiac sprue or sprue like intestinal disease. Gastroenterology 1990; 98:310-315.
4. Catassi, et al. Risk of non-Hodgkin lymphoma in celiac disease. JAMA 2002; 287:1413-1419.
5. Arranz E, Ferguson A. Intestinal antibody pattern of celiac disease: Occurrence in patients with normal jejunal biopsy histology. Gastroenterology 1993; 104: 1263-72.
6. Hill ID, et al. Celiac disease: Working group report of the first world congress of pediatric gastroenterology, hepatology, and nutrition. J. Pediatr Gastroenterol Nutr 2002; 35:S78-S88.
7. Rosario et al. J Pediatr Gastroenterol Nutr 1998; 27:191-195.
8. Vitoria JC, et al. Antibodies to gliadin, endomysium, and tissue transglutaminase for the diagnosis of celiac disease. J Pediatr Gastroenterol Nutr 1999; 29:571-4.
9. Rittmeyer C, Rhoads JM. IgA deficiency causes false-negative endomysial antibody results in celiac disease. J Pediatr Gastroenterol Nutr. 1996; 23:504-6.
10. Kumar V et al. Tissue transglutaminase and endomysial antibodies-diagnostic markers of gluten-sensitive enteropathy in dermatitis herpetiformis. Clin Immunol. 2001; 98:378-82; Lagerqvist, C et al. Screening for adult coeliac disease - which serological marker(s) to use? Journal Intern Med. 2001; 250:241-248.
11. Lilic D, Sewell WA. IgA deficiency: what we should-or should not-be doing. J Clint Pathol 2001; 54:337-8; Seidman EG, Hollander GA. Autoimmunity with immuno-deficiency: a logical paradox. J Pediatr Gastroenterol Nutr. 1999; 28377-9.
12. Sleasman JW. The association between immunodeficiency and the development of autoimmune disease. Adv Dent Res. 1996;10:57-61.
13. J. Paed. Gastroenterol. 1999:28:81-83.

Recognizing Celiac Disease Down the Endoscope

1. Bassotti G, Castellucci G, Betti C et al. Abnormal gastrointestinal motility in patients with celiac sprue. Dig Dis Sci 1994; 39: 1947-54,

2. Dickey W, Hughes DF. Erosions of the second part of duodenum in patients with villous atrophy. Gastrointestinal Endoscopy 2004; 59: 116-118.

3. Dickey W. Diagnosis of coeliac disease at open access endoscopy. Scandinavian Journal of Gastroenterology 1998; 33: 612-5.

4. Dickey W, Hughes DF. Prevalence of celiac disease and its endoscopic markers among patients undergoing routine endoscopy. American Journal of Gastroenterology: 1999; 94: 2182-6.

5. Shah VH, Rotterdam H, Kotler DP, Fasano A, Green PHR. All that scallops is not celiac disease. Gastrointest Endosc 2000; 51: 717-20.

6. Oxentenko AS, Grisolano SW, Murray JA et al. The insensitivity of endoscopic markers in celiac disease. Am J Gastroenterol 2002; 97: 933-8.

7. Dickey W, Hughes DF. Disappointing sensitivity of endoscopic markers for villous atrophy in a high-risk population: implications for celiac disease diagnosis during routine endoscopy. Am J Gastroenterol 2001; 96: 2126-8.

8. Green PHR, Murray JA. Routine duodenal biopsies to exclude celiac disease? Am J Gastroenterol 2003; 58: 92-5.

Sorbitol H2-Breath Test: A Simple, Non Invasive, Cheap and Effective Method to Assess Small Bowel Damage in Celiac Disease

1. Martucci S, Biagi F, Di Sabatino A, Corazza GR. Coeliac disease. Dig Liver Dis 2002; 34(suppl.2): S150-3.

2. Rostami K, Kerckhaert J, Tiemessen R, von Blomberg ME, Meijer JWR, Mulder CJJ. Sensitivity of antiendomysium and antigliadin antibodies in untreated celiac disease: disappointing in clinical practice. Am J Gastroenterol 1999; 94: 888-94.

3. Dickey W, Hughes DF, McMillan SA. Reliance on serum endomysial antibody testing underestimates the true prevalence of coeliac disease by one fifth. Scand J Gastroenterol 2000; 35: 181-3.

4. Tursi A, Brandimarte G, Giorgetti GM, Gigliobianco G, Lombardi D, Gasbarrini G. Low prevalence of antigliadin (AGA) and anti-endomysium (EMA) antibodies in subclinical/silent celiac disease. Am J Gastroenterol 2001; 96: 1507-10.

5. Abrams JA, Diamone B, Rotterdam H, Green PHR. Seronegative celiac disease: increased prevalence with lesser degrees of villous atrophy. Dig Dis Sci 2004; 49: 546-50.

6. Washüttl J, Reiderer P, Baucher E. A qualitative and quantitative study of sugar-alcohols in several foods. J Food Sci 1973; 38: 1262-3.

7. Ojetti V, Nucera G, Migneco A et al. High prevalence of celiac disease in patients with lactose intolerance. Digestion 2005; 71: 106-10.

8. Swagerty DL Jr, Walling AD, Klein RM. Lactose intolerance. Am Fam Physician 2002; 65: 1845-50.

9. Strocchi A, Ellis C, Levitt MD. Reproducibility of measurement of trace gas concentrations in expired air. Gastroenterology 1991;101: 175-9.

10. Corazza GR, Strocchi A, Rossi R, Sirola D, Gasbarrini G. Sorbitol malabsorption in normal volunteers and in patients with coeliac disease. Gut 1988;29: 44-8.

11. Pelli MA, Capodicasa E, De Angelis V, Morelli A, Bassotti G. Sorbitol H2-breath test in celiac disease. Importance of early positivity. Gastroenterol Int 1998;11: 65-8.

12. Tursi A, Brandimarte G, Giorgetti G. Prevalence of anti-tissue transglutaminase antibodies in different degrees of intestinal damage in celiac disease. J Clin Gastroenterol 2003; 36(3): 219-221.

13. Tursi A, Brandimarte G, Giorgetti GM. Sorbitol H2-breath test versus anti-endomysium antibodies for the diagnosis of subclinical/silent coeliac disease. Scand J Gastroenterol 2001;36: 1170-2.

14. Marsh MN. Gluten, major histocompatibility complex, and the small intestine. A molecular and immunologic approach to the spectrum of gluten sensitivity (celiac sprue). Gastroenterology 1992;102: 330-54.

15. Auricchio S, Mazzacca G, Tosi R, Visakorpi J, Maki M, Polanco I. Coeliac disease as familial condition: identification of asymptomatic patients within family groups. Gastroenterol Int 1988;1: 25-31.

16. Barry RE, Morris JS, Kenwright S, Read AE. Coeliac disease and malignancy. The possible importance of familial involvement. Scand J Gastroenterol 1971;6: 205-207.

17. Stokes PL, Prior P, Sorahan TM, McWalter RJ, Waterhouse JA, Cooke WT. Malignancy in relatives of patients with coeliac disease. Br J Prev Soc Med 1976;30: 27-21.

18. Holmes GKT, Prior P, Lane MR, Pope D, Allan RN. Malignancy in coeliac disease – effect of gluten free diet. Gut 1989;30: 333-8.

19. Corazza GR, Valentini RA, Frisoni M ETAL. Gliadin immune reactivity is associated with overt and latent enteropathy in relatives of celiac patients. Gastroenterology 1992; 103: 1517-22.

20. Maki M, Holm K, Lipsaen V, Hallstrom O, Viander M, Collin P et al. Serological markers and HLA genes among healthy first-degree relatives of patients with coeliac disease. Lancet 1991;338: 1350-3.

21. Vazquez H, Cabanne A, Sugai E, Fiorini A, Pedreira S, Maurino E et al. Serological markers identify latent coeliac disease among first-degree relatives. Eur J Gastroenterol Hepatol 1996;8: 15-21.

22. A. Tursi, G. Brandimarte, G.M. Giorgetti, C.D. Inchingolo. Effectiveness of sorbitol H2 breath test in detecting histological damage among relatives of coeliacs. Scand J Gastroenterol 2003;38: 727-31.

23. Bardella MT, Trovato C, Cesana BM, Pagliari C, Gebbia C, Peracchi M. Serological markers of celiac disease: is it time to change? Digest Liver Dis 2001;33: 426-31.

24. Valentini RA, Andreani ML, Corazza GR, Gasbarrini G. IgA endomysium antibody. A valuable tool in the screening of coeliac disease but not its follow-up. Ital J Gastroenterol 1994;26: 279-82.

25. Sategna-Guidetti C, Grosso SB, Bruno M, Grosso S. Is human umbilical cord the most suitable substrate for the detection of endomysium antibodies in the screening and follow-up of coeliac disease? Eur J Gastroenterol Hepatol 1997;9: 657-60.

26. Dickey W, Hughes DF, McMillan SA. Disappearance of endomysial antibodies in treated celiac disease does not indicate histological recovery. Am J Gastroenterol 2001;95: 712-4.

27. Dieterich W, Ehnis T, Bauer M et al. Identification of tissue transglutaminase as the auto-antigen of celiac disease. Nat Med 1997;3: 797-801.

28. Tursi A, Brandimarte G, Giorgetti GM. Sorbitol H2-breath test versus anti-endomysium (EMA) antibodies to assess histological recovery after gluten-free diet in coeliac disease. Dig Liver Dis 2002;34: 846-50.

29. Tursi A, Brandimarte G, Giorgetti GM. Lack of effectiveness of anti-transglutaminase antibodies in assessing histological recovery after gluten-free diet in celiac disease. J Clin Gastroenterol 2003;37: 381-5.

30. Tursi A, Brandimarte G. The symptomatic and histological response to a gluten-free diet in patients with borderline enteropathy. J Clin Gastroenterol 2003;36: 13-7.

31. Tursi A, Giorgetti GM, Brandimarte G, Elisei W. High prevalence of celiac disease among patients affected by Crohn's disease. Inflamm Bowel Dis 2005;11: 662-6.

32. Nucera G, Gabrielli M, Lupascu A et al. Abnormal breath test to lactose, fructose and sorbitol in irritable bowel syndrome may be explained by small intestinal bacterial overgrowth. Aliment Pharmacol Ther 2005;21: 1391-5.

How is Your Heartburn?

1. Katz PO. Gastroesophageal reflux disease and extraesophageal disease. Rev Gastroenterol Disord. 2005;5 Suppl 2:31-8.

2. Suzuki H, Iijima K, Scobie G, Fyfe V, McColl KE. Nitrate and nitrosative chemistry within Barrett's oesophagus during acid reflux. Gut. 2005 Nov;54(11):1527-35.

Endoscopy in Celiac Disease

1. Martucci S, Biagi F, Di Sabatino A, Corazza GR. Coeliac disease. Digest Liver Dis 2002;34 (suppl. 2): S150-S153.

2. When is a celiac a celiac? Report of a working group of the United European Gastroenterology Week in Amsterdam, 2001. Eur J Gastroenterol Hepatol 2001;13: 1123-8.

3. Tursi A, Giorgetti GM, Brandimarte G, Rubino E, Lombardi D, Gasbarrini G. Prevalence and clinical presentation of subclinical/silent coeliac disease in adults: an analysis on a 12-year observation. Hepato-gastroenterol 2001; 39: 462-4.

4. Brocchi E, Corazza G, Caletti G et al. Endoscopic demonstration of loss of duodenal folds in the diagnosis of celiac disease. N Engl J Med 1988;319: 741-4.

5. Mc Intere AS, Mg DP, Smith JA , Amoah J, Long RG. The endoscopic appearance of duodenal folds is predictive of untreated adult celiac disease. Gastrointest Endosc 1992;38: 148-51.

6. Corazza GR, Caletti GC, Lazzari R et al. Scalloped duodenal folds in childhood celiac disease. Gastrointest Endosc 1993; 29: 543-5.

7. Smith AD, Graham I, Rose JD. A prospective endoscopic study of scalloped folds and grooves in the mucosa of the duodenum as sign of villous atrophy. Gastrointest Endosc 1998;47: 461-5.

8. Stevens FM, McCarthy CF. The endoscopic demonstration of coeliac disease. Endoscopy 1976;8: 177-80.

9. Brocchi E, Corazza GR, Brusco G, Mangia L, Gasbarrini G. Unsuspected celiac disease diagnosed by endoscopic visualization of duodenal bulb micronodules. Gastrointest Endosc 1996;4: 610-1.

10. Vogelsang H, Hänel S, Steiner B, Oberhuber G. Diagnostic duodenal bulb biopsy in celiac disease. Endoscopy 2001;33: 336-40.

11. Tursi A, Grandimarte G, Giorgetti GM, Gigliobianco A. Endoscopic features of celiac disease in adults and their correlation with age, histological damage, and clinical form of the disease. Endoscopy 2002;34: 787-92.

12. Niveloni S, Fiorini A, Dezi R et al. Usefulness of videoduodenoscopy and vutal dye staining as indicators of mucosal atrophy of celiac disease: assessment of interobserver agreement. Gastrointest Endosc 1998;47: 223-9.

13. Dickey W, Hughes D. Disappointing sensitivity of endoscopic markers for villous atrophy in a high-risk population: implication for celiac disease diagnosis during routine endoscopy. Am J Gastroenterol 2001;96: 2126-8.

14. Shah VH, Rotterdam H, Kjotler DP, Fasano A, Green PH. All that scallops is not celiac disease. Gastrointest Endosc 2000;51: 717-20.

15. Dickey W, Hughes D. Prevalence of celiac disease and its endoscopic markers among patients having routine upper gastrointestinal endoscopy. Am J Gastroenterol 1999;94: 2182-6.

16. Cammarota G, Martino A, Pirozzi GA et al. Direct visualization of intestinal villi by high-resolution magnifying upper endoscopy: a validation study. Gastrointest Endosc 2004;60: 732-8.

17. Cammarota G, Cesaro P, Martino A et al. High accuracy and cost-effectiveness of a biopsy-avoiding endoscopic approach in diagnosing celiac disease. Aliment Pharmacol Ther 2006;23: 61-9.

18. Cammarota G, Martino A, Di Caro S et al. High-resolution magnifying upper endoscopy in a patient with patchy celiac disease. Dig Dis Sci 2005;50: 601-4.

19. Badreldin R, Barrett P, Wooff DA, Mansfield J, Yiannakou Y. How good is zoom endoscopy for assessment of villous atrophy in coeliac disease? Endoscopy 2005;37: 994-8.

20. Di Caro S, May A, Heine DG, Fini L et al. The European experience with double-balloon enteroscopy: indications, methodology, safety, and clinical impact. Gastrointest Endosc 2005;62: 545-50.

21. MacDonald WC, Brandiborg LL, Flick AL et al. Studies of celiac sprue. IV. The response of the whole length of the small bowel to a gluten-free diet. Gastroenterology 1964;47: 573-89.

22. Dickey W, Hughes DF. Histology of the terminal ileum in coeliac disease. Scand J Gastroenterol 2004;39: 665-7.

23. Eliakim R. Wireless capsule video endoscopy: three years experience. World J Gastroenterol 2004;10: 1238-9.

24. Cellier C, Green PH, Collin P et al. The role of capsule endoscopy in coeliac disease: the way forward. Endoscopy 2005;37: 1055-9.

25. Green PH, Fleichauer AT, Baghat G et al. Risk of malignancy in patients with celiac disease. Am J Med 2003;115: 191-5.

26. Cellier C, Delabasse E, Helmer C et al. Refractory sprue, coeliac disease and enteropathy-associated T-cell lymphoma. French Coeliac Disease Study Group. Lancet 2000;356: 203-8.

27. Green JA, Barkin JS, Gregg PA et al. Ulcerative jejunitis in refractory celiac disease: enteroscopic visualization. Gastrointest Endosc 1993;39: 584-5.

28. Gay G, Delvaux M, Fassler I. Outcome of capsule endosocpy in determining indication and route for push-and-pull enteroscopy. Endoscopy 2006;38: 49-58.

29. Yamamoto H, Kita H, Sunada K et al. Clinical outcomes of double-balloon endoscopy for the diagnosis and treatment of small-intestinal diseases. Clin Gastroenterol Hepatol 2004;2: 1010-6.

30. Tursi A, Brandimarte G, Giorgetti GM. Endoscopic and histological findings in the duodenum of adults with celiac disease before and after changing to a gluten-free diet: a 2-year prospective study. Endoscopy 2006; 38: in press.

Lung Disease, Celiac Disease, Gluten Sensitivity, and Smoking Tobacco

1. Stevens FM, Connolly CE, Murray JP, McCarthy CF. Lung cavities in patients with coeliac disease. Digestion. 1990;46(2):72-80.

2. Papadopoulos KI, Sjoberg K, Lindgren S, Hallengren B. Evidence of gastrointestinal immune reactivity in patients with sarcoidosis. J Intern Med. 1999 May;245(5):525-31.

3. Brightling CE, Symon FA, Birring SS, Wardlaw AJ, Robinson R, Pavord ID. A case of cough, lymphocytic bronchoalveolitis and coeliac disease with improvement following a gluten free diet. Thorax. 2002 Jan;57(1):91-2.

4. Robertson DA, Taylor N, Sidhu H, Britten A, Smith CL, Holdstock G. Pulmonary permeability in coeliac disease and inflammatory bowel disease. Digestion. 1989;42(2):98-103.

5. The Ketogenic Diet: A Complete Guide for the Dieter and Practitioner by Lyle McDonald. 1998.

6. Kwan RM, Thomas S, Mir MA. Effects of a low carbohydrate isoenergetic diet on sleep behavior and pulmonary functions in healthy female adult humans. J Nutr. 1986 Dec;116(12):2393-402.

7. Suman S, Williams EJ, Thomas PW, Surgenor SL, Snook JA. Is the risk of adult coeliac disease causally related to cigarette exposure? Eur J Gastroenterol Hepatol. 2003 Sep;15(9):995-1000.

8. Austin AS, Logan RF, Thomason K, Holmes GK. Cigarette smoking and adult coeliac disease. Scand J Gastroenterol. 2002 Aug;37(8):978-82.

9. Vazquez H, Smecuol E, Flores D, Mazure R, Pedreira S, Niveloni S, Maurino E, Bai JC. Relation between cigarette smoking and celiac disease: evidence from a case-control study. Am J Gastroenterol. 2001 Mar;96(3):798-802.

10. Snook JA, Dwyer L, Lee-Elliott C, Khan S, Wheeler DW, Nicholas DS. Adult coeliac disease and cigarette smoking. Gut. 1996 Jul;39(1):60-2.

Gluten's Inflammatory Role in Celiac and Other Chronic Diseases

1. Published In "Inflammation and Infection. The Golden Triangle: Food—Microflora—Host Defense". P.J. Heidt, Z. Midtvedt., V. Rusch, D. van der Waaij (Eds.) Old Herborn University Seminar Monography, 2007

Chapter 6

Misguided Government Food Guides

1. Hadjivassiliou M, Gibson A, Davies-Jones GA, Lobo AJ, Stephenson TJ, Milford-Ward A. Does cryptic gluten sensitivity play a part in neurological illness? Lancet. 1996 Feb 10;347(8998):369-71.

2. Fine, Kenneth. Personal communication.

3. Sahi T. Genetics and epidemiology of adult-type hypolactasia. Scand J Gastroenterol Suppl. 1994;202:7-20.

4. McCullough ML, Feskanich D, Stampfer MJ, Rosner BA, Hu FB, Hunter DJ, Variyam JN, Colditz GA, Willett WC Adherence to the Dietary Guidelines for Americans and risk of major chronic disease in women. Am J Clin Nutr. 2000 Nov;72(5):1214-22.

5. Howard BV, Van Horn L, Hsia J, Manson JE, Stefanick ML, Wassertheil-Smoller S, Kuller LH, LaCroix AZ, Langer RD, Lasser NL, Lewis CE, Limacher MC, Margolis KL, Mysiw WJ, Ockene JK, Parker LM, Perri MG, Phillips L, Prentice RL, Robbins J, Rossouw JE, Sarto GE, Schatz IJ, Snetselaar LG, Stevens VJ, Tinker LF, Trevisan M, Vitolins MZ, Anderson GL, Assaf AR, Bassford T, Beresford SA, Black HR, Brunner RL, Brzyski RG, Caan B, Chlebowski RT, Gass M, Granek I, Greenland P, Hays J, Heber D, Heiss G, Hendrix SL, Hubbell FA, Johnson KC, Kotchen JM. Low-fat dietary pattern and risk of cardiovascular disease: the Women's Health Initiative Randomized Controlled Dietary Modification Trial. JAMA. 2006 Feb 8;295(6):655-66.

Chapter 7

Who Should Follow a Gluten-free Diet?

1. Engber, D. Throwing out the Wheat. Are we being too tolerant of gluten-intolerance? http://www.slate.com/id/2223745/

2. Turner, B. Make sure gluten-free diet is what you really need. Galveston County Daily News, July 19, 2009 http://galvestondailynews.com/story.lasso?ewcd=577107179c002dc4

3. Dicke, W.K. Coeliac Disease. Ph.D. Thesis 1950. http://members.shaw.ca/dicke/

4. Hoggan, R., "Absolutism's Hidden Message for Medical Scientism" Interchange, 28(2-3): 183-189, 1997

5. Pappas 1999 CCA national conference Kitchener/waterloo

6. Toscano V, Conti FG, Anastasi E, Mariani P, Tiberti C, Poggi M, Montuori M, Monti S, Laureti S, Cipolletta E, Gemme G, Caiola S, Di Mario U, Bonamico M, Importance of gluten in the induction of endocrine autoantibodies and organ dysfunction in adolescent celiac patients. The American Journal of Gastroenterology. (2000) 95, 1742–1748; doi:10.1111/j.1572-0241.2000.02187

7. http://epilepsy.suite101.com/article.cfm/drug_resistant_seizures

8. Hadjivassiliou M, Gibson A, Davies-Jones GA, Lobo AJ, Stephenson TJ, Milford-Ward A. Does cryptic gluten sensitivity play a part in neurological illness? Lancet. 1996 Feb 10;347(8998):369-71.

9. Hadjivassiliou M, Grünewald RA, Kandler RH, Chattopadhyay AK, Jarratt JA, Sanders DS, Sharrack B, Wharton SB, Davies-Jones GA. Neuropathy associated with gluten sensitivity. J Neurol Neurosurg Psychiatry. 2006 Nov;77(11):1262-6. Epub 2006 Jul 11.

10. Lewey S, Gluten Sensitivity: A Gastroenterologist's Personal Journey down the Gluten Rabbit Hole. Cereal Killers, Celiac.com, 2009.

11. Anderson LA, McMillan SA, Watson RGP, Monaghan P, Gavin AT, Fox C, Murray LJ. Malignancy and mortality in a population-based cohort of patients with coeliac disease or 'gluten sensitivity'. World Gastroenterol 2007; Jan 7, 13(1): 146-151

12. Fasano A, Celiac Disease Insights: Clues to Solving Autoimmunity Study of a potentially fatal food-triggered disease has uncovered a process that may contribute to many autoimmune disorders. August 2009 Scientific American Magazine

Celiac Disease Versus Gluten Sensitivity: New Role for Genetic Testing and Fecal Antibody Testing?

1. Abrams et al. Seronegative celiac disease:increased prevalence with lesser degrees of villous atrophy. Dig Dis Sci 2004;49:546-550.

2. Alaedini A. and Green P.H.R. Narrative Review: Celiac Disease: Understanding a Complex Autoimmune Disorder. Ann Intern Med. 2005;142:289-298.

3. Arranz et al. Jejunal fluid antibodies and mucosal gamma/delta IEL in latent and potential coeliac disease. Adv Exp Med Biol. 1995; 371B:1345-1348.

4. Dewar D. and Ciclitira P. Clinical Features and Diagnosis of Celiac Disease. Gastroenterology 2005;128:S19.

5. Kappler et al. Detection of secretory IgA antibodies against gliadin and human tissue transglutaminase in stool to screen for coeliac disease in children:validation study. BMJ 2006; 332:213-214.

6. Kaukinen et al. HLA-DQ Typing in the Diagnosis of Celiac Disease. Am J Gastroenterol. 2002;97(3):695-699.

7. Fine KD and Rostami K. Don't throw the baby out with the bath water. BMJ February 13, 2006 rapid response editorial.

8. Fine K. Early diagnosis of gluten sensitivity before the villi are gone. Transcript of presentation to Greater Louisville Celiac Support Group, June 2003. http://www.enterolab.com/essay/ .

9. Picarelli et al. Antiendomysial antibody detection in fecal supernatants:in vivo proof that small bowel mucosa is the site of antiendomysial antibody production. Am J Gastroenterol. 2002 Jan;97(1):95-98.

10. Sbartati A. et al. Gluten sensitivity and "normal" histology: is the intestinal mucosa really normal? Dig Liver Dis 2003;35:768-773.

11. Sollid L. and Lie B. Celiac Disease Genetics:Current Concepts and Practical Applications. Clinical Gastroenterology and Hepatology 2005;3:843-851.

12. WGO-OMGE Practice Guideline Celiac Disease. World Gastroenterology News. 2005;10(2):supplement 1-8.

Newly Diagnosed Celiacs Need Bone Density Testing

1. Walters JR, Banks LM, Butcher GP, Fowler CR. Detection of low bone mineral density by dual energy x ray absorptiometry in unsuspected suboptimally treated celiac disease. Gut. 1995 Aug;37(2):220-4.

2. Pistorius LR, Sweidan WH, Purdie DW, Steel SA, Howey S, Bennett JR, Sutton DR. Coeliac disease and bone mineral density in adult female patients. Gut. 1995 Nov;37(5):639-42.

3. Fickling WE, McFarlane XA, Bhalla AK, Robertson DAF. The clinical impact of metabolic bone disease in coeliac disease. Postgrad Med J. 2001; 77:33-36

4. Vitoria JC, Arrieta A, Arranz C, Ayesta A, Sojo A, Maruri N, Garcia-Masdevall MD. Antibodies to gliadin, endomysium, and tissue transglutaminase for the diagnosis of celiac disease. J Pediatr Gastroenterol Nutr. 1999 Nov;29(5):571-4.

5. Marsh MN. Bone disease and gluten sensitivity: time to act, to treat, and to prevent. Am J Gastroenterol. 1994 Dec;89(12):2105-7.

6. Rude RK, Olerich M. Magnesium deficiency: possible role in osteoporosis associated with gluten-sensitive enteropathy. Osteoporos Int. 1996;6(6):453-61.

7. Hoggan R. http://www.celiac.com/st_prod.html?p_prodid=781

8. Kumar V, Valeski JE, Wortsman J. Celiac disease and hypoparathyroidism: cross-reaction of endomysial antibodies with parathyroid tissue. Clin Diagn Lab Immunol. 1996 Mar;3(2):143-6.

9. Kisakol G, Kaya A, Gonen S, Tunc R. Bone and Calcium Metabolism in Subclinical Autoimmune Hyperthyroidism and Hypothyroidism. Endocrine Journal Vol. 50 (2003) , No. 6 657-661

10. .Kemppainen T, Kröger H, Janatuinen E, Arnala I, Kosma VM, Pikkarainen P, Julkunen R, Jurvelin J, Alhava E, Uusitupa M. Osteoporosis in adult patients with celiac disease. Bone. 1999 Mar;24(3):249-55.

11. McFarlane XA, Bhalla AK, Robertson DA.Effect of a gluten free diet on osteopenia in adults with newly diagnosed coeliac disease. Gut. 1996 Aug;39(2):180-4.

12. Sategna-Guidetti C, Volta U, Ciacci C, Usai P, Carlino A, De Franceschi L, Camera A, Pelli A, Brossa C. Prevalence of thyroid disorders in untreated adult celiac disease patients and effect of gluten withdrawal: an Italian multicenter study. Am J Gastroenterol. 2001 Mar;96(3):751-7.

New Data on Used Oats

1. Hogberg L, Laurin P, Falth-Magnusson K, Grant C, Grodzinsky E, Jansson G, Ascher H, Browaldh L, Hammersjo JA, Lindberg E, Myrdal U, Stenhammar L. Oats to children with newly diagnosed coeliac disease: a randomised double blind study. Gut. 2004 May;53(5):649-54.

2. Peraaho M, Kaukinen K, Mustalahti K, Vuolteenaho N, Maki M, Laippala P, Collin P. Effect of an oats-containing gluten-free diet on symptoms and quality of life in coeliac disease. A randomized study. Scand J Gastroenterol. 2004 Jan;39(1): 27-31.

More on the Problems with Oats in the Gluten Sensitive

1. Storsrud S, Olsson M, Arvidsson Lenner R, Nilsson LA, Nilsson O, Kilander A. Adult coeliac patients do tolerate large amounts of oats. Eur J Clin Nutr. 2003 Jan;57(1):163-9.

2. Kilmartin C, Lynch S, Abuzakouk M, Wieser H, Feighery C. Avenin fails to induce a Th1 response in coeliac tissue following in vitro culture. Gut. 2003 Jan;52(1): 47-52.

3. Janatuinen EK, Kemppainen TA, Julkunen RJ, Kosma VM, Maki M, Heikkinen M, Uusitupa MI. No harm from five year ingestion of oats in coeliac disease. Gut. 2002 Mar;50(3):332-5.

4. Teschemacher H. Opioid receptor ligands derived from food proteins. Curr Pharm Des. 2003;9(16):1331-44. Review.

5. Yoshikawa M, Takahashi M, Yang S. Delta opioid peptides derived from plant proteins. Curr Pharm Des. 2003;9(16):1325-30. Review.

6. Horvath K, Graf L, Walcz E, Bodanszky H, Schuler D. Naloxone antagonises effect of alpha-gliadin on leucocyte migration in patients with coeliac disease. Lancet. 1985 Jul 27;2(8448):184-5.

7. Zioudrou C, Streaty RA, Klee WA. Opioid peptides derived from food proteins. The exorphins. J Biol Chem. 1979 Apr 10;254(7):2446-9.

8. Hoggan R. Considering wheat, rye, and barley proteins as aids to carcinogens. Med Hypotheses. 1997 Sep;49(3):285-8.

9. Fukudome S, Yoshikawa M. Opioid peptides derived from wheat gluten: their isolation and characterization. FEBS Lett. 1992 Jan 13;296(1):107-11.

10. Kuitunen P, Savilahti E, Verkasalo M. Late mucosal relapse in a boy with coeliac disease and cow's milk allergy. Acta Paediatr Scand. 1986 Mar;75(2): 340-2.

11. Holmes, et al. "Malignancy in coeliac disease - effect of a gluten free diet" Gut 1989; 30: 333-338

12. Holmes GK. Coeliac disease and malignancy.Dig Liver Dis. 2002 Mar;34(3): 229-37

13. Collin P, Pukkala E, Reunala T. Malignancy and survival in dermatitis herpetiformis: a comparison with coeliac disease. Gut. 1996 Apr;38(4):528-30.

14. Chartrand LJ, Russo PA, Duhaime AG, Seidman EG. Wheat starch intolerance in patients with celiac disease. J Am Diet Assoc. 1997 Jun;97(6):612-8.

INDEX

LaVergne, TN USA
25 July 2010
190854LV00006B/27/P